Interventional Radiology

Adjunctive Medication and Monitoring

Proceedings of an International Symposium
held in Basel, January 1992

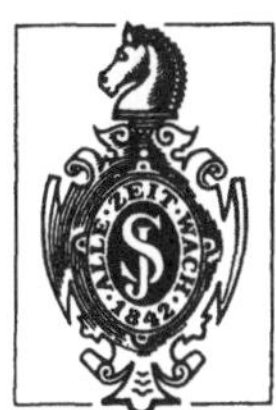

W. Steinbrich W. Gross-Fengels (Eds.)

Interventional Radiology

Adjunctive Medication and Monitoring

With Contributions by
P. Aspelin, R. F. Dondelinger, A. Essinger, F. J. Frei, E. Geller,
W. Gross-Fengels, H.-J. Hertfelder, U. Hörnchen, A. Jacob, K. Jäger,
S. Kadir, E. B. Keeffe, W. Kiowski, K. Lackner, A. Laurent,
C. Neuhaus, M. Pfisterer, E. W. Radü, G. Rudofsky, R. M. Walter,
E. Zeitler, C. L. Zollikofer and Co-workers

With 32 Figures

Springer-Verlag
Berlin Heidelberg GmbH

Prof. Dr. W. STEINBRICH
Departement
Medizinische Radiologie
der Universität Basel
Petersgraben 4

4031 Basel, Switzerland

Priv.-Doz. Dr. W. GROSS-FENGELS
Allg. Krankenhaus Harburg
Abt. für Klinische Radiologie
Eißendorfer Pferdeweg 52

2100 Hamburg 90, FRG

This International Symposium was funded by an educational grant from F. Hoffmann-La Roche Ltd. Basel, and Sintetica SA, Distributor for Bracco Contrast Media, Mendrisio, Switzerland

---

ISBN 978-3-662-01656-5 ISBN 978-3-662-01654-1 (eBook)
DOI 10.1007/978-3-662-01654-1

Library of Congress Cataloging-in-Publication Data. Interventional radiology : adjunctive [sic] medication and monitoring / W. Steinbrich, W. Gross-Fengels (eds.) p. cm. Includes bibliographical references and index.

1. Radiology, Interventional. I. Steinbrich, W. (Wolfgang) II. Gross-Fengels, W. [DNLM: 1. Radiology, Interventional–methods. WN 160 I6132] 617'.05–dc20

Originally published by Springer-Verlag Berlin Heidelberg New York in 1993

21/3130-543210 – Printed on acid-free paper

Preface

Over the years, interventional radiology has developed many effective and less invasive procedures. As the number and types of interventions increase, radiologists are becoming more and more involved in clinical patient care. This includes pre-interventional patient workup, sophisticated medical therapy and monitoring during interventions, regular inpatient rounds and complete follow-up management. Therefore interventional radiologists are faced with a broad spectrum of clinical and pharmacological questions.

Adjunctive medical therapy should increase the patient's comfort, should improve the success rates, and should further reduce the risks of the procedures. In order to fulfill our responsibility to the patients, a profound knowledge of certain drugs is indispensable. This includes, for example, sedatives, analgesics, cardiovascular drugs and agents to prevent infections, thromboembolic complications or restenoses. Moreover, a good monitoring system during complex procedures will increase the safety of radiological interventions. These topics and several more have been presented and discussed during an international symposium in Basel, Switzerland, in January 1992. It is the benefit of the authors, that all these results could be published shortly after the event. Connected with our thanks to all the co-workers the editors hope to find this publication assisting an increasing number of safe interventions.

W. Steinbrich W. Gross-Fengels

Contents

Monitoring

Clotting

Concomitant Drug Therapy During Radiologic Interventions

Contrast Media

Treatment of Emergencies During Radiologic Interventions

Postinterventional Drug Treatment

List of Contributors

ANTONUCCI F., Institut für Radiologie, Kantonsspital Winterthur, 8401 Winterthur, Switzerland

ASPELIN P., Karolinska Institute, Department of Diagnostic Radiology, Huddinge University Hospital, 14186 Huddinge, Sweden

AYMARD A., Service de Neuroradiologie, Hôpital Lariboisière, Faculté de Médecine, 2 Rue Ambroise Paré, 75010 Paris, France

BAILLY A. L., Service de Neuroradiologie, Hôpital Lariboisière, Faculté de Médecine, 2 Rue Ambroise Paré, 75010 Paris, France

CASASCO A., Service de Neuroradiologie, Hôpital Lariboisière, Faculté de Médecine, 2 Rue Ambroise Paré, 75010 Paris, France

CHRIST G., Medizinisches Zentrum für Radiologie, Abteilung Strahlendiagnostik, Philipps-Universität, Baldingerstraße, 3550 Marburg, FRG

DONDELINGER R. F., Service d'Imagerie Médicale, Centre Hospitalier Universitaire de Liège, Sart Tilman B 35, 4000 Liège 1, Belgium

EICHLISBERGER R., Abteilung für Angiologie, Departement Innere Medizin, Universität Basel, Petersgraben 4, 4031 Basel, Switzerland

ESSINGER A., CHUV – Centre Hospitalier Universitaire Vandois, Service de Radiodiagnostic, 1011 Lausanne, Switzerland

FISCHBACH R., Institut und Poliklinik für Radiologische Diagnostik der Universität zu Köln, Joseph-Stelzmann-Straße 9, 5000 Köln 41, FRG

FRAUCHIGER B., Abteilung für Angiologie, Departement Innere Medizin, Universität Basel, Petersgraben 4, 4031 Basel, Switzerland

FREI F. J., Departement Anästhesie, Universitätskliniken, Kinderspital Basel, 4005 Basel, Switzerland

FROELICH J., Medizinisches Zentrum für Radiologie, Abteilung Strahlendiagnostik, Philipps-Universität, Baldingerstraße, 3550 Marburg, FRG

GELLER E., Department of Anesthesiology and Critical Care Medicine, Tel-Aviv-Elias Sourasky Medical Center and the Sackler Faculty of Medicine, Tel-Aviv University, Tel-Aviv, Israel

GOBIN Y. P., Service de Neuroradiologie, Hôpital Lariboisière, Faculté de Médecine, 2 Rue Ambroise Paré, 75010 Paris, France

GROSS-FENGELS W., Allgemeines Krankenhaus Harburg, Abteilung für Klinische Radiologie, Eißendorfer Pferdeweg 52, 2100 Hamburg 90, FRG

HERTFELDER H. J., Institut für Experimentelle Hämatologie und Transfusionsmedizin der Universität Bonn, Sigmund-Freud-Straße 25, 5300 Bonn, FRG

HÖRNCHEN U., Institut für Anästhesiologie, Rheinische Friedrich-Wilhelms-Universität, Sigmund-Freud-Straße 25, 5300 Bonn 1, FRG

HOUDART E., Service de Neuroradiologie, Hôpital Lariboisière, Faculté de Médecine, 2 Rue Ambroise Paré, 75010 Paris, France

JACOB A., Institut für Diagnostische Radiologie, Departement Medizinische Radiologie, Universität Basel, Petersgraben 4, 4031 Basel, Switzerland

JÄGER K., Abteilung für Angiologie, Departement Innere Medizin, Universität Basel, Petersgraben 4, 4031 Basel, Switzerland

KADIR S., Saint Louis University, 10 Country Life Acres, St. Louis, MO 63131, USA

KEEFFE E. B., Liver Transplant Program, Division of Gastroenterology and Hepatology, California Pacific Medical Center, University of California, San Francisco, CA 94115, USA

KIOWSKI W., Abteilung für Kardiologie, Departement Innere Medizin, Universität Basel, Petersgraben 4, 4031 Basel, Switzerland

KLOSE K. J., Medizinisches Zentrum für Radiologie, Abteilung Strahlendiagnostik, Philipps-Universität, Baldingerstraße, 3550 Marburg, FRG

KUHN M., Institut und Poliklinik für Radiologische Diagnostik der Universität zu Köln, Joseph-Stelzmann-Straße 9, 5000 Köln 41, FRG

LACKNER K., Institut und Poliklinik für Radiologische Diagnostik der Universität zu Köln, Joseph-Stelzmann-Straße 9, 5000 Köln 41, FRG

LAUNAY F., Service de Neuroradiologie, Hôpital Lariboisière, Faculté de Médecine, 2 Rue Ambroise Paré, 75010 Paris, France

LAURENT A., Service de Neuroradiologie, Hôpital Lariboisière, Faculté de Médecine, 2 Rue Ambroise Paré, 75010 Paris, France

LAUVEN P. M., Institut für Anästhesiologie, Rheinische Friedrich-Wilhelms-Universität, Sigmund-Freud-Straße 25, 5300 Bonn 1, FRG

LEPPEK R., Medizinisches Zentrum für Radiologie, Abteilung Strahlendiagnostik, Philipps-Universität, Baldingerstraße, 3550 Marburg, FRG

MADER I., Institut für Diagnostische Radiologie, Departement Medizinische Radiologie, Universität Basel, Petersgraben 4, 4031 Basel, Switzerland

MATTIAS P., Institut für Radiologie, Kantonsspital Winterthur, 8401 Winterthur, Switzerland

MERLAND J. J., Service de Neuroradiologie, Hôpital Lariboisière, Faculté de Médecine, 2 Rue Ambroise Paré, 75010 Paris, France

NEUHAUS C., Medizinisches Zentrum für Radiologie, Abteilung Strahlendiagnostik, Philipps-Universität, Baldingerstraße, 3550 Marburg, FRG

PFISTERER M., Abteilung für Kardiologie, Departement Innere Medizin, Universität Basel, Petersgraben 4, 4031 Basel, Switzerland

POPOV-CENIĆ S., Institut für Experimentelle Hämatologie und Transfusionsmedizin der Universität Bonn, Sigmund-Freud-Straße 25, 5300 Bonn, FRG

RADÜ E. W., Institut für Diagnostische Radiologie, Departement Medizinische Radiologie, Universität Basel, Petersgraben 4, 4031 Basel, Switzerland

RAVUSSIN P., CHUV – Centre Hospitalier Universitaire Vandois, Service de Radiodiagnostic, 1011 Lausanne, Switzerland

RUDOFSKY G., Klinik und Poliklinik für Angiologie, Hufelandstraße 55, 4300 Essen, FRG

SCHUMACHER M., Sektion Neuroradiologie, Radiologische Universitätsklinik, Albert-Ludwigs-Universität, Hauptstraße 5, 7800 Freiburg, FRG

SIEMENS P., Institut und Poliklinik für Radiologische Diagnostik der Universität zu Köln, Joseph-Stelzmann-Straße 9, 5000 Köln 41, FRG

STEINBRICH W., Institut für Diagnostische Radiologie, Departement Medizinische Radiologie, Universität Basel, Petersgraben 4, 4031 Basel, Switzerland

STUCKMANN G., Institut für Radiologie, Kantonsspital Winterthur, 8401 Winterthur, Switzerland

URWYLER A., Departement Anästhesie, Universitätskliniken, Kinderspital Basel, 4005 Basel, Switzerland

WALTER R. M., Universität Wien, Abteilung für Diagnostische Radiologie, Allgemeines Krankenhaus Wien, Währinger Gürtel 18–20, 1090 Wien, Austria

ZEITLER E., Radiologisches Zentrum, Abteilung Diagnostik, Klinikum Nürnberg, Flurstraße 17, 8500 Nürnberg, FRG

ZOLLIKOFER C. L., Institut für Radiologie, Kantonsspital Winterthur, 8401 Winterthur, Switzerland

Analgesia, Sedation, and Anesthesia

Pharmacologic Bases of Sedatives, Analgesics, and Anesthetic Agents

E. GELLER

Introduction

Interventional radiologic procedures are being performed with increasing frequency, often replacing surgical interventions under general anesthesia. These complex radiologic procedures often require prolonged immobility and may be very uncomfortable and stressful to patients. Failure to alleviate pain and anxiety may not only make the procedure technically more difficult but may also jeopardize the condition of these often critically ill patients.

Intimate knowledge of the patients' history, their medical condition, as well as the plan of the proposed procedure go into formulating an adequate system for choosing either conscious or deep sedation, with or without systemic analgesia, or resorting to general anesthesia.

The rational and safe selection of anesthetic drugs and techniques is based on a thorough understanding of the pharmacology of the various sedatives, analgesics, and anesthetics, the interaction between them, and the effects of pharmacokinetic and pharmacodynamic factors.

In the following chapter a brief review is presented of the pharmacology of the most frequently used drugs.

Sedatives, Hypnotics, and Intravenous Anesthetics

Benzodiazepines

Benzodiazepines are among the most widely used drugs in clinical medicine. In anesthesiology they are utilized for premedication, sedation, hypnosis, and anesthesia. Comparative studies have shown benzodiazepines to be more effective in producing anxiolysis and amnesia, and more accepted by patients than barbiturates or butyrophenones.

The favorable characteristics of benzodiazepines include anxiolysis, amnesia, sedation/hypnosis, centrally mediated muscular relaxation, and anticonvulsant effects without inducing nausea or vomiting. Benzodiazepines exert their effects by binding to a benzodiazepine receptor that modulates the CNS effects of gamma-aminobutyric acid (GABA), the brain's major inhibitory neurotransmitter. Graded increases in benzodiazepine-receptor occupancy may be responsible for the dose-dependent transition from anxiolysis (20% occupancy) to sedation (25%–50%) and hypnosis (60%–90%, [1]). A specific, competitive benzodiazepine antagonist, flumazenil, capable of reversing all the CNS effects of benzodiazepines in a dose-dependent manner has recently been introduced into clinical practice [8].

In sedative doses benzodiazepines produce minimal respiratory depression. However, in large doses, or in the presence of chronic lung disease, or with the addition of opioids, or if unconsciousness ensues, apnea as well as airway obstruction may occur. Cardiovascular effects of benzodiazepines are also mild and often similar to those observed in natural sleep. In large doses, especially in hypovolemic patients and/or in the presence of opioids, significant decreases in systemic vascular resistance and hence in blood pressure may be observed.

Compared to other intravenous anesthetics, the onset of benzodiazepine effects is relatively slow (2–3 min). To avoid an overdose, therefore gradual titration with an adequate interval between doses is recommended. It should also be noted that the elderly are more sensitive to the effects of benzodiazepines.

Protein binding and volumes of distribution are not significantly different between diazepam and midazolam, the benzodiazepines most commonly used in anesthesia. The clearance rates and hence elimination half-lives are, however, significantly different: 20–50 h for diazepam (even longer for active metabolites) versus 1–4 h for midazolam. The elimination half-lives may be prolonged in the elderly, critically ill, and those with liver disease. The termination of the effect after a single dose of these benzodiazepines is not determined by metabolism, but is primarily a result of the redistribution of the lipid soluble drugs from the CNS to other tissues (muscle, fat). When given in repeated doses or as a continuous infusion, midazolam blood levels will decrease more rapidly than those of diazepam because of midazolam's greater hepatic clearance [12].

Diazepam

Diazepam is rapidly absorbed after oral administration but erratically absorbed after i.m. injection. Pain and thrombophlebitis may be associated with i.v. and i.m. administration due to the use of organic solvents. Oral administration of 10 mg diazepam produces amnesia in about 25% of patients beginning 20–30 min after ingestion and persisting for 90 min. A 5 mg i.v. injection produces amnesia in 50% of patients, the peak effect being at 2–3 min and persisting for approximately 30 min.

Midazolam

Due to its more favorable pharmacologic profile, midazolam is steadily replacing diazepam as the oral and parenteral benzodiazepine sedative and anesthetic of choice. Midazolam is the only benzodiazepine that is water soluble and therefore does not cause pain or venoirritation on injection. It is almost completely absorbed after intranasal and intramuscular administration. Midazolam is four to six times as potent as diazepam and produces more complete amnesia.

The bioavailability of midazolam after oral or rectal (0.3 mg/kg in children, [14]) administration is only 50%, probably due to liver first-pass effects. Intranasal administration of midazolam (0.1–0.2 mg/kg) appears to be a useful method for rapidly sedating children prior to the induction of anesthesia [15] and for the sedation of infants during painless diagnostic procedures [11].

The dose of midazolam for preoperative sedation is 0.05–0.1 mg/kg i.m., while for conscious sedation increments of 1–2.5 mg i.v. should be slowly titrated. For induction of anesthesia 0.1–0.4 mg/kg is necessary depending on whether premedication with opioids has been given. The dose of midazolam should be reduced with advancing age, thus patients over the age of 70 years need only half to one third the dose appropriate for younger patients.

The combination of midazolam with an opioid (e.g., meperidine, fentanyl, alfentanil) is a widely used sedative and anesthetic technique. Often the interaction is synergistic, producing unconsciousness with a fraction of the individual doses [3]. An increased incidence of apnea and hypoxemia with these combinations has also been reported [2].

Midazolam is frequently administered by continuous infusion for prolonged sedation. A loading dose of 0.025–0.1 mg/kg is slowly titrated to the desired level of sedation and then followed by a maintenance infusion of 0.25–1 µg/kg per minute.

Flumazenil

Flumazenil is a specific competitive antagonist of all benzodiazepines, with minimal intrinsic activity. By competing at the benzodiazepine receptor, flumazenil prevents or reverses in a dose-dependent manner the CNS effects of benzodiazepines. The onset of effect is very rapid, peak effect occurs within 3–5 min, and plasma half-life is only about 1 h. The recommended dose is 0.1–0.2 mg i.v. every minute, titrated to the desired effect (usually up to 1 mg). When antagonizing large doses of an agonist, resedation may occur, requiring close observation of the patients for signs of resedation, which may be treated with repeated doses or a continuous infusion of flumazenil. Giving flumazenil in small titrated increments is not associated with any adverse effects.

Barbiturates

Barbiturates have been the standard intravenous anesthetic for the last half century. For nighttime sleep, premedication, and sedation during procedures they have, however, largely been displaced by benzodiazepines because barbiturates have a lower therapeutic index, no anxiolytic properties, and occasionally cause disorientation and a lack of cooperation.

Barbiturates produce generalized CNS depression by interaction with the GABA-receptor complex. For the induction of anesthesia, the thiobarbiturate thiopental and the oxybarbiturate methohexital are most commonly used. Their dose-dependent effects range from mild sedation to unconsciousness. At low doses patients may become hyperalgesic with an exaggerated response to painful stimulation and heightened airway reflexes. The barbiturates cause central respiratory depression, venodilatation, and myocardial depression.

The ultrashort-acting barbiturates thiopental and methohexital are highly fat soluble and have a rapid onset and short duration of action (few minutes). Their duration of effect, when administered in an induction dose, is limited by redistribution from the brain back into other body tissues. The elimination half-life of thiopental is about 12 h versus about 4 h for methohexital. Both are biotransformed in the liver to inactive metabolites.

Thiopental is rarely used by infusion while methohexital is sometimes used by infusion for sedation; a loading dose of 0.25–1 mg/kg given over several minutes is followed by 0.6–3 mg/kg per hour.

Ketamine

Ketamine is a phencyclidine derivative producing a cataleptic-like state, often termed "dissociative anesthesia," in which the patients' eyes are open; they often verbalize and may move in this state. Ketamine is unique among i.v. anesthetics in that it produces intense somatic analgesia, the protective airway reflexes are partially preserved, and it causes respiratory and cardiovascular stimulation. Ketamine is also a potent bronchodilator. Since cerebral metabolism and blood flow are increased by ketamine, special care must be exercised in patients with intracranial mass lesions. Similarly, it may be contraindicated in patients with significant coronary artery disease or hypertension as it is known to cause cardiovascular stimulation.

The high incidence of hallucinations and nightmares associated with recovery from ketamine is a major drawback, especially in adults, but can be greatly attenuated by the administration of benzodiazepines. Pretreatment with an antisialagogue is also recommended.

The action of a single i.v. dose of ketamine (1–3 mg/kg) is usually terminated by rapid redistribution; elimination is primarily by the liver and clearance is relatively high, accounting for a short elimination half-life of 2–3 h.

In subanesthetic doses (0.2–0.8 mg/kg i.v. or 2–4 mg/kg i.m.) ketamine can be useful for sedation, especially in the pediatric age group in which it is probably the anesthetic most commonly used in children undergoing procedures outside the operating suite (cardiac catheterization, radiotherapy, etc.). It is also frequently used for the induction of anesthesia in children and uncooperative patients since it is rapidly absorbed after i.m. administration (5–10 mg/kg).

Propofol

Propofol is the latest i.v. anesthetic to be introduced into clinical practice. It is a phenol derivative formulated in a white aqueous emulsion containing soybean oil. Injection is associated with up to a 40% incidence of pain. Similar to other i.v. anesthetics it is highly lipid soluble with rapid onset and quick recovery due to redistribution (5–10 min after a single induction dose). Also contributing to this rapid recovery without residual sedation, which is propofol's major advantage, is the extremely high elimination clearance of propofol, making it also ideally suited for prolonged i.v. administration. The very high elimination clearance of propofol, exceeding liver blood flow, suggests that there is a significant extrahepatic component to its elimination. It has been suggested that propofol possesses antiemetic properties.

Propofol produces dose-dependent cardiovascular depression that is manifested by decreases in blood pressure caused by lowered cardiac output and systemic vascular resistance. Similar to other hypnotics it also causes dose-dependent respiratory depression and transient apnea.

Propofol is suitable as a means of sedation when given in subanesthetic doses. Published experience in this indication is, however, limited and centers around sedation of patients undergoing surgery under regional anesthesia or sedation in intensive care. In healthy patients the recommended loading dose is 0.25–1 mg/kg with a maintenance infusion of 0.6–3 mg/kg per hour, titrated to the desired level of sedation. In elderly or sick patients, and if opioids are added, the dose of propofol should be markedly reduced. The combination of midazolam-propofol has been suggested to offer advantages over either drug used alone for sedation [13].

General anesthesia is usually induced with a dose of 1–2.5 mg/kg followed by a maintenance infusion of 3–9 mg/kg per hour, depending on additional drugs used.

Opioids

The terms opioids, opiates, and narcotics are used to describe drugs that bind to opioid receptors in the spinal cord and brain. The clinically available agents range from the naturally occurring alkaloids (morphine, codeine, etc.) to the synthetic compounds (meperidine, fentanyl, etc.).

The analgesia produced by opioids is a complex effect of interfering with the rostral processing of pain information by suppressing the transmission of noxious stimuli, activating the inhibitory pathways in the brain stem, and altering mental responses. Besides analgesia, opioids produce sedation, depressed cough reflex, and nausea and vomiting through the stimulation of the chemoreceptor trigger-zone.

All narcotics produce dose-related respiratory depression and probably no one pure agonist is safter than any other. With small doses of opioids tidal volume is initially maintained while respiratory rate decreases, but with larger doses tidal volume also decreases. In addition, opioids significantly depress the response of the respiratory center to hypercapnea and hypoxemia [17]. This explains the hazards of administering narcotics to patients with intracranial pathology since CO_2 retention will result in cerebrovascular dilation and possible increased intracranial pressure. Respiratory depression may linger into the postoperative period when, due to lack of stimulation, sleep may ensue, reducing even further the response of the respiratory center to increases in CO_2 and to a reduction in oxygenation [7]. Preexisting respiratory illness, as well as concurrent disease and advanced age, all increase the potential for opioid-induced respiratory depression. The administration of other CNS-depressing drugs such as sedatives, tranquilizers, or potent inhalation anesthetics will also potentiate the respiratory-depressant action of the opioids. Ventilation may also be impaired due to narcotic-induced muscle rigidity. This centrally mediated effect is usually associated with large doses of opioids being injected rapidly, however, it has also been reported with small intravenous doses [9].

All opioids except meperidine produce a dose-dependent bradycardia which can be attenuated by atropine. At clinically relevant doses opioids do not depress myocardial contractility. Morphine and, to a lesser extent, meperidine cause arteriolar and venous dilatation, probably by histamine release. The newer synthetic agent fentanyl, and its congeners, are devoid of histamine release and have therefore a greater margin of cardiovascular safety. Patients with high sympathetic tone (i.e., marked anxiety, hypovolemia, etc.) may nevertheless become hypotensive due to reduced medullary sympathetic outflow caused by all opioids. Since patients differ greatly in their response to opioids it is recommended that small doses be titrated to the desired effect.

The opioids are rapidly distributed throughout the body after i.v. administration and have relatively large volumes of distribution (3–5 l/kg), except alfentanil (0.5–1 l/kg). Elimination is primarily via the liver with excretion of inactive metabolites by the kidneys.

Morphine

Morphine produces analgesia, sedation, euphoria, as well as nausea, vomiting, and ventilatory depression. It is more effective against continuous dull pain than sharp intermittent pain arising from either skeletal or visceral origin.

Morphine is well absorbed after i.m. injection with onset of effect at 15–30 min, reaching peak effect at 45–90 min and lasting 4–5 h. After i.v. administration peak analgesic effect is reached after 20 min. The typical perioperative dose is 0.05–0.2 mg given i.m. or i.v. in divided doses.

Due to its relatively poor lipid solubility and high degree of ionization, and in spite of low-protein binding, only a small amount of administered morphine gains access to the CNS.

Morphine is conjugated with glucuronic acid in hepatic and extrahepatic sites and metabolites are eliminated mostly by the kidneys. In patients with renal failure elimination of metabolites may be impaired, causing the prolongation of ventilatory depression.

Histamine release probably accounts for the urticaria and erythema commonly seen at the site of injection.

Meperidine

Meperidine is a synthetic opioid with about one tenth the potency of morphine. It has mild cholinergic effects accounting for the observed increase in heart rate associated with its use. Also, in contrast to other opioids, meperidine exerts a negative ionotropic effect on the heart when administered in large doses. Treatment with monamine oxidase inhibitors is an absolute contraindication to the use of meperidine due to the risk of precipitating life-threatening hyperpyrexia, convulsions, and coma [16]. Meperidine is more lipid soluble than morphine, accounting for a somewhat faster onset of action after both i.v. and i.m. administration. Duration of action is about 2–3 h.

Fentanyl

Fentanyl is a synthetic opioid structurally related to meperidine and 50–100 times more potent than morphine due to its high-lipid solubility. Even in large doses it does not release histamine and is therefore associated with hemodynamic stability leading to its use in large doses (50–150 µg/kg) as a sole anesthetic for cardiac surgery. Bradycardia and chest wall rigidity are potential side effects of high doses or rapid administration.

After i.v. injection of an analgesic dose (1–3 µg/kg) peak onset occurs after 5–6 min and clinical effects last for only 30–45 min due to fentanyl's large volume of distribution and the effects of redistribution. When larger or repeated doses are used, the highly lipid-soluble fentanyl is redistributed into fat and then released into the plasma to be metabolized by the liver with a half-life of about 4 h.

In the neonate, fentanyl's clearance seems comparable to that of older children and adults, while in premature infants it is markedly reduced.

Sufentanil

Sufentanil, an analogue of fentanyl, is the most potent opioid available for clinical use, being five to ten times more potent than fentanyl. It is highly lipophylic, is extensively bound to serum proteins, and has a smaller volume of distribution than fentanyl. Compared to fentanyl it has a slightly more rapid onset of effect, shorter duration of action, and an elimination half-life of 2.7 h. Sufentanil is useful in producing anesthesia in patients who require high-dose opioid techniques to maintain cardiovascular stability.

Alfentanil

Alfentanil is another analogue of fentanyl that is only one fifth to one tenth as potent but has entirely different pharmacokinetics and pharmacodynamic properties. The distinctive edge of alfentanil is its very rapid onset of action, 1–2 min, which is due to it being in a nonionized form at physiologic pH, thus readily crossing the blood-brain barrier. Alfentanil also has a short duration of effect and the shortest elimination half-life among opioids (1.5 h), which is mainly a function of its small volume of distribution (0.7 l/kg). This makes alfentanil more easily titratable with a more predictable duration of effect when administered in repeated doses of 5–10 µg/kg, or a continuous infusion (0.25–1 µg/kg per minute).

Naloxone

Naloxone is a pure competitive opioid antagonist capable of reversing the CNS effects of earlier administered opioids. It is practically devoid of agonist activity. In low titrated doses it may be possible to antagonize opioid-induced respiratory depression and excessive sedation without affecting analgesia.

The recommended i.v. dose of naloxone is 1–4 µg/kg given in divided doses. Onset is within 1 min with a duration of 30–45 min. Care must be taken to carefully observe the patient for signs of renarcotization and respiratory depression since the half-life of naloxone is shorter than that of many opioids. Side effects include severe hypertension, arrhythmias, and pulmonary edema.

Inhaled Anesthetics

General anesthesia is most commonly reserved for the pediatric age group undergoing interventional radiologic procedures. Most children are induced into an anesthetic state by a mask inhalation technique, thus avoiding the often traumatic experience of having to establish intravenous access in an awake child.

An anesthetic state is achieved when an appropriate partial pressure of an anesthetic gas has been established in the brain. Inhalation anesthetics enter the body through the lungs by establishing a series of gradients of anesthetic partial pressure from the anesthesia machine > inspired gas > alveolar gas > arterial blood > tissues (brain). The absorption of an anesthetic by the blood and its distribution to body tissues is determined by the solubility of the anesthetic in the blood and tissues, alveolar ventilation, cardiac output, and blood flow to the individual organs and their mass [5]. Except for adipose tissue, the tissue/blood solubility coefficients are generally similar to the blood/gas coefficients. The less soluble an anesthetic is in the blood, the more rapid a partial pressure will be established in the blood and, consequently, in the brain. Thus, among the commonly used anesthetic gases, nitrous oxide has the lowest blood/gas partition coefficient (0.47), leading to the most rapid onset of effect, as well as the fastest recovery. The potent inhalation anesthetics, in order of decreasing solubility are halothane (2.3), enflurane (1.9), isoflurane (1.4), and the newest agent sevoflurane (0.6).

The uptake of inhalation anesthetics is more rapid in infants and small children than in adults due to the major differences in blood/gas solubility, body composition, ventilation, and distribution of cardiac output.

The concept of minimum alveolar concentration (MAC) has been used to compare the potency of the inhaled anesthetic gases. MAC is defined as the alveolar concentration of an anesthetic that will prevent movement in 50% of subjects in response to painful stimulation [6]. Exceeding MAC by a factor of 1.25–1.3 will prevent most patients from moving in response to a surgical incision [10]. The addition of CNS-depressing drugs such as opioids, barbiturates, or benzodiazepines decreases MAC. With increasing age the relative MAC requirements decrease progressively, while infants are known to have greater anesthetic requirements than older children or adults.

Nitrous oxide is not a very potent anesthetic gas (MAC = 104%, which can only be achieved under hyperbaric conditions) and must therefore be supplemented with other potent inhalation agents or i.v. drugs, such as opioids. On the other hand it has analgesic properties, a concentration of 20% is equipotent to 15 mg morphine, and it has been reported to be effective in interventional radiologic procedures [4]. Nitrous oxide decreases the MAC of potent inhalation agents by about 1% for each volume percent concentration. At the usual anesthetic concentrations of over 60%, nitrous oxide has good amnesic and analgesic properties. When used alone, it exerts mild sympathomimetic effects on the cardiovascular system and has little effect on respiration. Its use should be avoided during procedures involving closed, gas-containing spaces (e.g., pneumoencephalography, risk of air emboli, etc.) and when high concentrations of inspiratory oxygen are necessary.

Halothane (MAC = 0.77%), the longest used potent inhalation agent is most popular in pediatric anesthesia due to its mild, nonirritating odor and facilitating mask inhalation induction. The other halogenated agents in common use are ethers: enflurane (MAC = 1.7%) and isoflurane (MAC = 1.15%).

All potent inhalation agents produce dose-related CNS depression, increased cerebral blood flow, exert negative inotropic and chronotropic effects on the heart, and reduce myocardial oxygen consumption. Halothane sensitizes the myocardium the most to the arrhythmogenic effects of epinephrine (i.e., in local anesthetic solutions) and to sympathomimetic agents. The potent inhalation agents cause a dose-related repiratory depression, primarily manifested by an increased respiratory rate and a decreased tidal volume. All three agents are bronchodilators and potent depressors of airway reflexes. Skeletal muscles are partially relaxed by the potent agents, reducing the dose of non-depolarizing muscle relaxants required.

Elimination of the potent anesthetic agents is mostly via the lungs, although about 20% of halothane, 2% of enflurane, and 0.2% of isoflurane undergo metabolization primarily by the liver. All inhalation agents may trigger malignant hyperthermia in susceptible individuals.

Conclusions

The clinician approaching the selection of drugs for sedation, analgesia, and anesthesia has a plethora of agents at his disposal with varied pharmacologic properties. To be used in an optimal and safe manner, intimate knowledge of the advantages and disadvantages of the individual drugs must be acquired. In addition, consideration of the age and general condition of the patient, concomitant diseases, especially respiratory and cardiovascular, as well as liver and kidney failure have a major impact on the patient's response to the drugs and doses selected.

It must not be forgotten that the added comfort, anxiolysis, amnesia, and analgesia provided to the patients by these drugs also imposes an additional element of risk. This added risk can only be justified if adequate supervision of the patients' response to the drugs is provided by an adequately trained and equipped individual, free of other duties. It is recommended that all locations at which these drugs are used be fully equipped with resuscitation equipment, drugs, and monitors, and that all medical personnel be proficiently trained in techniques of advanced life support.

References

1. Amrein R, Hetzel W (1990) Pharmacology of dormicum (midazolam) and anexate (flumazenil). Acta Anaesthesiol Scand 34 [Suppl 92]:6–15
2. Bailey PL, Pace NL, Ashburn MA, Moll JWB, Easat KA, Stanley TH (1990) Frequent hypoxemia and apnea after sedation with midazolam and fentanyl. Anesthesiology 73:826–830

3. Ben-Shlomo I, Abed-El-Khalim H, Ezry J, Zohar S, Tverskoy M (1990) Midazolam acts synergistically with fentanyl for induction of anaesthesia. Br J Anaesth 64:45–47
4. Braun SD, Miller GA Jr, Ford KK et al. (1985) Nitrous oxide: effective analgesic for vascular and interventional procedures. AJR 45:377–379
5. Eger EI II (1974) Anesthetic uptake and distribution. Williams and Wilkins, Baltimore, pp 77–94
6. Eger EI II, Saidman LJ, Brandstater B (1965) Minimum alveolar concentration: A standard of anesthetic potency. Anesthesiology 26:756
7. Forrest WH, Belville JW (1964) The effect of sleep plus morphine on the respiratory response to carbon dioxide. Anesthesiology 25:137
8. Geller E, Halpern P (1991) Benzodiazepine antagonists. Int Anesthesiol Clin 29:69–81
9. Janis KM (1972) Acute rigidity with small intravenous doses of Innovar: a case report. Anesth Analg 51:375
10. de Jong RH, Eger EI II (1975) MAC expanded: AD50 and AD95 values of common inhalation anesthetics in man. Anesthesiology 42:384
11. Latson LA, Cheatham JP, Gumbiner CH, Kugler JD, Danford DA (1991) Midazolam nose drops for outpatient echocardiography sedation in infants. Am J Cardiol 121:209–210
12. Reves JG, Glass PSA (1990) Nonbarbiturate intravenous anesthetics. In: Miller RD (ed) Anesthesia, 3rd edn. Churchill Livingstone, New York, pp 243–279
13. Taylor E, White PF (1991) Use of midazolam in combination with propofol for sedation during MAC. Anesth Analg 72:S 293
14. Saint-Maurice C, Meistelman C, Rey E, Eslève C, de Lauture D, Olive G (1986) The pharmacokinetics of rectal midazolam for preinduction in children. Anesthesiology 65:536–538
15. Walbergh EJ, Willis RJ, Eckhert J (1991) Plasma concentration of midazolam in children following intranasal administration. Anesthesiology 74:233–235
16. Wells DG, Bjorksten AR (1989) Monamine-oxidase inhibitors revisited. Can J Anaesth 36:64–74
17. Weil JV, McCullough RE, Kline JS et al. (1975) Diminished ventilatory response to hypoxia and hypercapnea after morphine in normal man. N Engl J Med 292:1103–1106

Recommended additional reading

Barash PG, Cullen BC, Stoelting RK (eds) (1989) Clinical anesthesia. Lippincott, Philadelphia

Miller RD (ed) (1990) Anesthesia, 3rd edn. Churchill Livingstone, New York

Stoelting RK (1991) Pharmacology and physiology in anesthetic practice, 2nd edn. Lippincott, Philadelphia

Analgesia and Sedation in the Hands of the Interventional Radiologist

A. Essinger and P. Ravussin

Since the end of the 1970s, interventional radiologists have been taking up their direct patient care responsibilities by performing interventions ranging from a simple dilatation to a life-saving recanalization of an occluded coronary artery or embolization for massive bleeding.

These types of procedures used to be done surgically under general anesthesia. Nowadays, interventional radiologic procedures, which often cause pain and anxiety, are generally performed under local anesthesia. However, caring for an agitated and anxious patient with difficulties in controlling his pain, in a darkened room, while attempting to perform an interventional procedure, is far from optimal. Thus, the aim of this chapter is to up-date the sedation and monitoring of patients scheduled for most radiologic interventions.

The aims of medication are:

- The relief of anxiety and apprehension
- Sedation
- Pain control
- Blood-pressure control
- Vagal-reflexes control
- Physical control of a quiet, calm, and cooperative patient

Prior to interventional procedures, patients should be maintained NPO for 4–5 h, but should be well hydrated, and oral medication such as beta blockers and calcium channel-blockers should be continued.

Before prescribing intravenous sedative and analgesic medication, which can lead to hypotension and respiratory depression, the physician must have some way of assessing the patient's respiration, heart rhythm, heart rate, blood pressure, peripheral oxygen saturation, and eventually end-tidal CO_2 (Table 1).

The physician in charge of such a patient must also respect the minimum safety standards required for medication and resuscitation equipment necessary for treatment, should any problem occur. Thus oxygen, suction, oral and nasal airways should be readily available. A functional bag and mask device (Ambu Bag) is invaluable when ventilation becomes necessary. In addition, laryngoscopes, endotracheal tubes, and other advanced life-support equipment must be located near the radiology suite. A certain number of drugs to initiate life support in case of life-threatening complications must also be present [1].

Table 1. Possible monitoring in invasive radiology

	Method of monitoring
Respiration	Observe patient's breathing and record respiratory rate and PET CO_2
Heart rhythm	Continuously displayed ECG (rhythm)
Heart rate	Continuously displayed ECG (rhythm)
Blood pressure	Automatic noninvasive blood pressure (NIBP) Arterial monitoring (IBP)
Peripheral oxygen saturation (Sa O_2)	
End-tidal capnometry (PET CO_2)	

Such standards for monitoring patients undergoing general anesthesia have been established by the American Society of Anesthesiologists [2, 3]; it seems appropriate to apply them to invasive radiologic procedures. In fact, the main goal in continuously monitoring the patient is to ensure his well-being and to be able to immediately treat any hypoxemia, the main cause of anesthetic-related injuries or deaths [4]. As there are not always extra people available to measure blood pressure or to watch the patients respiratory pattern in a radiology suite, the following minimum monitoring equipment is mandatory: pulsed-oximetry, ECG recording, and automated blood-pressure monitoring or arterial monitoring.

After having performed a baseline assessment of the patient's status and consulted laboratory results [5], most radiologic procedures can be performed under local anesthesia such as lidocaine, which provides rapid onset of anesthesia when injected locally. It is usually at this stage that the most frequently encountered cardiovascular complication arises; a bradycardia and hypotension are found, which indicate a vasovagal reaction. This can be managed by means of conservative measures, such as the administration of intravenous fluid, inducing a cough, and finally an intravenous injection of 0.5 mg atropine, which can be repeated if necessary until a normal rhythm is established [6].

Under the stress of any interventional vascular procedure, angina can appear in a patient with coronary artery disease (CAD) and can be relieved by the administration of nitrate derivatives. Usually we use an isosorbid dinitrate spray. Hypertension, present before the procedure, is very often aggravated by anxiety, pain, or both. If the patient's systolic blood pressure rises above 180 mmHg [6], moderate pressure reduction is advisable. A 20 mg capsule nifedipine retard can be given p.o. with a sip of water.

Interventional vascular procedures are usually not painful. An adequate patient/physician relationship, a reassuring conversation, and a musical background help in performing procedures with minimal analgesia and sedation.

If the patient is anxious and if the procedure is long and painful rending the patient uncomfortable, adequate sedation and pain relief using intravenous medication should be given, taking into account the age and weight of the patient and the duration of the procedure. Special caution should be given to patients over the age of 70, those with liver or renal disease, those with cardiovascular problems, and finally those with chronic obstructive pulmonary disease (COPD). Until now, routine premedication has not been given on the ward, but we might revise this by giving a small dose of a sedative p.o. when the patient is called from the radiologic suite, in order to reduce vasovagal reactions.

Since anesthetic coverage is not present for routine radiologic procedures, with the help of our colleagues in anesthesiology we have had to educate ourselves regarding anxiolytic agents and narcotics.

Those characteristics of an ideal agent for sedation in interventional radiology include:

- A short half-life
- Smooth action
- Rapid onset of action
- Easily titrable
- Easily reversed by an antagonist
- Little respiratory depression
- Painless on injection
- Sedative, anxiolytic, and/or analgesic properties

In radiologic literature there is no agreement on "the best" premedication or on an appropriate combination of drugs for sedation and analgesia based on solid pharmacologic background and clinical experience. In a recent publication [3] 12 different drugs were proposed for premedication along with their dosages, which were so huge that they would probably cause a heavy sleep if not more! Another article published in 1991 [6] suggests ten different sedatives, analgesic and antiemetic drugs for interventional radiologic procedures together with their dosages that may require intubation and ventilation of the patient and actually correspond to intravenous anesthesia.

Therefore in association with a colleague from the Department of Anesthesiology [7] a sedative protocol has been established using two drugs only: a narcotic and a sedative, which have, if used intravenously, a rapid onset of action, a short elimination half-life, a short recovery time, and no recurrent sedation for use in ambulatory patients. The drugs are water soluble, induce a minimal respiratory and cardiac depression, and can be reversed by an antagonist. The dosage of these medications has been kept at a low level on purpose and the initial dose can be repeated once. In case of difficult management or complications, the anesthesiologist on call is available and will be contacted.

In the radiologic literature, the most often mentioned sedative is diazepam, a benzodiazepine. This anxiolytic agent has different characteristics that make it far from the ideal sedative agent; the drug is not soluble in water, and, if mixed with saline, will produce a precipitate. According to the manufacturer, it must be dissolved in glycol which may cause pain on injection and result in phlebitis. It's terminal elimination half-life is very long (>48 h) and thus pro-

Table 2. Drugs and dosages commonly used for sedation

Class	Drug	Doses	Top up	Antagonist
Sedative	Midazolam (Dormicum)	2.5 mg i.v. = 0.5 cc	1.25 mg	Flumazenil (Annexate) 0.1 mg = 1 cc
Narcotics	Alfentanil (Rapifen)	0.25 mg i.v. = 0.5 cc	0.25 mg	Naloxon (Narcan) 0.2 mg = 0.5 cc
Anticholinergic	Atropine	0.5 mg i.v. = 1 cc	0.5 mg	
Vasodilators	Isosorbide-dinitrate (Isoket)	2 puffs	1 puff	
	Dihydralazine (Nepresol)	6.25 mg i.v. = 0.5 cc	–	
Calcium channel-blockers	Nifedipine (Adalat retard)	20 mg per os per lingual	–	
Amine	Ephedrine	5 mg i.v. = 0.5 cc		

longed sedation can be a problem, particularly in elderly patients. We have therefore stopped using it.

In order to make the patient comfortable, sedation is started not with a benzodiazepine but rather with a new narcotic, an opiate synthetic derivate, alfentanil (Rapifen), which produces pain relief and a certain degree of euphoria. In comparison to fentanyl to which it is connected, alfentanil has a much more rapid onset of action and also a shorter duration; in small doses it does not produce symptoms of stiff chest or board-like thorax rigidity to the same extent, nor does it induce a dose-dependent respiratory depression and hypotension. Maximum analgesia is effective 1 min after injection. Most of the negative effects of this synthetic narcotic can, if necessary, be reversed by the opioid antagonist naloxone (Narcan). As the action and negative effects of alfentanil are dose dependent, it should not be injected at a rate of more than 0.25 mg (0.5 cc). If the painful procedure lasts more than 10 min, the administration can be repeated once with minimal risk.

If the control of anxiety and pain is not sufficient with alfentanil, a sedative agent, midazolam (Dormicum) is added. It is a benzodiazepine with a faster onset of action and a much shorter elimination half-life than diazepam. A small dose of 2.5 mg (0.5 cc) is injected slowly at a rate of 1 mg per 30 s. Two minutes after the injection the sedation starts; with the present dose the midazolam sedation has never needed to be reversed with the benzodiazepine antagonist flumazenil (Anexate) administered at a dose of 0.1 mg (1 cc), which can be repeated. Because of flumazenil's short half-life, resedation can occur.

One has to be aware that a sedative and narcotic drug potentiate each other. Mild cardiac depression, which is often noticed, is especially helpful in hypertensive patients; a respiratory depression resulting in a severe drop in oxygen saturation measured by pulse oximetry can be a real problem. As a drop to 80% often happens in vascular patients, monitoring is mandatory and oxygen should be administered.

In general, with this drug regimen, we are able to manage most situations. Nevertheless, in one patient who had a renal transplant with very severe hypertension, the systolic blood pressure rose to 250 mmHg. An additional drug was necessary to render hemostasis possible after decannulation. Dihydralazine, in a dose of 6.25 mg (0.5 cc) was given by our nephrologist which brought the systolic value down to 150 mmHg.

In conclusion, interventional radiologists prescribing sedation and analgesia in adults undergoing vascular interventional radiologic procedure, should use only a limited number of drugs in order to become familiar with their effects and dosage, and their antagonists (Table 2). Two drugs, midazolam and alfentanil are recommended as they have a short onset and duration of action, few side effects in doses easy to remember, that is 0.5 cc alfentanil, plus, if necessary, 0.5 cc midazolam, and are close to the requirements of an ideal agent. No major side effects were encountered with this regimen over a 4-year period and it was never necessary to reverse the effect of the medication with any antagonist. Monitoring equipment is mandatory in order to evaluate the effect of the drug on the patient's cardiovascular and respiratory function, and this includes automated noninvasive blood-pressure monitoring, ECG, and pulse-oximetry.

References

1. Lind LJ, Mushlin PS (1987) Sedation, analgesia, and anesthesia for radiologic procedures. Cardiovasc Intervent Radiol 10:247–253
2. American Society of Anesthesiologists Committee on Standard of Care (1986) Standards for basic intraoperative monitoring (approved by ASA House of Delegates, 21 Oct 1986)
3. Hurlbert BJ, Landers DF (1987) Sedation and analgesia for interventional radiologic procedures in adults. Semin Intervent Radiol 4(3):151–160
4. Withers CE, Scheller MS, van Sonnenberg E (1988) Anesthesia for interventional radiologic procedures. Semin Intervent Radiol 5(2):125–131
5. Kadir S (1986) Preangiographic patient evaluation. Diagnostic angiography. Saunders, 78–81
6. Barth KH, Matsumoto AH (1991) Patient care in interventional radiology. Radiology 178:11–17
7. Ravussin P (1990) Neurological sedation and control of intracranial volume and pressure. Anaesth Rounds 22:4–15
8. Merry AF, Clapham GJ, Walker JS (1988) The reversal of midazolam sedation with the benzodiazepin antagonist flumazenil (annexate). NZ Med J 101:571–572

Sedation and Anesthesia in Radiologic Interventions

U. Hörnchen and P. M. Lauven

Introduction

Radiologic examinations and interventions are sometimes unpleasant and physically distressing for the patient. In addition, repeated treatment is often necessary. But heavy sedation or even full anesthesia is in general not required. On the contrary, the aim of (conscious) sedation during radiologic interventions is a patient who is only slightly sedated, but awake and cooperative on demand, amnestic, and free of anxiety and fear [18]. Furthermore the administration of sedatives and analgesics in itself should not demand the hospitalization of all patients.

Features of the Ideal Drug for Conscious Sedation

The ideal drug for conscious sedation should have a rapid and reliable onset followed by a predictable level of sedation preferably within one arm–brain circulation time and strictly depending on a well-defined and not too steep dose–effect relationship. Side effects should be minimal and calculable. For concscious sedation the drugs should ideally have the following features:

- Anxiolytic
- Antegrade amnestic
- Rapid onset of action
- Defined dose–effect relationship
- Broad therapeutic window
- Water soluble
- No venous irritation
- No pain on injection
- Rapid recovery
- No cardiovascular side effects
- No respiratory side effects

The first rapidly acting drugs capable of producing sedation up to loss of consciousness were hexobarbital and thiopental, both introduced into clinical practice in the 1930s. In particular thiopental has proved so useful in inducing sedation or loss of consciousness that it has developed into a "standard drug" against which all the more recently introduced hypnotic agents are compared, even if it is by no means the "ideal drug" for sedation.

When during the 1960s the benzodiazepines were introduced into clinical practice, diazepam rapidly evolved into an additional "gold standard" drug for sedation. In use as an intravenous sedative for nearly three decades, however, diazepam is also far from being the ideal drug for conscious sedation, although the problems of local venous irritation and thrombosis seem largely resolved with the lipid-emulsion formulation [13, 28, 29].

As only low doses should be used, a reliable and fast onset of action can only be achieved by administering the sedative intravenously. Therefore, the drug should be water soluble, or at least available in an injectable form, and there should be no pain on injection or local reactions.

Other features of an ideal drug for conscious sedation should be that the desired effect must occur without causing airway obstruction or respiratory and cardiovascular depression.

Anxiolysis and antegrade amnesia should be induced for the whole procedure so that the patient will be prepared to accept repeated testing. No residual effects should be present in the postinterventional period, even after short procedures. As long as low doses of sedative drugs are used, pharmacokinetic considerations play only a minor role in conscious sedation, as drug action is limited by a distribution process into muscle and fat rather than by elimination. However, if repeated and/or higher doses are administered, modern drugs, e.g., midazolam, propofol, and alfentanil, with high plasma clearances of 500–2000 ml/min and short elimination half-lives in the range of 1–3 h should be preferred over drugs like diazepam, thiopental, or morphine that exhibit a much slower pharmacokinetic profile with total plasma clearances of 25–500 ml/min and elimination half-lives of 5–50 h [23, 24, 28, 29].

Drugs Used for Conscious Sedation

A variety of drugs in low doses have been investigated for use in conscious sedation. Among these are phenothiazines, butyrophenones, barbiturates and non-barbiturate hypnotics, benzodiazepines, and the hypnoanalgesic ketamine, as well as the opioid alfentanil.

Phenothiazines and butyrophenones may also be addressed as neuroleptic drugs. Their main field of therapeutic administration is the treatment of psychiatric disorders. Neuroleptics, when used as sedatives, will normally not induce a loss of consciousness but produce a tendency to sleep and a lack of interest in the environment. Accordingly they reduce the patients' display of emotions and affect and impair complex behavior. There are reports that many patients feel imprisoned and unable to move after premedication with neuroleptic drugs. Therefore nowadays, these drugs are only seldom used as premedicants or perioperative sedatives.

Barbiturates and nonbarbiturate hypnotics reliably induce sedation when used in small doses [5, 9]. In particular some of these agents, e.g., methohexital or propofol, demonstrate a fast onset of action as well as a rapid recovery [29]. However, their therapeutic window with respect to loss of consciousness and subsequent apnea and hypotension is very small. This has been demonstrated by Lauven et al. [15] for methohexital. The therapeutic window of methohexital, obtained from young volunteers, exhibits a lower threshold concentration of induced sleep and recovery of approximately 4 μg/ml and an upper threshold of 9–10 μg/ml for deep coma, when the electrical activity of the cortex is so far synchronized that suppression periods of varying duration combined with sudden bursts were observed (burst-suppression pattern of the EEG). The deep coma threshold is thereby only twice as high as that of light sedation.

Doses of 0.5–1.0 mg methohexital/kg may therefore induce conscious sedation for a few minutes, whereas less than 1.0–2.0 mg/kg may lead to deep coma with apnea and hypotension, especially in older patients or patients at risk. Similar findings have been reported for thiopental, etomidate, and propofol [14, 24, 28, 29].

Barbiturates and nonbarbiturate hypnotics should therefore only be administered when trained personnel is present and the patient is continuously monitored by pulsoximetry and noninvasive blood pressure measurements. In view of the small therapeutic window, equipment for ventilatory and circulatory resuscitation must be available at all times.

Due to respiratory depression, the same holds true when opioid drugs like alfentanil or pethidine are administered for sedation, whether they are used alone or in combination with hypnotics. The threshold concentration of alfentanil for sedation and spontaneous respiration is about 100–200 ng/ml which can easily be achieved by small doses of less than 1.0 mg alfentanil [23].

Of the hypnoanalgesics, only ketamine offers minimal respiratory depression and virtually no cardiovascular depression when used in sedative doses of 0.5–1.0 mg/kg. However, ketamine induces dissociative anesthesia which is extremely difficult to relate to the traditional signs of sedation. Nystagmus and myoclonic movements after ketamine dosage make it very difficult to judge the depth of sedation or anesthesia. Thus, the use of ketamine is no substitute for good airway management. Due to its stimulating effects on the cardiovascular system, ketamine is contraindicated in patients with poorly controlled hypertension or coronary heart disease.

In addition, the use of ketamine in patients with psychiatric disorders should be avoided as postsedation emergence reactions like nightmares occur frequently, even if the incidence of these postsedation reactions is decreased when benzodiazepines are given prior to ketamine [1, 28].

As benzodiazepines offer not only sedative but also profound amnestic and anxiolytic effects, these drugs are administered worldwide for conscious sedation and are sometimes considered as the "gold standard" of sedation [18, 30]. In general, these drugs exhibit only minor effects on the cardiovascular system in particular when used in small doses. Their dose-effect curves are not very steep and demonstrate a ceiling effect when higher doses are administered. These drugs are therefore considered very safe drugs for sedation [16, 21, 29]. For example, midazolam doses of less than 3 mg up to doses of 15 mg may safely induce conscious sedation. It has to be considered, however, that the high midazolam dose of 10 mg may affect the memory for about 3 h, even though the patient is perhaps no longer sedated 1 h after the dosage [21, 30]. In addition, dosage requirements decrease with age. Patients of more than 60 years of age should receive only half or even a third of the dose required by a young patient. It is strongly recommended that particularly in elderly patients or patients at risk, no fixed dosage regimen based on milligrams per kilogram calculations is applied, but the desired level of sedation is achieved by titrating the total dose individually required for conscious sedation [2, 3, 19].

Side Effects of Sedation

Even safe drugs must be handled with caution as profound drug–drug interactions are possible and some patients may demonstrate adverse effects even after a low dosage. Side effects of sedatives include:

- Oversedation
- Decrease in blood pressure
- Bradycardia
- Respiratory depression
- Histamine liberation
- Venous and tissue sequelae
- Thrombophlebitis
- Pain on injection
- Psychomimetic reactions

According to dosage, sedative drugs may induce all degrees of depression of the central nervous system, ranging from mild sedation, through undue and long-lasting drowsiness, to coma in combination with cardiovascular and respiratory depression. The hazards of hypoxia are even more likely to occur when a variety of drugs, including very low doses of local anesthetics, are given concomitantly [4].

What are the most important side effects? Caplan [8] found in a closed claims analysis of 14 cases of unexpected cardiac arrest after conscious sedation during spinal anesthesia that the initial clues of cardiac arrest were bradycardia, hypotension, and cyanosis (Table 1). Only in one case was loss of consciousness the first clue prior to arrest. One of the patterns of management recurring in all cases was the use of sedation with very low doses of sedative drugs (Table 2).

How can these mishaps be explained in terms of the pharmacology of drugs for conscious sedation? Because benzodiazepines are the most important drugs for conscious sedation [18], this class of agents shall shortly be reviewed with respect to important drug–drug interactions.

Table 1. Clinical signs observed prior to cardiac arrest during spinal anesthesia (data from [8])

	1st clue	2nd clue	Combined incidence
Bradycardia	7	2	9
Hypotension	2	6	8
Cyanosis	4	3	7
Loss of consciousness	1	1	2
Asystole	0	2	2

Table 2. Doses of drugs administered prior to cardiac arrest during spinal anesthesia (data from [8])

Drugs	*n*	Amount administered	
		Average ± SD	Range
Fentanyl	9	108 ± 64 µg	25–200 µg
Diazepam	8	3 ± 2 mg	2–10 mg
Droperidol	5	3 ± 2 mg	1.25–7.5 mg
Thiopental	5	95 ± 62 mg	50–200 mg
Other	2	–	–

Drug–Drug Interactions of Sedatives

Tverskoy [25] could demonstrate that low doses of 10–20 mg methohexital will shift the dose-response curve of midazolam for sedation in young adults from 10 mg to doses of only 3 mg. Similar findings were reported by Vinik [27] who observed a marked shift in the dose-response curve of alfentanil to one fifth of the original dose when combined with low doses of midazolam (3–5 mg).

Profound drug–drug interaction could be demonstrated between all sedative drugs and local anesthetics or analgesics, as well as following a combination of sedative drugs acting at different receptor sites like benzodiazepines at the gamma-aminobutyric acid (GABA) system and phenothiazines or barbiturates at the cholinergic system [10, 17, 20, 26]. The benzodiazepine receptor is closely related to barbiturate-binding sites and may also be modulated synergistically by opioids or local anesthetics. If administered in combination, even small doses of sedatives and analgesics or combinations of different sedative drugs may induce such profound sedation and respiratory depression that artificial ventilation may be necessary.

In addition, for some drugs histamine liberation and anaphylactic reactions (barbiturates), venous and tissue sequelae, thrombophlebitis, and pain on injection (due to solubilizer "Cremophor EL"; etomidate, thiopentone, methohexitone, diazepam) have been reported. The combination of benzodiazepines and ketamine has achieved greater popularity during procedures that are painful because of the lack of respiratory depression during adequate sedation. However, if benzodiazepine sedation is not adequate before ketamine administration, marked cardiovascular stimulation may occur and the patient may experience unpleasant psychomimetic emergence reactions. In addition, light sedation may provoke sexual sensations and fantasies [6, 7, 11, 12, 22]. The present evidence suggests that these are much more likely to occur when large doses ($\geq$0.1 mg/kg midazolam) have been given.

Although rare (an incidence of about 1 in 200), unpleasant sequelae can occur and one must be aware of this effect. It seems that morbidity following the use of intravenous sedation with benzodiazepines (diazepam), barbiturates (thiopental, methohexital), and analgesics (fentanyl) is more frequent in women than in men. Since there is clear evidence that sedation can sometimes induce psychomimetic reactions, physicians are well advised not to sedate a woman without a third person being present.

Conclusion

To achieve a fast and reliable onset of action the sedative drug of choice should be injectable. One should avoid combinations of sedative drugs. If combinations are used, enhanced monitoring of the patient is mandatory as profound respiratory and/or cardiovascular problems may arise. Drugs with a rapid decline in action and/or drugs that can be antagonized should be preferred. One should always bear in mind that the dose necessary for sedation decreases with age. In patients over 60 years of age the dose should be half or only a third of the dose for patients of 20–30 years of age. To avoid hazards of oversedation the drug should be administered by careful intravenous titration to find the minimal effective dose for the individual patient. Patients will then be satisfied and will not experience pain or discomfort while being cooperative.

If sedation is too deep, e.g., by drug–drug interaction or overdose, after stabilizing blood pressure and ventilation, it can be useful to administer antagonists, e.g., flumazenil against benzodiazepines or physostigmine against anticholinergic drugs like phenothiazines or tricyclic antidepressants, to overcome the hazards of such a situation.

If one compares the pharmacologic actions of drugs used for conscious sedation, one will find that benzodiazepines, especially midazolam fits most of the desired features [18, 30]. Cardiovascular and respiratory side effects are minimal in the dose range proposed. In addition, its effects can be counteracted reliably by flumazenil which is a unique feature when compared to other classes of sedatives.

References

1. Baldessarini RJ (1985) Drugs and the treatment of psychiatric disorders. In: Goodman Gilman A, Goodman LS, Rall TW, Murad F (eds) The pharmacological basis of therapeutics, 7th edn. Macmillan, New York, pp 339–371
2. Bell GD, Spickett GP, Reeve PA, Morden A, Logan RF (1987) Intravenous midazolam for upper gastrointestinal endoscopy: a study of 800 consecutive cases relating dose to age and sex of patient. Br J Clin Pharmacol 23:241–243
3. Bell GD, Reeve PA, Moshiri M (1987) Intravenous midazolam: a study of the degree of oxygen desaturation occurring during upper gastrointestinal endoscopy. Br J Clin Pharmacol 23:703–708
4. Bernards CM, Carpenter RL, Rupp SM, Brown DL, Morse BV, Morell RC, Thompson GE (1987) Effect of midazolam and diazepam premedication on central nervous system and cardiovascular toxicity of bupivacaine in pigs. Anesthesiology 70:318–323
5. Blake DW, Donnan G, Novella J, Hackman C (1988) Cardiovascular effects of sedative infusions of propofol and midazolam after spinal anaesthesia. Anaesth Intensive Care 16:292–298
6. Brahams D (1989) Benzodiazepine sedation and allegations of sexual assault. Lancet ii:1339–1340
7. Campbell RL, Satterfield SD, Dionne RA (1980) Postanesthetic morbidity following fentanyl, diazepam and methohexital sedation. Anesth Prog 2:45–48
8. Caplan RA, Ward RJ, Posnerk, Cheney FW (1988) Unexpected cardiac arrest during spinal anesthesia: a closed claims analysis of predisposing factors. Anesthesiology 68:5–11
9. Dubois A, Balatoni E, Peeters JP, Baudoux M (1988) Use of propofol for sedation during gastrointestinal endoscopies. Anaesthesia 43:75–80
10. Duvoisin, Katz R (1968) Reversal of central anticholinergic syndrome in man by physostigmine. JAMA 206:1963–1965
11. Dundee JW (1986) Do fantasies occur with intravenous benzodiazepines? SAAD Dig 6:173–176
12. Gastak JD, Malamed SF (1980) Nitrous oxide sedation and sexual phenomena. J Am Dent Assoc 101:38–40
13. Harvey SC (1985) Hypnotics and sedatives. In: Goodman Gilman A, Goodman LS, Rall TW, Murad F (eds) The pharmacological basis of therapeutics, 7th edn. Macmillan, New York, pp 339–371
14. Knill RL, Bright S, Manninen P (1984) Hypoxic ventilatory responses during thiopentone sedation and anesthesia in man. Can Anaesth Soc 25:366–372
15. Lauven PM, Schwilden H, Stoeckel H (1987) Hypnotic threshold concentrations of methohexitone. Eur J Clin Pharmacol 33:261–265
16. Lauven PM, Stoeckel H (1986) Venous threshold concentrations of midazolam. Eur J Anaesthesiol 3:64–65
17. Lauven PM, Stoeckel H (1988) Flumazenil (Ro 15-1788) and physostigmine. Resuscitation 16:41–48
18. Lauven PM, Hörnchen U (1991) Techniques used for conscious sedation. Curr Opin Anesthesiol 4:530–533
19. Mora CT, Torjman M, White PF (1989) Effects of diazepam and flumazenil on sedation and hypoxic ventilatory response. Anesth Analg 68:473–478
20. Peele R, von Loetzen IS (1973) Phenothiazine deaths: a critical review. Am J Psychiatry 130:306–309
21. Persson MP, Nilsson A, Hartvig P (1988) Relation of sedation and amnesia to plasma concentrations of midazolam in surgical patients. Clin Pharmacol Ther 43:324–331
22. Reyes-Guerra A (1984) Erotic complications in the dental office under anesthesia. Dent Anaesth Sedat 13:68–69
23. Schüttler J, Stoeckel H (1982) Alfentanil (R 39209), ein neues kurzwirkendes Opioid. Pharmakokinetik und erste klinische Erfahrungen. Anaesthesist 31:10–14

24. Schüttler J, Schwilden H, Stoeckel H (1986) Pharmacokinetic – dynamic modeling of propofol (Diprivan). Anesthesiology 65 [Suppl]: A549
25. Tverskoy M, Ben-Shlomo I, Ezry J, Finger J, Fleyshman G (1989) Midazolam acts synergistically with methohexitone for induction of anaesthesia. Br J Anaesth 63: 109–112
26. Tverskoy M, Fleyshman G, Braley EL jr, Kissin I (1987) Midazolam–thiopental anesthetic interaction in patients. Anesth Analg 67: 342–345
27. Vinik HR, Bradley EL, Kissin I (1989) Midazolam–alfentanil synergism for anesthetic induction in patients. Anesth Analg 69: 213–217
28. Way WL, Trevor AJ (1986) Pharmacology of nonnarcotic anesthetics. In: Miller RD (ed) Anesthesia, vol 2. Churchill Livingstone, New York, pp 799–833
29. White PF (1986) Outpatient anesthesia. In: Miller RD (ed) Anesthesia, 2nd edn: vol 3. Churchill Livingstone, New York, pp 1895–1919
30. Whitwham JG (1990) The use of midazolam and flumazenil in diagnostic and short surgical procedures. Acta Anaesthesiol Scand 34 [Suppl 92]: 16–20

Special Aspects of Analgesia, Sedation, and Anesthesia in Children

F. J. FREI and A. URWYLER

Description of the Problem

"Fortunately, relatively few complications occur with pediatric sedation. Unfortunately they tend to be ignored, and although not able to prove it, I think these complications are dramatically underreported" [2].

Procedures

Recent years have witnessed an increase in radiologic procedures performed in pediatric patients. It is helpful to divide these procedures into (1) painless examinations such as computed tomography (CT), magnetic resonance imaging (MRI), and scintigraphy, and (2) painful examinations such as cardiac catheterization [18–20], intravascular procedures, e.g., angiography and/or embolizations [1, 9], CT or ultrasound-guided intervention, e.g., puncture of a liver abscess of percutanous nephrostomy in the newborn, and neuroradiologic investigations, e.g., myelography. For these painful procedures, patients need sedation and analgesia or sometimes anesthesia. Children above the age of 5–7 years may not need sedation for painless examinations if they are well informed as to what to expect. However, due to a lack of cooperation, infants and small children below this age require some form of sedation for painless examinations.

Infants and Small Children: How Do They Differ from Adults?

Children, and especially infants only a few months old, differ markedly from adults. Many of the most important differences, however, are not obvious. Although the most apparent is a contrast in size, physiologic differences relating to general metabolism and to immature function of various organ systems (including the brain, heart, lungs, kidneys, and liver) are of major importance.

Psychology

The most intense fear of an infant or young child is created by separation from the parents. Toddlers (children between 2 and 3 years of age) are at a stage when they find they can master their surroundings most of the time and can get instant attention by crying. Preschool children are at a very vulnerable stage of development, being more aware of reality than toddlers but not yet having the defense mechanisms, experience, and knowledge of older children. These psychologic characteristics sometimes makes it difficult to perform a radiologic procedure without traumatizing the child.

Pharmacology

Although from a theoretical point of view, body surface area is probably the most accurate parameter to use as a basis for calculating fluid requirements and drug dosages, for practical purposes we use body weight in kilograms. The differences between children and adults in response to pharmacologic agents are most pronounced in the first few months after birth due to the immaturity of various organs.

Pharmacodynamics

The response to drugs may differ between the various age groups [10]. The sedative effect of midazolam, for instance, is less pronounced and shows a larger variation in small children compared to school-age children. On the other hand, small infants may react with increased respiratory depression to the administration of morphine [17, 28].

Gas Exchange

Unquestionably, the most feared complication in a deeply sedated child is severe undetected hypoxemia, which may lead to bradycardia, cardiac arrest, and death. Oxygen consumption in an infant is about twice as much as in an adult; in addition, the ratio between alveolar minute ventilation and functional residual capacity is much larger in infants. Therefore, oxygen reserve is much less in the young and hypoxemia will appear much earlier if gas exchange is not guaranteed. Upper airway obstruction due to muscular hypotonia with or without central hypoventilation occurs quite frequently in sedated patients and, if undiagnosed and untreated, may lead – in its most serious form – to the sequence of events described above.

Intravenous Access

Orally administered sedatives or analgesic drugs may prove to be ineffective and intravenous augmentation may be necessary. Intravenous access in a well-nourished, 6-month-old infant may be a real challenge and may be very time consuming.

Organization

Radiologic examinations may be performed at pediatric hospitals, adult hospitals, teaching hospitals, free-standing institutions, etc. In an extensive survey of 834 hospitals in the United States, 47% of the respondents reported that the radiologist decides the sedation regimen and assumes responsibilities for it, while 37% reported that the primary physician is in charge [14]. Anesthesiologists (or nurse anesthetists) were only involved in 4% of the institutions. Less than a fourth of the hospitals have a separate room for sedation and 29% have a separate room for recovery. Other organizational aspects include obtaining informed consent or providing a nothing by mouth (NPO) order.

Definition of Terms

To ensure that safe recommendations are prescribed, definitions are important. The American Academy of Pediatrics, Section on Anesthesiology, Committee on Drugs uses the following definitions [3]:

1. *Conscious sedation* is a minimally depressed level of consciousness that retains the patients ability to maintain a patent airway independently and continuously, and respond appropriately to physical stimulation and/or verbal command, e.g., "open your eyes". "For the very young or handicapped individual, who is incapable of the usually expected responses, a minimally depressed level of consciousness should be maintained. The caveat that the loss of consciousness should be unlikely is a particularly important part of the definition of conscious sedation, and the drugs and techniques used should carry a margin of safety broad enough to render unintended loss of consciousness unlikely.
2. *Deep sedation* is a controlled state of depressed consciousness or unconsciousness from which the patient is not easily aroused. It may be associated with partial or complete loss of protective reflexes, including the ability to maintain a patent airway independently and respond purposefully to physical stimulation and verbal command.
3. *General anesthesia* is a controlled state of unconsciousness accompanied by a loss of protective reflexes including the ability to maintain a patent airway independently and respond purposefully to physical stimulation and verbal command.

Approach at Our Institution

Background

Twelve years ago, a 16-month-old male had to undergo a jejunal biopsy during the diagnostic work-up of a suspected celiac sprue at the Children's Hospital of Basel. The patient was premedicated with chlorprothixene (Taractan) and pethidine (Dolantin), both drugs given intramuscularly. A gastroenterologist and a nurse were present during the procedure, which was done in a darkened room. The patient suffered a cardiac arrest during the procedure and was successfully resuscitated, but survived with persistent signs of hypoxic brain damage. After this occurrence, the medical administrative staff of the hospital decided to appoint anesthetists for most radiologic procedures that require conscious sedation, deep sedation, or anesthesia in pediatric patients.

Conscious sedation for painless examinations is performed by the radiologist in charge using chloral hydrate (Chloralhydrat-Rectiole) rectally or promazine (Prazine) orally.

Techniques Used by the Anesthesiologist

Personnel

There are always two persons present who sedate or anesthetize the patient.

Preprocedural Evaluation

We (physicians from the department of anesthesia) always see the patient before the examination takes place. We obtain a medical history, do a short physical examination, and prescribe drugs to be administered in the late morning, as radiologic procedures are usually scheduled in the early afternoon. Approximately 1.5 h before the procedure begins, the patient receives an oral premedication consisting either of midazolam or chlorprothixene. In addition, we apply a local anesthetic cream (EMLA) on suitable places for venipuncture. When the patient arrives in the radiology department, we usually insert an intravenous line.

NPO Orders

Patients may eat or drink milk up to 6 h (above 1 year of age) or up to 4 h (less than 1 year of age) before the procedure. All are allowed to drink unlimited amounts of clear fluids up to 2 h before the procedure begins.

Monitoring

We monitor the patient according to our minimal safety standards [13], which are an electrocardiogram, a pulse oximeter, and a device for measuring blood pressure noninvasively.

Drugs

For nonpainful examinations, it is possible that no further drugs may be needed; when required, propofol or midazolam is titrated intravenously according to the needs of the patient. Conscious sedation is the ideal; however, deep sedation or even general anesthesia with or without endotracheal intubation may be necessary.

For painful examinations, several drug combinations are routinely used: midazolam with an opioid such as alfentanil or fentanyl; propofol with or without an opioid; ketamine with or without midazolam; general anesthesia with inhalational anesthetics.

Patients who undergo magnetic resonance imaging (MRI) always receive general anesthesia with endotracheal intubation (except for infants below 5 kg body weight, who receive chloral hydrate).

Comment

Due to a bad experience in the past, our approach is very cautious and expensive but we think very safe.

It is evident that with this organization the failure rate – due to movement of the patient – for a nonpainful examination such as a CT or a MRI is almost nil. With every other less cautious organization the failure rate will probably increase [25].

In addition, with our approach, painful procedures can be optimally managed in that each patient will receive the required amount of drugs to be in a state of analgesia and, hopefully, amnesia.

Each institution has to decide what failure rate – caused by movement or intolerable pain – it is willing to accept. This decision will have a profound impact on the amount of personnel needed, what skills they should have, and how extensive the monitoring has to be in order to guarantee maximal safety. For example, if only conscious sedation is performed, it is not necessary to have two persons experienced in airway management present.

Recommendations and Discussion

The purpose of this section is to give recommendations. There is no uniform established approach to the problem of analgesia, sedation, and anesthesia in children [14]. Certainly many different approaches are possible depending on the characteristics of the institution and the experience of the health-care professionals involved. The recommendations outlined in Table 1 are a combination of our own experience and published data.

Table 1. Administration of sedatives and analgesics

Recommendations for pediatric patients without significant pulmonary, cardiac or neurological diseases		
Sedation	Painless examinations	Painful procedures
Conscious sedation (No combination of drugs)		
Definition: minimally depressed level of consciousness, ability to maintain airway, and airway reflexes present		(patients age > 3 months)
Personnel: One operator and one assistant trained to monitor appropriate physical parameter	Midazolam 0.4 mg/kg orally Chlorprothixen 1.5 mg/kg orally Chloral hydrate 80 mg/kg orally or rectally	Morphine 0.05–0.1 mg/kg i.v. Pentazocin 0.3–0.5 mg/kg i.v. Pethidine 0.5–1 mg/kg i.v.
Equipment: pulse oximetry, intravenous line not mandatory	Promazine 2 mg/kg orally or intramuscularly	
Deep sedation		
Definition: depressed consciousness or unconsciousness, not easily arousable, and partial or complete loss of protective reflexes including ability to maintain a patent airway independently and respond purposefully to physical stimulation		
Personnel: One operator, one qualified physician to direct sedation, and one assistant whose only responsability is observation and monitoring of the patient. One person responsible for sedation has both training and experience in pediatric airway management including endotracheal intubation	Propofol initially 2–3 mg/kg i.v. followed by 6–10 mg/kg/h (continuous infusion) Midazolam 0.1–0.2 mg/kg i.v. followed by midazolam boluses of 1–2 mg according to age and need	Midazolam 0.1–0.2 mg/kg i.v. combined with alfentanyl 10–20 μg/kg i.v. or pethidine 0.25–1 mg/kg i.v. or fentanyl 1–2 μg/kg i.v.
Equipment: ECG, pulse oximetry, capnography, noninvasive blood pressure measurement, intravenous line present		

Facility

The radiology facility should have an emergency cart or kit that is readily accessible. All the necessary drugs and equipment for resuscitation must be available. In addition, the room must be equipped with an oxygen delivery system and a suction apparatus.

Personnel

Responsible persons must be familiar with the use of the emergency equipment. Recommendations concerning the required personnel during conscious sedation specify the need for the presence of a member of the health-care team who is appropriately trained in monitoring a patient and managing his/her airway [8]. This is an issue of controversy because it might be difficult and expensive to have such a person available for every CT or MRI [2, 14, 22].

For deep sedation or general anesthesia, two persons should be present [8]. The reason for this lies in the definition of the term "deep sedation" (see definition of terms). We think that two persons are required to manage a patient without protective airway reflexes who is unable to maintain a patent airway.

Preprocedural Examination

There are four groups of patients in whom sedation should be used with extreme caution: (1) Those with upper airway abnormalities causing obstruction, including obstructive sleep apnea syndrome, (2) those with abnormalities of the respiratory center, (3) those with abnormalities of metabolism or excretion (kidney and liver diseases, neonates), and (4) those with (potentially) increased intracranial pressure. It is absolutely mandatory to obtain a medical history and a physical status of every patient who receives sedative or analgesic drugs.

NPO Status

There is no consensus on NPO orders between radiologic institutions [14]. However, if routine practice consists of the augmention of conscious sedation to a level where partial or complete less of protective reflexes may occur (deep sedation), NPO order are mandatory to avoid aspiration of gastric contents. In this case, patients should receive no solids or milk for longer periods (e.g., 4 h for patients less than 1 year of age and 6 h for patients above 1 year of age). Patients may drink clear fluids up to 2 h before the examination [4, 21].

This approach interferes with the ingestion of oral contrast material for abdominal CT. In cooperative patients, most radiologists administer the oral contrast material 30–60 min prior to the examination. In a deeply sedated child, the amount of contrast material would put the individual at an increased risk of pulmonary aspiration. Therefore, we intubate the patient after ensuring that the examination is really indicated and necessary and administer the contrast material through a nasogastric tube. Theoretically, it might be possible for the child to ingest the contrast material 2 h before the examination takes place. However, there are two uncertainties with this technique; it is not known whether oral contrast material behaves like clear fluids, nor is it known whether 120 min between the ingestion of contrast material and CT examination is an appropriate amount of time to give optimal CT results. Finally, the easiest approach would be to avoid deep sedation; this would result in an examination failure rate of about 10%–20% [22, 25].

Monitoring

Besides clinical monitoring of respiration and cardiac functions, the continuous measurement of oxygen saturation should be available in every situation where sedatives and analgesics are administered for a radiologic examination. If deep sedation or anesthesia is required, noninvasive blood-pressure monitoring, electrocardiogram, and capnography are appropriate monitors. For long-lasting procedures, especially in a cold environment, body temperature must be recorded. A special situation exists for MRI where visual assessment of the airways is nearly impossible, even to an observer in the imaging room. The techniques for general anesthesia and sedation for MRI have been described [11, 12, 15, 22]. Pulse oximeters are available which also function during MRI without disturbing the image (NONIN Pulse Oxymeter, Modell 8604D, Nonin Medical Inc, Plymouth MN 55441, US). Electrocardiogram, noninvasive blood-pressure monitoring, and capnography are all possible during MRI.

Drugs

Oxygen is the optimal drug. Its benefits are effective, it is inexpensive, and it is not toxic. Consequently, oxygen should be administered to all patients receiving sedative medications, with the possible exception of neonates who are at risk from retinopathy because of prematurity and, more rarely, the patient with an abnormal ventilatory response. The benefit of oxygen lies in the reserve that it provides for the patient with apnea or an obstructed airway. In pediatric patients, the concept of this reserve is even more important because they have a decreased oxygen reserve.

There are no rules about the amount of supplemental oxygen that a patient requires; rather, administration of any amount of oxygen improves the margin of safety. Administration of oxygen does not need to be complicated; simple devices such as nasal prongs or a mask can be used. Thus, oxygen should be routinely administered when patients are sedated.

Numerous drugs in different dosages, alone or in combination, have been recommended in the literature [5–7, 16, 22–24, 26, 27]. In experienced hands they all may work. In inexperienced hands most of them are dangerous.

For conscious sedation, orally or rectally administered drugs which are in routine use for preoperative sedation can be recommended (Table 1). It is our opinion that, if possible, intramuscular injections should be avoided in pediatric patients. For painful procedures, opioids should be given intravenously in patients above the age of 3 months. Augmentation of sedation always bears the danger of a transition from conscious to deep sedation. This is especially true for painful procedures where relatively high doses of sedatives and analgesics may be required and – after the painful episode is over – hypoventilation, airway obstruction, and apnea may occur [29].

Generally speaking, if deep sedation is desired, drugs (alone or in combination) should be titrated intravenously to the desired effect.

References

1. Bidabe AM, Greselle JF, Gin AM, Floras P, Caille JM (1990) Protocol for preparation, anesthesia and monitoring in therapeutic angiography. Agressologie 31:280–283
2. Cohen MD (1990) Pediatric sedation. Radiology 175:611–612
3. Committee on Drugs, section on anesthesiology (1992) Guidelines for Monitoring and Management of Pediatric Patients During and After Sedation for Diagnostic and Therapeutic Procedures. Pediatrics 89:1110–1115
4. Coté CJ (1990) NPO after midnight for children – a reappraisal. Anesthesiology 72:589–592
5. Coventry DM, Martin CS, Burke AM (1991) Sedation for paediatric computerized tomography – a double-blind assessment of rectal midazolam. Eur J Anaesthesiol 8:29–32
6. Diament MJ, Stanley P (1988) The use of midazolam for sedation of infants and children. AJR 150:377–378
7. Ferrer-Brechner T, Winter J (1977) Anesthetic considerations for cerebral computer tomography. Anesth Analg 56:344–347
8. Fisher DM (1990) Sedation of pediatric patients: an anesthesiologist's perspective. Radiology 175:613–615
9. Graziano DV, Gifuni D, Ruggiero R, Bandieramonte G, Ruggiero C, Ruggiero A (1990) Anesthesia in the diagnostic stages of cerebral arteriovenous malformations in children under 3 years of age. Agressologie 31:284–286
10. Greene CA, Gillette PC, Fyfe DA (1991) Frequency of respiratory compromise after ketamine sedation for cardiac catheterization in patients less than 21 years of age. Am J Cardiol 68:1116–1117
11. Groh J, Weber W, Baierl P, Seiderer M, Peter K (1988) Anaesthesie zur Magnetresonanz-Tomographie. Anaesthesist 37:384–386
12. Hipp R, Nusser K, Eisler K, Tempel G, Kolb E (1987) Anaesthesie bei der Kernspintomographie. Anaesthesist 36:19–22
13. Kaufmann M, Scheidegger D (1991) Minimal Safety Standards in der Anästhesie. Schweiz Arzteztg 72:1065–1066
14. Keeter S, Benator RM, Weinberg SM, Hartenberg MA (1990) Sedation in pediatric CT: National survey of current practice. Radiology 175:745–752

15. Kuharik MA (1990) Sedation, anesthesia and patient monitoring. In: Cohen MD, Edwards MK (eds) Magnetic resonance imaging of children. Decker, Philadelphia, pp 75–81
16. Magnin G, Pelikan MC, Kobtane R, Couaillier JF, Foissac J, Wilkening M (1981) Anaesthesia for computerised axial tomography in children. Anesth Analg 38:475–477
17. Mitchell AA, Louik C, Lacouture P, Slone D, Goldman P, Shapiro S (1982) Risks to children from computed tomographic scan premedication. JAMA 247:2385–2388
18. Morray JP, Lynn AM, Stamm SJ, Herndon PS, Kawabori I, Stevenson JG (1984) Hemodynamic effects of ketamine in children with congenital heart disease. Anesth Analg 63:895–899
19. O'Higgins JW (1988) The anaesthetist and paediatric cardiac catheterization. Br J Hosp Med 40:58–63
20. Ruckman RN, Keane JF, Freed MD (1980) Sedation for cardiac catheterization: a controlled study. Pediatr Cardiol 1:263–266
21. Schreiner MS, Treibwasser A, Keon TP (1990) Ingestion of liquids compared with preoperative fasting in pediatric outpatients. Anesthesiology 72:593–597
22. Shepherd JK, Hall-Crags MA, Finn JP, Bingham RM (1990) Sedation in children scanned with high-field magnetic resonance; the experience at the Hospital for Sick Children, Great Ormond Street. Br J Radiol 63:794–797
23. Strain JD, Harvey LA, Foley LC, Campbell JB (1986) Intravenously administered pentobarbital sodium for sedation in pediatric CT. Radiology 161:105–108
24. Strain JD, Campbell JB, Harvey LA, Foley LC (1988) IV Nembutal: safe sedation for children undergoing CT. AJR 151:975–979
25. Thompson JR, Schneider S, Ashwal S, Holden BS, Hinshaw DB, Hasso AN (1982) The choice of sedation for computed tomography in children: a prospective evaluation. Radiology 143:475–479
26. Valtonen M (1989) Anaesthesia for computerized tomography of the brain in children: a comparison of propofol and thiopentone. Acta Anaesthesiol Scand 33:170–173
27. Varner PD, Ebert JP, McKay RD, Nail CS, Whitlock TM (1985) Methohexital sedation of children undergoing CT scan. Anesth Analg 64:643–645
28. Way WL, Costley EC, Way EL (1965) Respiratory sensitivity of the newborn infant to meperidine and morphine. Clin Pharmacol Ther 6:454–461
29. Yaster M, Nichlos DG, Deshpande JK, Wetzel RC (1990) Midazolam – fentanyl intravenous sedation in children: case report of respiratory arrest. Pediatrics 86:463–467

Discussion

on the papers by E. GELLER, A. ESSINGER, U. HÖRNCHEN, and F. J. FREI

It became clear in the discussion that sedation is not necessary in every radiological intervention. In general, though, the number of sedations is increasing with the aim of making the interventions more tolerable and therefore better accepted. This means that even in quantitative terms it is not practicable for anesthetists to regularly carry out each sedation. Essinger pointed out that in most institutions anesthetists were at best only available for radiological interventions in the afternoon.

The differentiation between conscious and deep sedation had by now been widely accepted, even if the borders remained somewhat fluent (Hörnchen). Hörnchen furthermore preferred the term "anesthesia" with deep sedation and stressed that only the anesthetist should cross the dividing line between conscious and deep sedation. It was generally accepted that conscious sedation represented a safe method of adjunctive medication in the hand of the interventional radiologist. While Essinger suggested that, generally, only conscious sedation was needed for radiological interventions, even for such painful procedures as embolization or chemoembolization, Hörnchen pointed out that deep sedation could be necesary in both uncooperative patients and children under 5 years of age. The presence of either a pediatrician with anesthetic experience or an anesthetist is then usually required. This holds for purely diagnostic procedures such as CT or MRI, too. The way these procedures were carried out in uncooperative patients – under deep sedation or narcosis – differed from institution to institution, but in any case suitable monitoring was mandatory (Frei).

While Frei generally kept a combination of a narcotic with a sedative for deep sedation, according to Geller, with suitable dosages a combination medication could also be used for conscious sedation. In general, however, the risks of respiratory depression and circulatory disturbances are higher with combined medications. Appropriate titration of the medications used is important. Geller drew attention to the time taken for benzodiazepines to have their maximum effect, which is only reached after several circulations. It is important to first define the goal of the sedation and to approach this in small titration steps over 10 min, is the depth of sedation also because depending on the amount of internal and external stimulation the patient is receiving. Procedures that are stressful to the patient require a correspondingly higher dosage in order to reach the same depth of sedation, and the response is also subject to individual variations. Essinger thought that it is necessary to determine the maximum dosage. In his experience, a dose of, for instance 2.5 mg midazolam should not be exceeded, titration occurring in 1-mg steps.

If paradoxical reactions occur, an increase in the dosage is contraindicated. Rather, slow injection of an antagonist would frequently both eliminate the paradoxical effect and at the same time maintain light sedation. Before the antagonist is given, however, one had to ensure that it really is a paradoxical reaction that is in fact occurring. Pain can lead to uncontrolled defense reactions under sedation, as the sedation alone did not produce analgesia. Consequently, for painful procedures combination with analgesics is preferable.

When combining a sedative with an analgesic, said Geller, the order of administration could vary. He recommended first starting with the sedative, titrating this to the desired level of sedation. Only for painful procedures an analgesic would also be required. The dose of this needed then often is much lower than if the medications had been given in the opposite order. This method of proceeding is particularly beneficial when opiates are being given because of the respiratory depression they cause.

There was general agreement that suitable observation is always needed for sedation. Apparative monitoring [see chapter on monitoring] makes observation easier. In Essinger's view, the levels of the alarm functions should be preset by each hospital's own anesthetists. Having one particular person exclusively responsible for monitoring appeared not to be necessary if the correct equipment is available. Monitoring of the sedation can usually be satisfactorily carried out by the whole team, provided that they had had suitable training. Since more complicated procedures are often carried out jointly by two radiologists, responsibility for patient monitoring could be taken by one of the two. Training had to include experience in intubation, reanimation, and defibrillation. Furthermore, a reanimation team had to be on call in the hospital.

Geller pointed out further that complications of sedating can also appear in the phase after the procedure, when the reduced external stimulation can bring about deepening of the sedation. Correspondingly, continuous observation of the patient is necessary, particularly after combination sedation, and this can best be done in the holding unit of the radiology department.

Hemodynamics and Circulation

Pathopysiologic Aspects of Blood-Pressure Dysregulation, Hypovolemia, and Microcirculation

G. RUDOFSKY

Introduction

Increasing technical possibilities combined with pharmacologic support have broadened the range of indications for interventional vascular techniques. More multilocated complex occlusions or stenoses located before long occlusions, e.g., iliac stenosis proximal to a complete long femoral obliteration, can be safely and successfully treated. This means on the one hand that these patients are usually older than the ideal candidate for percutaneous transluminal angioplasty (PTA) with single short stenosis but the older the patient is the higher are the risks of concomitant diseases and limitations in physiologic body functions. On the other hand the local situation with regard to blood supply and nutrition is also quite different to the ideal for PTA as these complex occlusions often lead also to a decompensated blood flow under resting conditions. Often patients with this kind of lesions have rest pain, gangrene, or acute ischemic syndromes. Therefore a wide spectrum of different pathophysiologic mechanisms that may interfere with revascularization has to be considered.

Systemic Disturbances

According to many investigations, 60%–90% of all patients with severe POAD also have coronary heart disease. In most of them this is combined with left ventricular failure and often a long history of hypertension. The resulting general low-flow state in decompensation is predisposing for arterial and venous thrombotic complications [2, 6, 11, 13, 14].

The concomitant hypervolemia due to fluid retention may even be increased if ionic or nonionic contrast media are given during intervention and induce acute left ventricular failure and pulmonary edema [10].

Especially poorly controlled arrythmia should be carefully monitored during and after treatment because it can be aggravated by hypervolemia, pain, or psychologic stress and endanger the patient not only by leading to cardiac arrest but also to a low output.

In the elderly a physiologic reduction in renal function characterized by a reduced clearance of creatinine can be found [1, 5, 12]. In a group of 400 patients with POAD, 15% showed pathologic renal clearance [6]. The administration of hyperosmotic drugs as contrast media and plasma-expanding fluid replacements lead to an osmotic impairment of tubuli function and a further decrease in renal function that could make transient or permanent dialysis necessary, especially in diabetics. Although it is very rare, with increasing age silent plasmocytoma may develop and accompany and even aggravate preexisting POAD. An uncontrolled application of contrast media will, in these situations, dramatically reduce renal function.

In the elderly, body fluid content is reduced by 40% compared to younger people [3]. This is often further aggravated by a reduced fluid uptake because of a reduced thirst sensation [4]. In this condition the patient develops hypovolemia with resulting hypocirculation [5].

The orthostatic dysregulation that can even occur in the aged in the supine position is mostly of the hyposympathicotonic or asympathicotonic type. As in sustained hypotension, the mean arterial pressure and resulting perfusion pressure in POAD can be dramatically reduced and a normalization of or mild elevation in blood pressure (BP) will often increase peripheral blood flow (induced hypertension) in such conditions [13].

In contrast, untreated hypertension with BP more than 180 mm Hg produces turbulent blood flow and leads to a flow reduction.

Hematologic diseases such as thrombocytosis, erythrocythemia, and plasmocytoma though rare conditions, may occur in the older patients. Thrombophilia, hyperviscosity, and late-stage renal impairment may endanger the patient with POAD [5].

Hyperfunction of the thyroid gland in elderly patients can be asymptomatic or monosymptomatic, and may lead to thyrotoxic crisis when contrast media are given unknowingly. These patients also have a reduced blood volume which may further increase the risk.

A critical situation that demands careful monitoring is the dilatation of a renal artery stenosis causing hypertension. The normalization of renal blood flow results in a reduction in the vasopressor substances and vasodilatation with the possibility of a critical fall in BP. As these patients often have concomitant occlusive diseases in other regions of the vascular system, they are at risk of developing acute aggravations or new occlusions in preexisting stenoses [9].

Local Disturbances

Blood-flow reduction depends on the extension of obliterations and existing collaterals. The more extensive the occlusions are the higher the additional loss of kinetic energy is and the lower the remaining energy for the perfusion of postocclusive tissues will be [15, 16]. As the oxygen supply is reduced more and more, local acidosis develops because energy production is shifted to anaerobic metabolization, with an increased production of lactate and pyruvate and

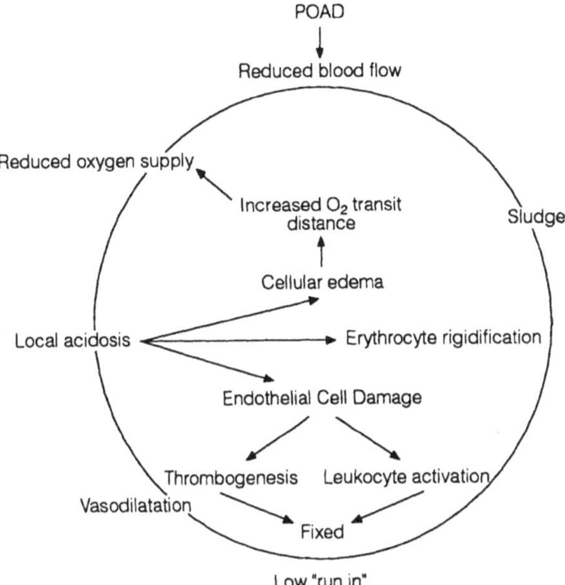

Fig. 1. Vicious circle of reduced blood supply, local metabolic disturbance, and further local circulatory worsening

a resulting decrease in pH value. This local acidosis causes a vasodilatation in the concerned region. As a result of the restricted blood supply, the flow is further decreased in the vascular bed together with the oxygen supply. In the low-flow areas, erythrocytes can aggregate especially in high levels of fibrinogen [8]. These aggregates cannot pass the nutritive capillaries and are shunted to the venous side or lead to prestasis and stasis in the arterial tree. The local acidosis increases the osmotic pressure in the cells and impairs membrane function, so fluid leaks into the tissues and a local edema results in an increase in the oxygen transit distance from the capillary to the cell organelles. Not only the oxygen supply is further diminished but also the blood itself is concentrated due to the fluid loss into the tissues, resulting in increased hematocrit on the venous side of the vascular tree.

The nutritional deficit also induces damage to the endothelial layer with the liberation of thrombogenic and chemotactic agents and the desquamation of endothelial cells inducing thrombosis and myocyte proliferation. Leukocytes are activated and stick to the denudated vessel walls or block the nutritional capillaries [13, 14].

Tissue acidosis also passes into the vessels. This acts in two ways on the blood cells: erythrocytic deformability is reduced and leukocytes are activated (Fig. 1). The rigidification of erythrocytes increases blood viscosity, which is further raised due to fluid loss into the tissues, systemic hemoconcentration, and reactive hyperfibrinogenemia. Vessel resistance is therefore not only increased by alterations in the vessel wall but also by the content of the vessel

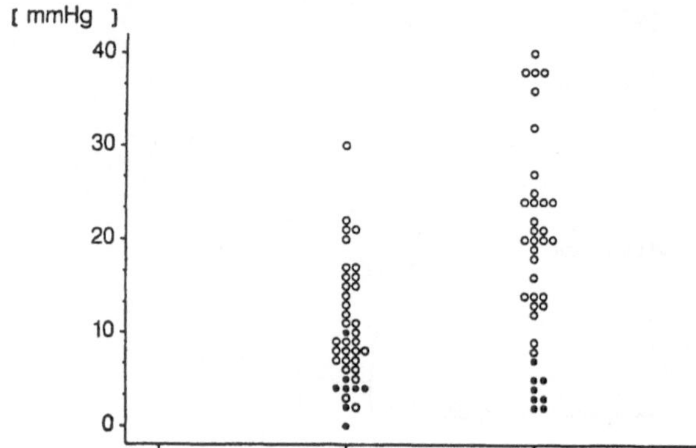

Fig. 2. Transcutaneous oxygen pressure ($tcPO_2$) before (*left*) and on the day after (*right*) treatment (PTA + PTA with lysis) in 40 patients with advanced POAD. Note the low pressure values (mean of 10 mmHg) before treatment. ● ● ●, Unsuccessful; ○ ○ ○, successful

which diminishes the run off. Results of our own prospective study on the influence of interventional treatment on microcirculatory parameters as transcutaneous oxygen pressure (tcP O_2), capillary density, and laser Doppler flux showed the tremendous decrease of the initial values on the forefoot after the treatment (Fig. 2, [7]).

Preexisting low-flow state in advanced stages of POAD probably aggravates the often bad outcome of interventions by repetitive balloon occlusions with hemodynamic (vasodilatation) disorders, metabolic (acidosis) decompensations with associated consequences of cellular edema, rigidification of erythrocytes, stress reaction of endothelial cells with leukotaxis, induction of thrombosis, and desquamation of endothelial cells.

So the pathophysiologic aspects of circulation in patients can be manifold and only careful analysis, broad pre- and aftertreatment, and conscientious monitoring will make interventional treatment safe.

References

1. Coper H, Schulze G (1986) Altersbedingte Änderungen in der Empfindlichkeit für Arzneimittel. Internist 27:53–60
2. Ettinger WH (1989) Immobility. In: Kelley WN (ed) Textbook of internal medicine. Lippincott, Philadelphia
3. Fülöp T Jr, Worum I, Csongor J, Foris G, Leövey A (1985) Body composition in elderly people. Gerontology 31:6
4. Ganten D, Mann JFE (1989) Durst. In: Resch RD (ed) Endokrinologie. Urban and Schwarzenberg, Munich
5. Goldstein S (1989) The biology of aging. In: Kelley WN (ed) Textbook of internal medicine. Lippincott, Philadelphia
6. Graf T (1985) Aspekte der Multimorbidität bei Patienten mit einer arteriellen Verschlußkrankheit der Beine. Dissertation, University of Ulm

7. Huang G (1992) Korrelation zwischen mikrozirkulatorischen Untersuchungsmethoden und dem klinischen Verlauf bei Patienten mit peripheren arteriellen Verschlußkrankheiten. Medical dissertation, University of Essen
8. Kiesewetter H, Jung F, Witt R, Kotitschke G, Winkelhog C, Nüttgens HP, Gerhards M, Roebruck P, Waterloh E (1987) Prävalenz der peripheren arteriellen Verschlußkrankheit, Risikofaktoren und rheologisches Profil: Ergebnisse der Eingangsuntersuchung der Aachen-Studie. Vasa Suppl 20:266–269
9. Mahler F (1990) Katheterinterventionen in der Angiologie (Periphere Arterien, Nierenarterien, PTA und Thrombolyse). Thieme, Stuttgart
10. Michel D (1984) Biorheuse des kardiovaskulären Systems. Internist 25:478–484
11. Müller-Bühl U, Diehm C, Sieben U, Berger B, Schuler G, Zimmermann R, Scheuermann W, Heuck CC, Mörl H, Kübler W, Schettler G (1987) Prävalenz und Risikofaktoren von peripherarterieller Verschlußkrankheit und koronarer Herzkrankheit. Vasa Suppl 21:11–14
12. Overhagen St, Ranft J, Rudofsky G (1991) Stumme Myokardischämien und Arrhythmien bei Patienten mit AVK Stadium II–IV. Vasa Suppl 33, Huber Verlag, Bern
13. Platt D (1984) Pharmakotherapie und Alter. Internist 25:491–500
14. Rudofsky G (1989) Kompaktwissen Angiologie, 2nd edn. Perimed, Erlangen
15. Rutherford RB (1989) Vascular surgery, vol I. Saunders, Philadelphia
16. Vollmar J (1982) Rekonstruktive Chirurgie der Arterien, 3rd edn. Thieme, Stuttgart

Huang [illegible] Korrelation zwischen mikroskopischen [illegible] Untersuchungsmethoden und dem klinischen Verlauf bei Patienten mit ambulant erworbener [illegible] Pneumonie. [illegible] medical dissertation, University of [illegible]

8. Kaiser [illegible] H, Lode [illegible], Schaberg T, Schlecht [illegible], [illegible] Ertel [illegible] Lorbeck [illegible] [illegible] (1987) [illegible] versus [illegible] Verschluss [illegible] Bakteriologische [illegible] Ergebnisse der Fluor [illegible] Untersuchung [illegible] Aachen-Studie [illegible] Suppl 26: 276–284

9. Mathur [illegible] (19[illegible]) [illegible] Infektiologie der Pneumonie [illegible] Thieme, Stuttgart

10. Müller [illegible] (19[illegible]) [illegible] 15: 477–484

11. Müller-Spinn [illegible] Berger S, Schuh [illegible], Zimmermann R, Schulenberg [illegible] Schuster [illegible] Müller W, Schlicht [illegible] (1987) Prävalenz und [illegible] der Keime [illegible] und [illegible] Suppl [illegible]

12. Ortqvist [illegible] Kalin [illegible], Lejdeborn L, Lundberg B (1990) Diagnostic fiberoptic bronchoscopy and protected brush culture in patients with community-acquired pneumonia. Chest 97: 576–582

13. Pond [illegible] (1986) [illegible] Respiratory infections [illegible] 1: 1–[illegible]

14. Rodnitzky [illegible] (19[illegible]) [illegible] Chest [illegible]

15. Schiller [illegible] (1987) [illegible]

16. Schmidt [illegible] (19[illegible]) [illegible]

Treatment of Disturbances in Blood-Pressure Regulation, Volume Homeostasis, and Microcirculation During Interventional Radiologic Procedures

W. Kiowski

Introduction

The development of interventional radiologic procedures has considerably changed the task of the physicians involved. In particular, the treatment of multimorbid and severely sick patients requires not only the mastering of the respective procedure but also a good working knowledge of the management of associated conditions and potential complications arising from the procedure. Among the potential problems encountered during acute interventions, disturbances in blood pressure, volume homeostasis, and microcirculation are of considerable importance. In order to handle such situations promptly and appropriately operators must be familiar both with the pathophysiology of associated or underlying conditions as well as the pharmacology of the most frequently used cardiovascular drugs and their particular indications and also contraindications. The present review focuses on these aspects and discusses general guidelines for the management of such situations. It is, however, obvious that a complete discussion of all details of these problems is beyond the scope of this brief review.

Mechanisms and Treatment of Hypertension

Primary hypertension is a frequent disease afflicting approximately 15%–20% of the adult population in western nations. Accordingly, preexisting hypertension is the most frequent cause of hypertension observed during interventional procedures. The elevation in blood pressure may not have been known before and the patient may have been untreated or poorly controlled. Frequently, the patient has not taken his usual medication because it was ordered that he should have nothing orally. In addition, the uncertainty and unfamiliarity with the procedure as well as the surroundings may lead to marked anxiety which can increase blood pressure considerably, especially in patients with preexisting and untreated or poorly controlled hypertension. Furthermore the triggering of visceral reflexes by pain, contrast agents or, e.g., the distention of the bladder due to the diuretic effects of contrast agents, may increase sympathetic tone and blood pressure considerably. An increase in intravascular volume, particularly through the use of hyperosmolaric contrast agents may also contribute to an increase in blood pressure.

General Considerations in the Treatment of Hypertension

In patients with preexisting treated hypertension it is mandatory for most procedures to ensure that the regular medication is also given on the day of the investigation. An exception to this rule may be renal-vein renin-sampling for the estimation of renin dependency of hypertension in patients undergoing renal angiography. If blood pressure in such patients appears to be too high and complications, e.g., at the puncture site, are anticipated, antihypertensive therapy can be administered after the completion of blood sampling according to the guidelines given below.

Since elevated blood pressure is frequently caused or aggravated by sympathetic stimulation due to the anxiety of the patient, it is of the utmost importance that the patient receives good and detailed information concerning the procedure that he is about to undergo. Even though this might alleviate the problem in many patients, it may not suffice in all and in those the administration of a minor tranquilizer, e.g., 10 mg diazepam 1 h prior to the investigation, should be considered. For patients who continue to suffer from high-grade anxiety the i.v. administration of small doses of a short-acting drug, such as 1–3 mg midazolam, usually eliminates the problem without any depression of the respiratory function. This approach offers the additional advantage of retrograde amnesia and unforeseen respiratory depression can be easily reversed by the diazepam receptor antagonist flumazenil. Also, the use of adequate local anesthesia or of i.v. analgesics including opiates can help to avoid pain-induced increases in blood pressure associated, e.g., with manipulations at puncture sites. Finally, it should always be ensured that the patient has an empty bladder prior to the study and that his wish to empty it during a procedure is readily followed.

Drug Therapy for Hypertension

Before an investigator considers acute drug therapy for hypertension it is essential that he decides what he considers the maximal tolerable blood pressure for the intended procedure. No general guidelines can be given but aspects like the patients' age, the use of oral or i.v. anticoagulants, a history of a previous cerebrovascular accident, or the presence of myocardial ischemia should be taken into consideration as to what level of blood-pressure elevation should be treated. If the decision for acute drug therapy is made, the drug employed should have a rapid and reliable onset of action and should be easy to administer. It should have a good steerability and, importantly, there should be no excessive antihypertensive effect. If there are concomitant diseases it might desirable to choose a drug with a respective positive effect and,

Table 1. Pharmacologic profiles of drugs used for acute treatment of hypertension

	Administration efficacy	Onset of action	Steerability	Excessive hypotension	Other beneficial effects	Contraindications
β Blockers	i.v. ±/+	++	±	–	CAD; diss. aneur.	Asthma; AV block; CHF
Ca antagonists	s.l./i.v. ++/+++	+/+++	±/++	–	CAD	–
Nitrates	s.l./i.v. ±/+	+++	++	–	CAD	–
Na^+-nitroprusside	i.v. +++	+++	+++	++	CAD	–
Hydralazine	i.v./++	++	+	++	–	CAD
Clonidine	i.v./++	++	+	–	–	AV block

s.l., sublingual; i.v. intravenous; CAD, coronary artery disease; AV, arteriovenous; CHF, congestive heart failure; diss. aneur, dissecting aneurysm.

almost needless to say, there should be no contraindications. A variety of drugs are available to acutely reduce blood pressure and Table 1 lists those with a more or less rapid onset of action either when given i.v., sublingually or, as in the case of some calcium antagonists, when given orally.

Beta blockers, when given acutely, usually do not lower blood pressure [17], perhaps with the exception of patients in whom an increase in sympathetic tone as a consequence of marked anxiety is responsible for the increase in pressure. However, beta blockers have antiischemic effects [5] and are essential for the treatment of dissecting aneurysms (see below). However, they are also contraindicated in patients with a history of asthma and in the presence of AV block or signs or symptoms of congestive heart failure.

Calcium antagonists, in particular nifedipine, show good efficacy when given sublingually [7] and orally [1], and excellent efficacy when given i.v. as is possible, e.g., with nifedipine [18], isradipine [3], and nicardipine [19]. The onset of action is rapid with i.v. administration which also provides good steerability of the effect, but sublingual administration also has an onset of action measuring 10–15 min, and a hypotensive effect after oral administration of a dihydropyridine calcium antagonist like nifedipine is usually seen after 30 min. In addition, these compounds also have pronounced antiischemic effects and there are virtually no contraindications. As shown in Fig. 1 the administration of 10 mg nifedipine sublingually in patients with hypertension significantly reduced blood pressure after 15 min and reduced it further up to the 30th min. This decrease in blood pressure was caused by a decrease in systemic vascular resistance. Although there is usually some reflex-mediated increase in heart rate after the administration of dihydropyridine calcium

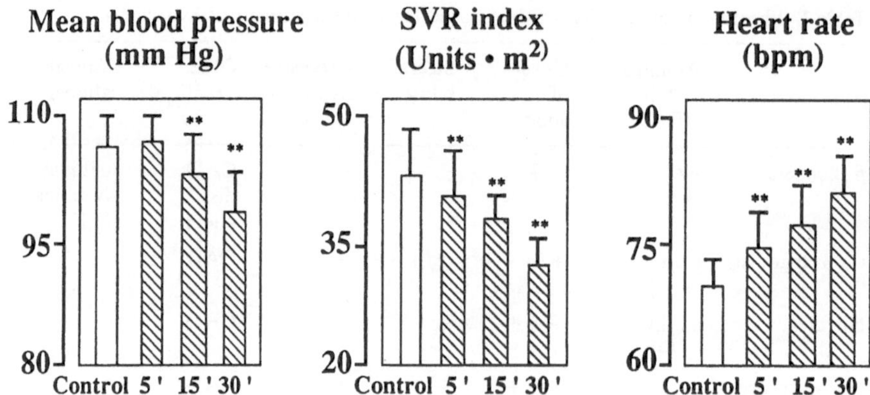

Fig. 1. Acute hemodynamic effects of nifedipine in patients with hypertension. Nifedipine (10 mg) was administered sublingually to 13 patients and systemic hemodynamics measured 5, 15, and 30 min later. Means + standard error of mean. ** $p < 0.01$ vs control measurements

antagonists, it rarely poses a problem with respect to the aggravation of myocardial ischemia.

Even though nitrates have a rapid onset of action their efficacy as antihypertensive agents is rather limited since they do not dilate arterial resistance vessels but rather the large conduit vessels which have little influence on blood-pressure regulation [16]. However, due to their beneficial effects in patients with coronary artery disease, the weak antihypertensive effect of either sublingual or i.v. nitroglycerine may be utilized in patients with mild blood-pressure elevation and concomitant coronary artery disease.

Sodium nitroprusside has long been known as a potent, rapidly acting antihypertensive drug [12] which due to its short half-life of a few minutes is characterized by a good steerability. However, when the dosage is increased too much there may be excessive hypotension which in most patients should be avoided at all cost. Due to the reduction in both pre- and afterload, it also has a beneficial effect on the balance between myocardial oxygen demand and supply in patients with coronary artery disease.

Intravenous hydralazine is also effective with a reasonably fast onset of action but the steerability is not as good and excessive hypotension may be encountered [10]. Due to the marked reflex tachycardia, it should not be used alone in patients with coronary artery disease because the increase in heart rate increases myocardial oxygen consumption and may lead to active ischemia or a worsening of preexisting ischemia.

Finally, the centrally acting agent clonidine is also effective when given i.v. with a fairly rapid onset of action and with little risk of excessive hypotension [20]. However, it should probably not be used in patients with underlying AV block.

Taken together, sodium nitroprusside and calcium antagonists are probably the most efficacious drugs; however, the ease of use of either orally or sublingually administrated calcium antagonists and the fact that blood pressure rarely has to be reduced within minutes make them the drug of choice in many situations. However, if a more rapid decrease in blood pressure is required the i.v. administration of a calcium antagonist or sodium nitroprusside must be considered, but continuous blood-pressure monitoring is advocated in these cases.

Treatment of Special Hypertensive Situations

Treatment of hypertension in patients with myocardial ischemia may be tried by the sublingual administration of nitroglycerin. This may suffice to reduce elevated blood pressure and also to improve the myocardial demand/supply ratio. If this should not suffice, i.e. beta blockade may be given in addition and, finally, a calcium antagonist might be added. In this context, it should be noted that the combination of verapamil and a beta blocker should be avoided because of the increased likelihood of experiencing marked hypotension and/or concomitant AV-conduction problems.

Dissecting aortic aneurysm requires immediate i.v. beta blockade to reduce myocardial contractility and diminish shear forces at the site of dissection [21]. If blood pressure should not respond to beta blockade alone, then i.v. sodium nitroprusside as a very fast acting agent [2] or, alternatively a calcium antagonist, should be administered to decrease the blood pressure to an acceptable, but not necessarily normal level.

In case of a suspected or documented pheochromocytoma, the i.v. administration of the combined alpha- and beta blocker labetalol is the preferred mode of therapy [14]. If this does not lower blood pressure sufficiently, combination with a calcium antagonist often leads to the desired goal.

Finally, increased blood pressure in patients with congestive heart failure should be aggressively treated to avoid a worsening of the congestive heart failure. In this situation, a second generation calcium antagonist like nisoldipine [8] or felodipine without a negative inotropic effect would be the preferred drug. In most cases it might be prudent to also give a fast-acting diuretic to improve the filling conditions of the heart. In case of pulmonary edema, sublingual administration of nitroglycerine or i.v. sodium nitroprusside should also be considered.

Mechanisms and Treatment of Hypotension

When considering treatment of hypotension it is crucial to consider the patients usual blood pressure. This is of particular importance since, e.g., the lower limit of cerebral and renal autoregulation is increased in patients with hypertension and their cerebral circulation may not tolerate low blood pressure as well as that of normotensive patients [13]. The potential consequences of hypotension are obvious: reduced organ perfusion, particularly of organs supplied by stenotic vessels and in combination with negative effects of contrast agents. Thus, e.g., kidney function may be impaired and, if hypotension is prolonged may progress to acute renal failure. Myocardium ischemia may cause further impairment of myocardial pump function and potentially life-threatening arrhythmias. Hypotension may also alter the level of consciousness and, in the worst case, may even lead to stroke. Thus, the management of hypotension, even more than that of hypertension, is a critical point in the management of patients undergoing interventional procedures.

The causes of hypotension are numerous but the most frequent one is the triggering of reflexes leading to an increase in vagal tone and to a vasovagal-vasodepressor reaction. The loss of blood from the puncture site may be considerable and should always be considered as a cause of hypotension. The risk of an allergic reaction to contrast agents with the stimulation of histamine release and the vasodilating kinin system is increased approximately two and a half to four times in high-risk patients (general allergies, previous reaction, [11]) and cardiac failure due to a negative inotropic effect of contrast agents can also lead to hypotension. Accordingly, the management of hypotension has to be familiar to all physicians responsible for the administration of contrast agents.

Treatment of Hypotension

Vasovagal syncope is characterized by hypotension together with sinus bradycardia or sinus arrest, rarely with high-grade AV block, and general malaise. The therapy of choice is the i.v. administration of 0.5–1 mg atropine and an increase in venous return, using either head-down tilt or an elevation of the legs. In rare cases, it might be necessary to administer fluids rapidly, i.v. and usually non-colloidal fluids such as saline or 5% dextrose suffice.

In acute left-sided pump failure there is no real alternative to inotropic support by i.v. infusions of either dopamine or dobutamine [6]. Dopamine increases myocardial inotropy through the stimulation of β_1 adrenoceptors and has the advantage at low dosages ($<2-4$ µg/min per kilogram body weight) of also stimulating renal-dopaminergic receptors which mediate splanchnic and renal vasodilation, thereby improving renal perfusion and function. However, high-dose dopamine infusions also stimulate peripheral vascular alpha receptors and thereby increase afterload, an unwanted effect when the heart is failing and afterload should be kept low. In this situation dobutamine has the advantage of stimulating vascular beta receptors, thereby leading to vasodilatation and a reduction in after-load [15]. Very often, if not always, a rapidly acting, high-ceiling diuretic should be administered to promptly relieve pulmonary congestion and dyspnea.

In contrast to left-sided pump failure, diuretics are usually not indicated in right-sided pump failure as exemplified by acute cor pulmonale caused by pulmonary embolism or right ventricular infarction. In these situations fluids should rapidly be given i.v. to allow the venous side of the circulation and the right ventricle to act as a conduit for the left ventricle. If inotropic support is needed i.v. norepinephrine infusion is the treatment of choice, since it constricts the arterial resistance vessels allowing systemic pressure to become higher than pulmonary pressure. Thereby, perfusion of the right ventricle, which for the most part occurs during systole, is restored.

Allergic reactions require the immediate i.v. administration of an antihistaminic and norepinephrine. Steroids are usually also given even though their value in the acute situation is somewhat questionable. Furthermore, if capillary leakage occurs, the rapid administration of large amounts of fluids may be necessary to restore blood pressure.

Treatment of Hypovolemia

Hypovolemia during interventional procedures is usually attributable to either a loss of blood from arterial puncture sites or to a bleeding lesion for which the patient has to be treated by, e.g., embolization. However, allergic reactions with an increased extravasation of plasma into the interstitium can also result in marked hypovolemia.

The principles of treatment are simple. In case of blood loss the elimination of the site of bleeding is the ultimate solution, but until this is achieved replacement of intravascular volume is necessary. As an intermediary measure, rapid i.v. infusion of large quantities of noncolloidal fluids (physiologic saline or 5% dextrose in water) may alleviate the problem, but this effect is usually of short duration. Infusions of plasma-protein solution or fresh frozen plasma are usually preferable because of their ability to stay in the vascular compartment. Ultimately, replacement of erythrocytes by infusion of erythrocyte concentrates is usually needed. If blood losses are gross, the replacement of whole blood also containing components of the coagulation cascade and platelets or erythrocyte concentrates and fresh-frozen plasma may become necessary. Reversal of oral anticoagulation by sodium warfarin derivates may also be necessary and can be achieved by the infusion of fresh-frozen plasma or commercially available factor VII concentrates. In these cases, the cooperation of someone experienced in the management of coagulation disorders should probably be sought.

Treatment of Disturbances of the Microcirculation

Of the mechanisms involved in disturbances of the microcirculation sludging of erythrocytes, platelet activation with the formation of microthrombi, and possibly a disturbance of endothelial function lend themselves to therapeutic interventions. However, it must be recognized that in contrast to the easily measurable effects of, e.g., the treatment of blood-pressure disturbances, the assessment of therapeutic effects aiming at an improvement in the microcirculation is difficult.

Treatment of the sludging phenomenon and the formation of microthrombi aims at an improvement in the rheologic properties of the blood without compromising oxygen delivery. Thus, it has been documented that hemodilution sufficient to bring hematocrit down to 35%–37% significantly reduces the sludge phenomenon in low-flow situations and improves oxygen delivery to the tissues. This effect is usually achieved by venesection of 300–500 ml blood together with the replacement of the same amount of dextran solution and administration of a further 500 cc dextran. Besides the reduction in hematocrit, dextran reduces platelet adhesiveness and aggregation, which thereby counteracts the formation of microthrombi. Furthermore, low-molecular dextran causes a desaggregation of erythrocytes reducing sludge directly and improving microcirculatory flow, but due to its low molecular weight and renal excretion it has a shorter duration of action than dextran. The antiaggregatory effects of antiplatelet therapy by cyclooxygenase inhibitors, such as acetylsalicylic acid, are well established and the effects of heparin also do not need comment. However, it should be remembered that the effects of cyclooxygenase inhibition are different in platelets and the vascular wall. Thus, aspirin irreversibly inhibits cyclooxygenase both in platelets and endothelium. However, nonnucleated platelets cannot synthesize new cyclooxygenase and vasoconstricting thromboxane will be produced only by new platelets not exposed to aspirin. In contrast, endothelium is able to continuously synthesize new cyclooxygenase and thereby continue to produce vasodilating prostacyclin. Accordingly, it has been shown that low doses of aspirin, e.g., 100 mg/day, usually completely block platelet cyclooxyenase but allow the endothelium to recover and continue to produce prostacyclin. This phenomenon has been described also in man [4] and stresses the usefulness of low-dose aspirin (50–100 mg) with respect to the inhibition of platelet activation. However, if a rapid onset of action is required it might be prudent to give a higher dose, e.g., 150–300 mg.

Beyond the production of prostacyclin, the endothelium is increasingly recognized as an organ with numerous functions serving to regulate vascular tone and prevent platelet aggregation and the formation of thrombus [9]. So far, specific therapeutic interventions are rare, but it may for instance be possible in the future to specifically stimulate endothelial release of endothelial-derived relaxing factor (EDRF) and thereby cause vasodilation, an effect which so far is only mimicked by the administration of nitrovasodilators such as nitrates or sodium nitroprusside. It may also be possible to selectively counteract the vasoconstrictor effects of endothelin-1, an endothelium-derived potent vasoconstrictor polypeptide. While this is not possible now, it is of interest that calcium antagonists seem to effectively prevent endothelin-1-induced vasoconstriction. Thus, endothelin-1 induces a marked increase in vascular resistance

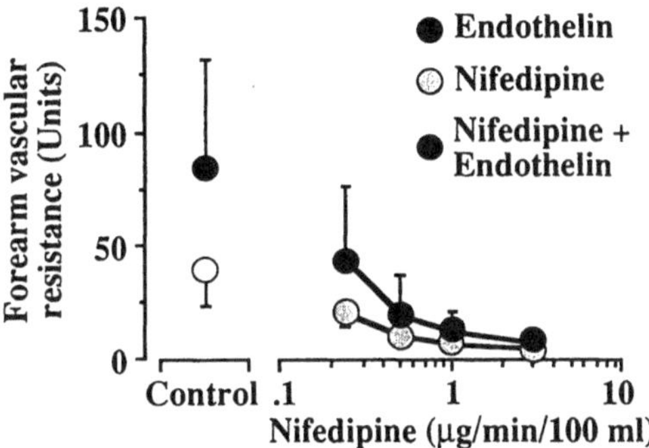

Fig. 2. Reversal of endothelin-induced vasoconstriction by slow calcium-channel blockade by nifedipine. Endothelin (50 ng/min per 100 ml forearm tissue) was infused into a brachial artery in ten normal volunteers resulting in marked vasoconstriction during control conditions. Infusion of nifedipine together with endothelin completely reversed vasoconstriction for the lowest dose and resulted in additional vasodilation for the higher nifedipine dosage. There was no difference in the vasodilator response to nifedipine alone or the combined endothelin and nifedipine. Means ± SD

when infused directly into the forearm of human volunteers (Fig. 2), but the intraarterial administration of nifedipine completely blocked this effect resulting in additional vasodilation for the higher dosages. However, the role of these systems in man in vivo is not yet clearly defined, neither in the normal nor in the diseased state, and the value of the interventions with respect to the improvement in microcirculatory function will have to be proven.

Conclusions

Attention to the maintenance of normal blood pressure during radiologic interventional procedures is of considerable importance and necessary measures require both the knowledge of the existence as well as of the pathophysiology of associated conditions since these may influence the therapeutic approach. In order to promptly and appropriately handle such situations the interventionist must be familiar with the pharmacology of the most frequently used cardiovascular drugs and their particular indications and also contraindications. Disturbances in the microcirculation are difficult to assess and therapeutic means more limited. Better understanding of the abnormalities and their underlying pathophysiology, e.g., the platelet–vessel wall interactions, may ultimately provide better treatment than the rather crude modalities available for therapy today.

References

1. Bertel O, Conen D, Radu EW, Muller J, Lang C, Dubach UC (1982) Nifedipine in hypertensive emergencies. BMJ 286:19–21
2. Cohn JN (1976) Nitroprusside and dissecting aneurysms of aorta. N Engl J Med 295:567–571
3. Edouard A, Dartayet B, Ruegg C, Samii K (1991) The use of calcium antagonists to treat intra-operative hypertension-evaluation of efficacy and safety of a new dihydropyridine derivative, intravenous isradipine, during abdominal surgery. Eur J Anaesthesiol 8:351–358
4. FitzGerald GA, Oates JA, Hawiger J (1983) Endogenous biosynthesis of prostacyclin and thromboxane and platelet function during chronic administration of aspirin in man. J Clin Invest 71:676–688
5. Frishman WH, Smithen C, Befler B et al. (1975) Non-invasive assessment of clinical response to oral propranolol. Am J Cardiol 35:635–640
6. Goldberg LI, Hsieh YY, Resnekov L (1977) Newer catecholamines for treatment of heart failure and shock: an update on dopamine and a first look at dobutamine. Prog Cardiovasc Dis 4:327–333
7. Kiowski W, Bertel O, Erne P, Bolli P, Hulthén UL, Ritz R, Bühler FR (1983) Hemodynamic and reflex responses to acute and chronic antihypertensive therapy with the calcium entry blocker nifedipine. Hypertension 5:I-70–I-74
8. Kiowski W, Erne P, Pfisterer M, Müller J, Bühler FR, Burkart F (1987) Arterial vasodilator, systemic and coronary hemodynamic effects of nisoldipine in congestive heart failure secondary to ischemic or dilated cardiomyopathy. Am J Cardiol 59:1118–1125
9. Kiowski W (1991) Endothelial function in humans: studies of forearm resistance vessels. Hypertension 18 [Suppl II]:84–89
10. Koch-Weser J (1974) Hypertensive emergencies. N Engl J Med 290:211–215
11. Lasser EC, Berry CC, Talner LB, Santini LC, Lang EK, Gerber FH, Stolberg HO (1987) Pretreatment with corticosteroids to alleviate reactions to intravenous contrast material. N Engl J Med 317:845–849
12. Page IH, Corcoran AC, Dustan HP et al. (1955) Cardiovascular actions of sodium nitroprusside in animals and hypertensive patients. Circulation 11:188–194
13. Paulson OB, Waldemar G, Schmidt JF, Strandgaard S (1989) Department of Neurology, Rigshospitalet, Copenhagen, Denmark. Cerebral circulation under normal and pathologic conditions. Am J Cardiol 63:2C–5C
14. Reach G, Thibonnier M, Chevillard C et al. (1980) Effect of labetalol on blood pressure and plasma catecholamine concentrations in patients with pheochromocytoma. Br Med J 1:1300–1303
15. Robie NW, Goldberg LI (1975) Comparative systemic and regional hemodynamic effects of dopamine and dobutamine. Am Heart J 90:340–345
16. Schnaar RL, Sparks HV (1972) Response of large and small coronary arteries to nitroglycerin, $NaNO_2$ and adenosine. Am J Physiol 223:223–228
17. Tarazi RC, Dustain HP (1972) Beta-adrenergic blockade in hypertension: practical and theoretical implications of long-term hemodynamic variation. Am J Cardiol 29:633–639
18. Walley TJ, Heagerty AM, Woods KL, Bing RF, Pohl JE, Barnett DB (1988) The haemodynamic effects of intravenous nifedipine in normotensive and hypertensive subjects. J Hum Hypertens 2:199–202
19. Wallin JD (1991) Intravenous nicardipine hydrochloride: treatment of patients with severe hypertension. Am Heart J 119:434–437
20. Weber MA, Graettinger WF, Drayer JIM (1987) The adrenergic inhibitors. Med Clin North Am 71:1
21. Wheat MW Jr (1973) Treatment of dissecting aneurysms of the aorta: current status. Prog Cardiovasc Dis 16:87–93

Discussion

on the papers by G. RUDOFSKY and W. KIOWSKI

Expanding on his paper, Rudofsky pointed out again the importance of hematocrit for the microcirculation and emphasized how important it is, before vascular interventions, to adjust the hematocrit to between 35% and 38%, or in patients with coronary heart disease between 40% and 42%. Compensation of the fluid balance using orally or intravenously administered fluids is often not sufficient, as the effect is not maintained for long enough. The use of low molecular weight dextrans could also not be recommended because of the low half-life (3 h) and the danger of subsequent hypovolemia. Furthermore, the risk of kidney failure, when low molecular weight dextrans are combined with larger amounts of contrast medium, was reported. More suitable are high molecular weight dextrans, plasma, or human albumin. The limit of the hematocrit beyond which PTA should not be carried out was set by Rudofsky at 45%.

If hemodilution was necessary, it was considered to be part of preparing patient for vascular intervention and has to be carried out by the responsible department. Further necessary preparatory measures he recommended are compensation of disturbances of cardiac performance, normalization of blood pressure to between 140 and 160 mm Hg, correction of fluid balance, and if necessary administration of vasocative drugs, especially prostaglandins.

When asked how the microcirculation could be checked, Rudofsky referred to a comparative study of his own, which showed measurement of the transcutaneous oxygen saturation to be as good as capillaroscopy, with laser Doppler methods coming out worse. In this context, Rudofsky also pointed out how important fibrinogen is with regard to the microcirculation. He said that fibrinogen levels could be reduced moderately to between 300 and 400 mg%, for instance by titration with urokinase, without increasing the risk of bleeding.

In the discussion on the talk given by Kiowski, a recommendation for treatment of high blood pressure in the context of vascular interventions was requested. Kiowski suggested oral calcium antagonists as the means of choice, such as nifedipine, because of its quick but not abrupt onset of action within 10–15 min and the low risk of side effects. A dosage of 20 mg generally suffices, although if necessary increases up to 40–60 mg are well tolerated. Kiowski recommended, however, that the need for a reduction in blood pressure always has to be critically examined, also with regard to the necessity of a compensatory high pressure, for instance in the presence of high-grade carotid stenosis.

Only rarely are fast reductions in blood pressure requiring intravenous medication necessary for interventional procedures. Here, too, nifedipine is useful. The very effective sodium nitroprusside should only be used if the radiologist has extensive experience with it. Kadir added a warning against using hydralazine, above all in older patients, as there had been reports of severe complications resulting from blood pressure dysregulation.

Monitoring

Equipment and Training of Staff for Patient Monitoring in Interventional Radiology

S. KADIR

Introduction

Recent years have seen a rather dramatic change in the practice of interventional radiology. There has been a rapid evolution from a primarily technique-oriented speciality to one actively involved in the clinical management of patients. This has brought with it the increased responsibilities of managing problems related intimately, or even remotely, to the interventional procedures. These added responsibilities have frequently transformed the role of the interventional radiologist from that of a consultant to one of a primary-care provider. In fact, under such circumstances the interventional radiologist may be better positioned to provide specific care for a given patient problem. Frequently, this responsibility falls upon the interventional radiologist as a result of the patient's choosing, confirming patient confidence.

Not all interventional radiologists feel the need for providing comprehensive patient care. Nevertheless, there are certain basic requirements for a safe and successful interventional practice. Problems with the delivery of interventional patient care are compound by the lack of understanding amongst general radiologists of the nature of interventional radiology (especially in the nonuniversity setting), and the lack of resources available to the interventionalists in private practice.

Interventional radiologic patient care is an around-the-clock service. It begins with a preprocedural evaluation; for an elective procedure, this is frequently an outpatient interview. For an inpatient procedure, this takes the form of a visit to the patient floor. It continues through the interventional procedure and hospitalization, and after the patient is discharged it is followed by a clinical visit or telephone call for follow-up. In addition, continuous contact is necessary with the outpatient under ongoing treatment or observation. Thus, for the interventional practice to be successful, a team of individuals is needed to render the service. The following describes some of the equipment and personnel requirements for a safe and successful interventional practice.

Equipment

Most diagnostic angiography suites are equipped with the basic emergency equipment (crash cart and cardiopulmonary resuscitation equipment, oxygen, suction, etc.). Most interventional practices require some additional monitoring equipment which is needed to assure patient safety and comfort. This should include a cardiac rhythm monitor, a pulse oximeter, a Doppler instrument, emergency power, and arterial pressure transducer. Optional equipment might include an automated blood-pressure cuff and a coagulometer.

Cardiac Monitoring

All patients undergoing interventional procedures should have cardiac monitoring. The device should be able to provide a 3-lead ECG and print a rhythm strip.

Oximetry

Adequate analgesia and sedation are important (1) to provide optimal patient comfort, (2) to avoid complications, and (3) to avoid negative patient perceptions about percutaneous interventional procedures.

Many of the interventional procedures, e.g., biliary intervention, can be associated with significant discomfort and pain. Past experience has shown that pain control becomes extremely difficult once the patient feels pain with every move of the interventionalists. Maintaining a heavy sedation and analgesia level from the beginning, i.e., before the painful segment of the procedure is begun, circumvents the problems associated with completing procedures on patients that have become agitated. Experience shows that once that patient feels pain, successful completion of the procedure may be in jeopardy, despite large doses of medication. In addition, there is a likelihood that this procedure is remembered by the patient as having been painful and intolerable, with the conclusion "never another percutaneous interventional radiologic procedure."

Current methods to monitor patients under heavy sedation, i.e., periodic blood pressure (BP), pulse, respiration, are not sensitive. Oximetry, on the other hand, is routinely used by the anesthesiologist. It provides a sensitive means to monitor the patient under heavy medication and alerts the interventionalist to an impending problem before it actually occurs, permitting timely action.

Doppler

Portable Doppler instruments are essential for an interventional practice. Assessment of the status of the peripheral vessels is made prior to and after intravascular intervention. In addition, Doppler-derived ankle-arm indices are used to document the success of the therapy, the detection of failures, and the recognition of problems that may require immediate attention.

Personnel

While most equipment requirements have already bean met with the establishment of angiographic suites, personnel requirements frequently remain undefined. The sustained success of an interventional practice depends, to a large extent, upon the establishment of a team comprising of individuals with the desire and motivation for interventional procedures beyond the regular work hours. This concept may be new to the mainstream radiologist but is common practice in other specialties. This team consists of the interventionalists, radiologic technologists with training and experience in interventional procedures, a registered nurse with experience in vascular and nonvascular interventional procedures, and a physician's assistant. Personnel requirements for interventional procedures suites are either two technologists per room together with one nurse per two rooms, or one technologist and nurse per room with one physician's assistant. Once a dedicated team is assembled, the interventional service is guaranteed a smooth operation.

The Interventional Physician's Assistant

The interventional physician's assistant (IPA) is a key player in the interventional team. This individual's role stretches from the preprocedure care, through the procedure, and into the postprocedure period. In interventional radiology, this position was established to fill a need created by an increasing work demand, and for the continuity of patient care. This position is not dissimilar to the physician's assistants in other clinical specialties.

The IPA's role is twofold: direct patient care and nonpatient care-related activities. Individuals best suited for this job should have the following qualifications:

1. Be a registered technologist or registered nurse with special competence in vascular and nonvascular interventional procedures
2. Must have a basic knowledge of commonly used pharmaceuticals
3. Must be able to start and manage intravenous lines
4. Must be certified to perform cardiopulmonary resuscitation
5. Must have compassion and care beyond the performance of the procedure

PROCEDURE: ______________________

CLINICAL PURPOSE FOR EXAM: ________ NAME:
HISTORY NO.:
______________________ DATE:
D.O.B.:
REFERRING M.D. ______________

PERTINENT HISTORY: ______________________

____

PRE-ANGIO VITAL SIGNS	MENTAL STATUS	ALLERGIES: ____
B.P.		LAB VALUES: ____
PULSE		____
RESP.		PREMEDICATION: ____

M.D. ORDERING MEDICATION ____________ NURSE ADMINISTERING MEDS ________

MEDICATION	DOSAGE	ROUTE	TIME	MEDICATION	DOSAGE	ROUTE	TIME

ARTERY CATHETERIZED: ______________________

PUNCTURE TIME: ____________ REMOVAL TIME: ____________

CONTRAST USED: ____________ AMOUNT: ____________

I.V. FLUID: ____________ AMOUNT: ____________

EMBOLIZING AGENT USED: ______________________

CATHETER USED: ______________________

M. D. (1) ____________ R.N. ____________

M. D. (2) ____________ R.T. ____________

Fig. 1. Interventional Procedures Form

The responsibilities of the IPA are:

1. Activities directly related to patient care (see below)
2. To maintain contact with the patient after completion of the procedure and discharge from the hospital
3. Educational: teach noninterventional personnel (in particular the nursing department) how to handle drainage catheters, wound-site care, make them aware of procedure-related problems (what to expect and what to do)

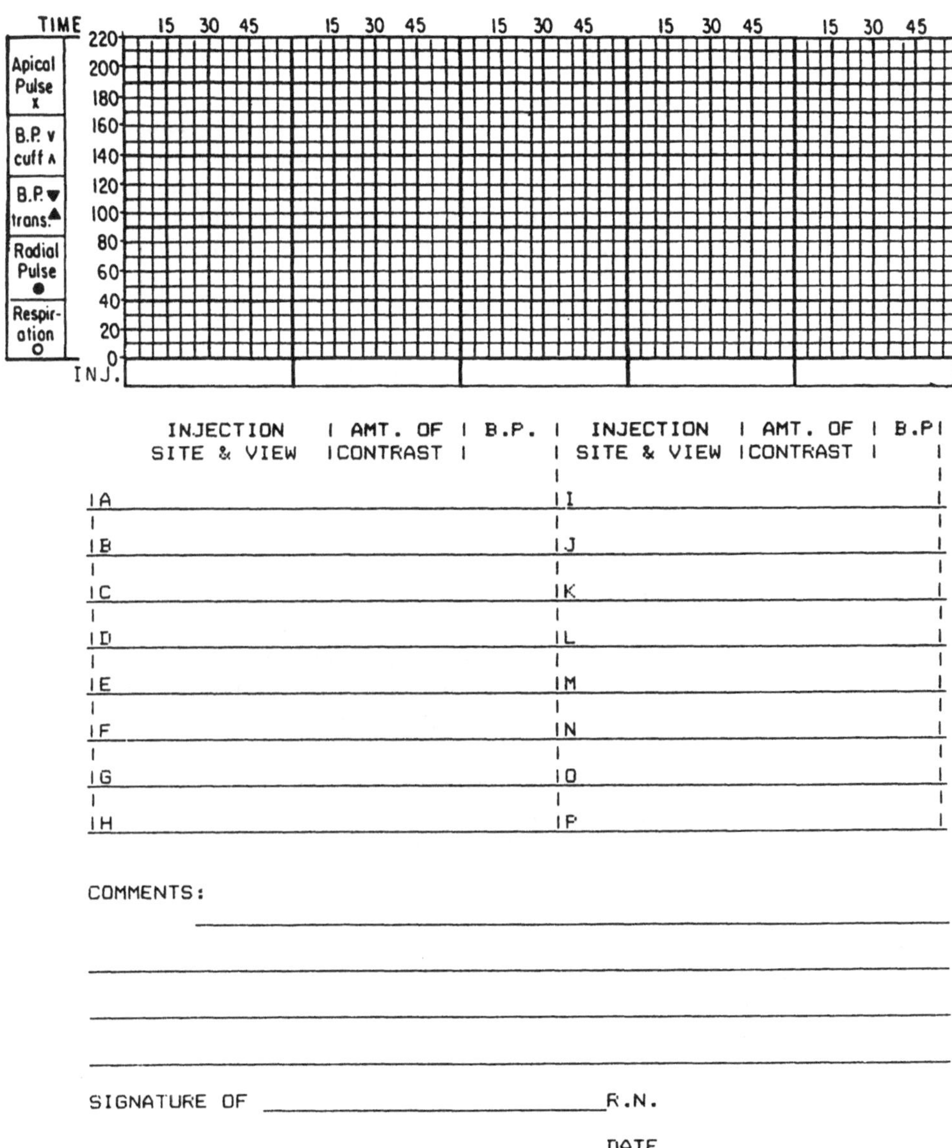

TIME 15 30 45 15 30 45 15 30 45 15 30 45 15 30 45

Apical Pulse x

B.P. v cuff ʌ

B.P. ▼ trans. ▲

Radial Pulse ●

Respiration O

220 200 180 160 140 120 100 80 60 40 20 0

INJ.

	INJECTION SITE & VIEW	AMT. OF CONTRAST	B.P.		INJECTION SITE & VIEW	AMT. OF CONTRAST	B.P.
A				I			
B				J			
C				K			
D				L			
E				M			
F				N			
G				O			
H				P			

COMMENTS: ______________________________

____

____

____

SIGNATURE OF ______________________________ R.N.

______________________________ DATE

The IPA interviews the patients, reviews the patient chart, orders blood work etc. In addition, the IPA discusses elective procedures with the patient (and family), thus laying the ground work for the interventionalist, who later obtains the informed consent. The preinformed patient (family) is in a better position to seek answers to specific questions. The additional advantages of this approach are the appropriate preparation and scheduling of patients for interventional procedures and avoidance of delays. Furthermore, an informed patient is frequently less apprehensive. The IPA follows the patient through the procedure, the postprocedure hospitalization, and subsequently in the postdischarge period.

The IPA makes daily rounds on hospitalized interventional patients, makes sure that the drainage or intraarterial infusion catheters etc. are functioning, changes dressings, and schedules these patients for follow-up contrast studies as indicated. Following completion of the interventional treatment, the IPA continues to follow these patients during the course of their hospitalization and provides them with verbal and written instructions, e.g., on catheter and wound-site care for patients with drainage catheters, and graduated exercise programs for patients who have undergone arterial recanalization. In addition, a contact telephone number is provided to schedule clinical visits and in case of emergencies (catheter blockage, dislodgement, etc.).

The Interventional Nurse

The interventional nurse (IN) plays a key role during the procedure itself. The qualifications are similar to those of an IPA and should include compassion and care beyond the performance of the procedure. Individuals best qualified for this position are nurses who have had intensive care experience.

As the patient comes to the interventional suite, the IN takes charge of the patient. The following steps are carried out as a matter of routine: a quick review of the floor nurse's notes, laboratory values, and baseline status assessment. The patient is asked about medical problems, diet restrictions, medication, and allergies. If an intravenous line is not present, one is inserted; if one is already present, the patency of the line is established. The patient is attached to the monitors and the IN immediately reports any abnormal findings to the interventionalist. Subsequently, the patient is premedicated according to the interventionalist's instructions. In many practices, the nurse (or IPA) prepares and drapes the patients in preparation for the procedure.

During the procedure, the nurse evaluates the patient every 15 min; more frequently if indicated for any reason. The evaluation includes BP, pulse, respiration, ECG, oxygenation, level of sedation, signs of discomfort, and any complications. Such an evaluation is repeated after every intravenous administration of sedatives, analgesics, or narcotic medication. The nurse watches for signs of discomfort/pain and reports this immediately to the interventionalists to permit timely administration of additional medication. With the use of the pulse oximeter, it is now possible to safely administer larger doses of sedatives and narcotics. In essence, the nurse becomes the eyes and ears of the interventionalist. This is an important task as it frees the interventionalist to concentrate on the procedure itself. All findings and the administration of medication are recorded on the special procedures form (Fig. 1).

Following the procedure, the patient undergoes a final assessment. Dressings, drainage bags, etc. are attached. The patient is given instructions on what not to do and what to expect. Finally, the patient is accompanied to the floor and a report is given to the receiving nurse on the floor. These tasks can be completed by either the IN or the IPA.

Conclusions

The increasing complexity of interventional procedures requires strict patient monitoring during procedures and necessitates a more comprehensive patient-care requirement in interventional radiology. This includes closely following patients undergoing in-hospital treatment, as well as those who have been discharged after the completion of the interventional treatment. Alone, interventional radiologists are not in a position to provide such patient care. However, a properly selected and trained interventional team consisting of interventional radiologists, radiologic technologists, IN, and IPA can not only facilitate a smooth operation during the procedure but also provide the appropriate follow-up of the interventional patient.

References

1. Adams P (1991) The physician's assistant in interventional radiology. In: Kadir S (ed) Current practice of interventional radiology. Decker, Philadelphia, pp 21–23
2. Land M, Carver D (1991) The role of the nurse in interventional radiology. In: Kadir S (ed) Current practice of interventional radiology. Decker, Philadelphia, pp 18–21
3. Lynch-Nyhan MA (1991) Interventional radiology inpatient service. In: Kadir S (ed) Current practice of interventional radiology. Decker, Philadelphia, pp 5–6

Technical Monitoring During Radiologic Interventions – What Can Be Done and What Must Be Done

E. B. Keeffe

Introduction

Most diagnostic invasive procedures require the use of some form of premedication for sedation. The use of sedation has become standard in the performance of gastrointestinal endoscopy by gastroenterologists and interventional radiologic procedures by radiologists. Even though the use of intravenous medications immediately prior to these procedures is routine, the exact types and dosages of medications used, either alone or in combination, are highly individualized by practicing physicians. The use of intravenous medications to achieve the production of sedation and amnesia, most often utilizing benzodiazepines and/or narcotics, is termed conscious sedation. The goal in using these medications is not to induce anesthesia; however, there is an overlap between conscious sedation and anesthesia such that anesthesia with the loss of protective reflexes may be induced in individual patients. The variable use of sedative medications and unpredictable patient response to intended light conscious sedation make monitoring an important and inseparable partner to sedation. In this review, basic information regarding physiologic patient monitoring systems is provided (i.e., what can be done). In addition, the politics and science of monitoring the sedated patient undergoing gastrointestinal endoscopy are summarized to highlight lessons that may be applicable to the use of conscious sedation during interventional radiologic procedures (i.e., what must be done).

Any physician who employs conscious sedation must be aware of the possibility of untoward responses that may include (1) respiratory depression, (2) allergic reactions, (3) paradoxical reactions, and (4) local reactions. It is incumbent upon the operating physician to provide for the appropriate monitoring, both clinical and technical, and to diagnose and respond to such complications early in their development. The most frequent complication during procedures utilizing conscious sedation is oxygen desaturation and respiratory depression. As an example, more than 50% of deaths associated with gastrointestinal endoscopy are related to cardiopulmonary problems [4]. Standard clinical monitoring of all patients undergoing gastrointestinal endoscopy or any invasive procedure is reviewed elsewhere in this monograph and should include clinical assessment by a nurse of the patient's tolerance to the procedure and the determination of vital signs at several different junctures during and after the procedure. There should be a designated nurse whose sole responsibility is patient monitoring, i.e., not an individual whose responsibilities are divided between monitoring the patient and assisting the operating physician. The degree of technical monitoring employed during invasive procedures is variable, but the standard practice is evolving towards monitoring more physiologic patient parameters with automated equipment.

What is the definition of monitoring? A generic definition of monitoring is "to watch, observe, or check on a person or thing." Monitoring in a general medical sense is the assessment of the patient's clinical status, e.g., degree of sedation, respiratory rate, skin color and temperature, and general tolerance to the procedure. A more specific definition of monitoring is the determination of physiologic parameters such as heart rate, blood pressure, oxygen saturation, or the electrocardiogram (ECG). Finally, a broader quality assurance definition of monitoring refers to the assessment of the quality of care as defined by certain indicators for a given procedure.

Technical Monitoring

What Can Be Done

There are two basic types of physiologic patient-monitoring systems: modular and configured. These monitors differ only in how they are constructed and in their flexibility, not in their monitoring capabilities. Modular monitors are larger and heavier, more expensive, and more flexible in that monitored parameters can be changed or added. Configured monitors are smaller and portable, less expensive, and have less flexibility. Technology has made possible a number of changes in patient monitoring devices over the past 20 years, primarily in the number and types of parameters that can be monitored, the reduced size of the equipment, the availability of continuous monitoring, electronic charting, and the capability for networking and storage.

Continuous monitoring of vital physiologic parameters is now standard in the operating room, postanesthesia care unit, intensive care unit, emergency department, and during the transport of critically ill patients. In recent years, there has been expanded use of technical monitors in the endoscopy unit, radiology suite, and labor and delivery areas. A number of factors have influenced the standard of care for monitoring during anesthesia; examples include: (1) the Joint Commission on Accreditation of Healthcare Organizations (JCAHO) standards for anesthesia care (found in the Surgical and Anesthesia Services chapter of the *Accreditation Manual for Hospitals*) [10], (2) the American Society of Anesthesiologists' (ASA) standards for basic intraoperative monitoring [2], (3) state regulations in the United States of America, (4) minimal standards of insurance carriers, and (5) other professional society standards. The specific parameters that are monitored are different during general anesthesia compared with intravenous conscious sedation. For general anesthesia, the following physiologic parameters are routinely monitored: ECG, heart rate, oxygen saturation (pulse oximetry), end-tidal carbon dioxide concentration (capnography), blood pressure, and temperature where changes are anticipated [2]. During conscious sedation, by contrast, monitoring practices are not standardized and generally fewer parameters are monitored: ECG (selective or universal), heart rate, oxygen saturation (pulse oximetry), and blood pressure (manual or automated). The use of pulse oximetry during conscious sedation appears to be particularly useful and is now commonly used in many diverse hospital settings [1].

The proliferation of physiologic patient monitoring and the increased practice to monitor more parameters has created the dilemma of how to respond to abnormalities that are identified. For example, do any baseline aberrations preclude proceeding with a procedure? At what threshold values should alarms be set? If physiologic abnormalities beyond these threshold values occur, do all or only some of these abnormalities warrant an intervention? How should staff respond? Should the physician individualize, or should there be a published unit protocol that is followed? Finally, when should a procedure be abandoned? The practice that has evolved in many endoscopy units is to perform simple interventions to correct physiologic abnormalities. For example, patients whose oxygen saturation falls below 90% are encouraged by the nurse to take deep breaths or given supplemental oxygen. Hypotension is treated by increasing the rate in intravenous saline infusion. More troublesome issues are when to administer additional drugs, such as reversal agents or atropine, and when to address identified ECG abnormalities (e.g., premature ventricular contractions). The answers to these questions have usually been individualized, but unit protocols may be useful, particularly for physicians not skilled in the pharmacologic treatment of arrhythmias.

What Must Be Done

A number of political issues have influenced monitoring in the practice of gastrointestinal endoscopy, and these lessons are likely to be applicable to sedation and monitoring practices in interventional radiology. The rapid growth in the performance of gastrointestinal endoscopy in the United States led to the routine practice of using conscious sedation. Although endoscopy, particularly upper endoscopy, can be performed without conscious sedation, surveys from the United States [11] and United Kingdom [7] indicate that both endoscopists and patients prefer some form of premedication. Another political issue that fueled attention to monitoring was confusion regarding the policies of the JCAHO regarding responsibility for sedation and monitoring policies in the hospital setting. Previous standards had implied that hospital-wide responsibilities for anesthesia services were the sole responsibility of the director of anesthesia services; these standards were revised in 1989 to state that "the responsibility for the provision of anesthesia services rests with the directors of the department/service in which the anesthesia care is provided" [10]. In other words, the director of the endoscopy unit or the interventional radiology unit is primarily responsible for anesthesia policies within that given unit. In addition, the JCAHO mandate to have operational quality assurance programs in all hospital units, necessitated documentation of patient monitoring during endoscopic procedures.

A further political issue that heightened awareness of monitoring was the introduction of midazolam for conscious sedation during gastrointestinal endoscopy and the initial concerns regarding its safety. Traditionally, endoscopists have limited their use of medications to a few drugs, particularly diazepam and meperidine. For the first time in over a decade, endoscopists began to use a new drug, midazolam, following its introduction in the United States in 1986. Following initial confusion regarding proper dosage and potency of midazolam verses diazepam, Roche Laboratories in November, 1987 sent a letter to all physicians advising "continuous monitoring of the cardiovascular and respiratory functions ... by personnel other than the person doing the procedure." This letter did not make specific recommendations whether monitoring should be clinical versus technical. The desire of the physicians to use midazolam, lingering concern regarding safety issues, and medicolegal concerns prompted many endoscopists for the first time to explore the routine use of technical monitoring with pulse oximetry and/or ECG. At approximately the same time, pulse oximetry became more widely available and was aggressively marketed to endoscopists. Later, further physiologic monitoring equipment was developed with the capability of measuring not only pulse oximetry, but also heart rate, blood pressure, and ECG on a continuous basis. Finally, national medical societies such as the American Society for Gastrointestinal Endoscopy (ASGE) and the British Society of Gastroenterology (BSG), which had been quiet regarding the issue of sedation and monitoring, published guidelines providing specific recommendations [5, 13]. The recommendations for standards of sedation and patient monitoring during gastrointestinal endoscopy were particularly strong in the guidelines published by the Endoscopy Committee Working Party of the BSG [5]. For example, while the ASGE stated that monitoring techniques such as pulse oximetry might be useful in certain high-risk patients and/or for high-risk procedures, the BSG specifically recommended pulse oximetry during all procedures.

In order to understand the controversies and politics of technical monitoring of patients undergoing gastrointestinal endoscopy, some background information is required. A number of studies have indicated that the safety record with endoscopy is quite good with the predominant use of clinical monitoring [3, 11]. Arrowsmith et al. studied cardiorespiratory complications during endoscopy by retrospectively analyzing a large computerized data base of the ASGE. An analysis of data from over 20000 procedures revealed that serious cardiorespiratory complications occurred at a rate of 5.4/1000 and death at a rate of 0.3/1000. There was no difference in the frequency of serious cardiorespiratory complications whether midazolam or diazepam was used for conscious sedation. An increased risk for cardiorespiratory complications was only associated with the concomitant use of narcotics or the performance of emergent procedures. Cardiopulmonary sedation-related complications were also very low in the survey by Keeffe and O'Connor, with only 9.1% reporting a patient death associated with endoscopy over an average 12.4-year career.

A number of studies have addressed the physiologic changes that occur during gastrointestinal endoscopy, and these data were recently reviewed [9]. The conclusions of Dr. Fleisher from the analysis of these studies are that: (1) oxygen saturation decreases during upper endoscopy and colonoscopy; (2) no correlation exists between the fall in oxygen saturation and the type or dose of medication used, and the age or sex of the patient; (3) data are conflicting regarding oxygen saturation and the importance of the length of the procedure, whether sedation is used or not, and if preprocedure pulmonary function tests are useful; and (4) a fall in oxygen saturation is related to the use of larger diameter endoscopes for upper endoscopy, the additive effect of a narcotic with a benzodiazepine, and the presence of preexisting pulmonary disease. More recent studies using automated equipment to monitor patients undergoing endoscopy with conscious sedation have demonstrated a common theme, i.e., physiologic abnormalities are common but appear to be clinically insignificant. In the study by DiSario et al., hemodynamic aberrations were noted in 71% of 618 patients having automated blood pressure and heart-rate monitoring (hypertension in 30%, hypotension in 6%, tachycardia in 32%, and bradycardia in 26%) [8]. In two other studies, the incidence of oxygen desaturation (SaO_2 <90%) was 41% and 45%, but no untoward clinical events were noted [6, 12].

As background for the development of a society guideline on sedation and monitoring, the ASGE sponsored a membership survey of current monitoring practices in the United States by mail during March and April 1989 [11]. This survey confirmed the fact that most American endoscopists routinely use sedation for endoscopic procedures, including meperidine (87%), midazolam (73%), diazepam (49%), and naloxone (30%). The majority of endoscopists provided for intravenous access to be available during endoscopy. Premedications for endoscopy were administered by a physician/endoscopist (83%) or by a registered nurse (43%). Only 3% stated that premedications were given by a physician/anesthesiologist.

The survey indicated that clinical monitoring during endoscopy was fairly, standard, with vital signs monitored before and after the procedure. One nurse was present during routine procedures, and a second nurse was present during more advanced procedures such as endoscopic retrograde cholangiopancreatography. At the time of the survey, 65% of endoscopists used pulse oximetry and 55% used continuous ECG monitoring. However, most technical monitoring was done in hospitals (99.5%) rather than in private offices (27%). While the majority of endoscopists used technical monitoring selectively for high-risk patients, 42% used it universally for all patients. An argument can certainly be made that automated physiologic monitoring should be used universally, since a cardiorespiratory complication or a death is equally or more tragic in a young, fit patient compared with an elderly patient with identified risk factors.

The availability of the resuscitation equipment and the qualifications of endoscopists and nurses in basic life support and advanced cardiac life support were also surveyed. A surprising finding from this survey was that only 76% of endoscopists were certified in basic life support techniques and 30% in advanced life support techniques.

After lengthy study, two large medical societies, the ASGE and the BSG, published specific recommendations regarding sedation and monitoring practices for their memberships. The key elements of the ASGE guideline entitled *Monitoring of Patients Undergoing Gastrointestinal Endoscopic Procedures* [13] are as follows:

1. The use of special monitoring equipment may be a useful adjunct to patient surveillance but it is never a substitute for clinical assessment.
2. Standard clinical monitoring should include the determination of heart rate, blood pressure, and respiratory rate before sedation, immediately after the procedure, and at the time of discharge from the gastrointestinal unit.
3. The proper role of pulse oximetry and continuous ECG monitoring during endoscopic procedures is controversial and evolving.
4. Pulse oximetry and ECG monitoring may be beneficial for certain high-risk patients and/or procedures.

The BSG recommendations regarding sedation and monitoring during gastrointestinal endoscopy are stronger and more specific [5]. A summary of these recommendations is as follows:

1. Safety and monitoring should be a part of a quality assurance program.
2. Resuscitation equipment and drugs must be available in endoscopy and recovery areas.
3. All endoscopy staff should be trained in resuscitation methods.
4. A qualified nurse should monitor the patient's condition during procedures.
5. Risk factors should be identified prior to endoscopy by a check list.
6. Dosage of drugs used for sedation should be kept to a minimum.
7. Antagonists for benzodiazepines and opioids should be available.
8. Intravenous access should be established for "at risk" patients.
9. Supplemental oxygen is recommended for "at risk" patients.
10. Monitoring techniques such as pulse oximetry are recommended.
11. Clinical monitoring of the patient must be continued into the recovery area.

Personal experience and informal surveys of colleagues in the United States indicate that monitoring practices have evolved since the ASGE guidelines and survey on sedation and monitoring practice were published. It is now likely that more than 90% of patients undergoing routine endoscopy in hospitals and receiving conscious sedation have some form of technical monitoring, most commonly pulse oximetry. The widespread availability of physiologic monitoring equipment and its likelihood to enhance the safety of conscious sedation, as well as a number of pressures, such as the recommendations of the JCAHO and medical societies, and also medicolegal considerations are leading to the routine rather than selective use of technical monitoring during endoscopy.

In spite of the recommendations of medical societies, there is significant skepticism regarding whether the use of physiologic monitoring equipment, such as pulse oximetry, will have any impact on the safety record of gastrointestinal endoscopy. Large surveys indicate that the safety record during endoscopy, with standard monitoring of clinical status by nurses, is quite good. Moreover, pulse oximetry equipment and monitoring equipment is expensive, ranging from US $ 3000 to US $ 8000. Another major unanswered question is how frequently oxygen desaturation is clinically significant. Studies reviewed above indicate that a fall in oxygen saturation does not appear to be associated with adverse clinical events. Finally, the most important question is whether pulse oximetry will improve the safety record of endoscopy.

Summary

In the opinion of the author, appropriate sedation and monitoring practices with the use of conscious sedation for invasive procedures should include the following in 1992:

1. Standard quality assurance program
2. Written unit protocol regarding sedation and monitoring
3. Patient check list for adverse risk factors
4. Physician and one to two nurses in attendance, including one nurse continuously responsible for clinical monitoring
5. Running intravenous line
6. Routine clinical monitoring
7. Automated physiologic monitoring with pulse oximetry and possibly also blood pressure, heart rate, and ECG
8. Code cart in procedure area with equipment and drugs, including antagonist
9. Personnel trained in cardiopulmonary resuscitation and advanced cardiac life support
10. Standard postprocedure protocol for monitoring and discharge

In summary, the question of what can be done and what must be done in terms of technical physiologic monitoring during the use of conscious sedation for interventional radiologic procedures should probably be supplanted by "what monitoring appears reasonable and meets the local standard of care." The rationale for technical monitoring is to a large part based on common sense and the mandate of published guidelines that the overall safety record of invasive procedures, although already quite good with standard clinical monitoring, may be improved further by the addition of automated physiologic monitoring systems.

References

1. Alexander CM, Teller LE, Gross JB (1989) Principles of pulse oximetry: theoretical and practical considerations. Anesth Analg 68:368–376
2. American Society of Anesthesiologists (1990) ASA standards for basic intraoperative monitoring. American Society of Anesthesiologists, Park Ridge
3. Arrowsmith JB, Gerstman BB, Fleischer DE, Benjamin SB (1991) Results from the American Society for Gastrointestinal Endoscopy/U.S. Food and Drug Administration collaborative study on complication rates and drug use during gastrointestinal endoscopy. Gastrointest Endosc 37:421–427
4. Bell GD (1990) Review article: premedication and intravenous sedation for upper gastrointestinal endoscopy. Aliment Pharmacol Ther 4:103–122
5. Bell GD, McCloy RF, Charlton JE, Campbell D, Dent NA, Gear MWL, Logan RFA, Swan CHJ (1991) Recommendations for standards of sedation and patient monitoring during gastrointestinal endoscopy. Gut 32:823–827
6. Bilotta JJ, Floyd JL, Waye JD (1990) Arterial oxygen desaturation during ambulatory colonoscopy: predictability, incidence, and clinical significance. Gastrointest Endosc 36:S5–S8
7. Daneshmend TK, Bell GD, Logan RFA (1991) Sedation for upper gastrointestinal endoscopy: results of a nationwide survey. Gut 32:12–15
8. Disario JA, Waring JP, Talbert G, Sanowski RA (1991) Monitoring of blood pressure and heart rate during routine endoscopy: a prospective, randomized, controlled study. Am J Gastroenterol 86:956–960
9. Fleischer D (1989) Monitoring the patient receiving conscious sedation for gastrointestinal endoscopy: issues and guidelines. Gastrointest Endosc 35:262–266
10. Joint Commission on Accreditation of Healthcare Organizations (1989) Accreditation manual for hospitals, 1990. Joint Commission on Accreditation of Healthcare Organizations, Chicago
11. Keeffe EB, O'Connor KW (1990) 1989 ASGE survey of endoscopic sedation and monitoring practices. Gastrointest Endosc 36:S13–S18
12. O'Connor KW, Jones S (1990) Oxygen desaturation is common and clinically underappreciated during elective endoscopic procedures. Gastrointest Endosc 36:S2–S4
13. Standards of Practice Committee. American Society for Gastrointestinal Endoscopy (1991) Monitoring of patients undergoing gastrointestinal endoscopic procedures. Guidelines for clinical application. Gastrointest Endosc 37:120–121

Monitoring of Vital Functions in the Course of Interventional Radiology Procedures

C. Neuhaus, R. Leppek, G. Christ, J. Froelich, and K. J. Klose

Introduction

During the past years interventional radiology (IR) has established itself increasingly as an independent field. Wilkins et al. [50] have shown in a survey conducted in 102 British hospitals that from 1981 to 1986 there was a remarkable increase of interventional procedures (Table 1).

Table 1. The expansion of interventional radiology within a 5-year period [49]

Procedure	Number of procedures		
	1981	1986	% change
Angioplasty	998	3782	+279%
Abscess drainage	275	1299	+372%
Liver and biliary procedures	561	2231	+298%

Not only did the number of procedures increase, but these interventions have become more complex and technically sometimes challenging procedures. IR offers patients a viable option to surgery. Often it is necessary to substitute strong analgesics and sedatives and in this case IR takes on an intermediary position between radiology, surgery and anesthesiology.

Within this context, it is also necessary to question the necessity to monitor significant vegetative parameters during an interventional procedure [37, 48]. Because IR deals mostly with people who are either severely ill or multimorbid patients, the striking question is whether patient monitoring conditions should be organized the same as for other minimally invasive therapy forms [3, 20]. IR monitoring has been recommended in the USA [37, 48] for a long time.

In this study we investigated the changes in vital functions which can appear in the course of an interventional procedure.

Material and Methods

Demographical Data

Between August 91 and March 92 we examined 107 individual patients from the routine program of our department. Altogether 130 examinations related to establishing changes of the vital functions in these patients were done. In order to create a comparative field of observation we divided the patients into four groups (Table 2).

The patients of the first three groups were on average 65 years old, while the fourth group was collectively 10 years younger on average. In the groups "peripheral angiography," "PTA" (percutaneous transluminal angiography) and "liver intervention" there were more men than women on each group; however, in the case of "visceral angiographies" the same number of men and women was investigated (Table 3).

Vital Functions

In this study we investigated the mentioned patient groups in relation to changes in blood pressure, heart rate, transcutaneous oxygen saturation, body temperature and ECG. Blood pressure was measured with the help of an

Table 2. Summary of the four investigation groups and number of supervised procedures per group

Group	Type of intervention	Subdivision	Number of supervisions
I	Peripheral angiography	Upper extremity Lower extremity	30
II	Visceral angiography	Renal arteries Carotid arteries Mesenteric artery Celiac trunk Abdominal aorta	30
III	PTA	Upper extremity Lower extremity Renal arteries	35
IV	Liver intervention	PTC PTCD Internal splinting Stent implantation Stone extraction Liver abscess drainage	35

PTA, percutaneous transluminal angioplasty; PTC, percutaneous transhepatic cholangiography; PTCD, percutaneous transhepatic cholangiodrainage.

Table 3. Patients and their demographical data according to the four groups

Group	Age (years)	Men (*n*) (%)	Women (*n*) (%)	Total patients (*n*)
I	66±10 years	22 (73)	8 (27)	30
II	64±14 years	15 (50)	15 (50)	30
III	65±14 years	21 (60)	14 (40)	35
IV	59±11 years	11 (61)	7 (39)	18

Table 4. Course of measurements in this study

Arteriography	PTA	Liver interventions
	Measurements three times before the intervention	
Injection of local anesthetics	Injection of local anesthetics	Injection of local anesthetics
Puncture	Puncture	Puncture
First contrast medium injection 2 min after first injection 5 min after first injection 10 min after first injection	First contrast medium injection 2 min after first injection 5 min after first injection 10 min after first injection First Dilatation	Contrast medium injection ↓ Catheter manipulations in the region of the biliary system ↓
↓	↓ Last Dilatation	Dilatations in the region of the biliary system ↓
Last contrast medium injection 2 min after last injection 5 min after last injection 10 min after last injection	Last contrast medium injection 2 min after last injection 5 min after last injection 10 min after last injection	Stent release ↓ Installation of a drainage catheter
		3 min after the intervention

PTA, percutaneous transluminal angioplasty.

automatic "Dinamap 1846 SX" blood pressure measuring instrument (Critikon Co., Norderstedt, Germany). A fitted "Oxytrak" pulsoximetry module helped to register the transcutaneous oxygen saturation (SaO_2) and the heart rate. A finger clip oxygen saturation detector with red/infrared light (600 and 805 nm) was used. The temperature was measured sublingually with a simple digital thermometer (Becton-Dickinson, Heidelberg, Germany). The ECG registration was made with a three-channel register "Cardiostat 5T" (Siemens, Erlangen, Germany). Limb leads were used according to Goldberger. Every individual measuring point was recorded by an ECG strip of 20-s duration and a paper assistance of 25 mm/s. The ECG evaluation was limited to the classification of arising extrasystoles.

The range of measurements for the individual groups is depicted in Table 4. Data were collected three times before the procedure, so as to maintain a possible representative initial value.

Data Evaluation

To determine the difference between the recorded preoperative initial value and the individual measuring points collected in progress levels, we used Wilcoxon's two-sided signed rank test. All statistical calculations were made with the help of the statistical programm "Wistat PC" (Wissoft. S. Franzen, Marburg, Germany).

Moreover, we analyzed minimum and maximum (minimax-) values of all parameters under investigation to avoid omission of significant individual changes. Those values were compared to already given critical minimal and maximal levels taken from the literature.

Results

Systolic Blood Pressure

The measuring point at which significant variations of the systolic blood pressure could be established as well as their significance level are illustrated in Tables 5–8. In addition to all patients with preprocedural pressure values over 160 mm Hg, blood pressure values increased significantly in all four groups during the procedure. The greatest increase was in the group "Liver interventions." The number of people with a systolic blood pressure lower than 100 mm Hg increased only in a small percentage (Fig. 1).

Table 5. Significant changes of vital functions in the course of peripheral angiography

Peripheral angiography (time →)	↑ LAI	↑ 1 CMI	↑ 2′p 1. CMI	↑ 2 CMI	↑ 3 CMI	↑ 2′p 3. CMI	↑ 4 CMI	↑ 5 CMI	↑ 6 CMI	↑ 7 CMI
Systolic RR	↑↑	–	–	↓	–	–	–	–	–	–
Diastolic RR	–	–	–	↓	–	–	–	–	–	–
Heart rate	–	–	–	↑↑	–	↑	–	–	–	–
SaO_2	–	↓↓	↓↓	–	–	–	↓	↓↓	↓	↓
Temperature	–	–	–	–	–	–	–	–	–	–

↑↑, The average measurement of data at this point is larger than the preinterventional measurement, and the significance level shows $p < 0.01$; ↑, the average measurement of data at this point is larger than the preinterventional measurement, and the significance level shows $p<0.05$; ↓↓, the average measurement of data at this point is smaller than the preinterventional measurement, and the significance level shows $p < 0.01$; ↓, the average measurement of data at this point is smaller than the preinterventional measurement, and the significance level shows $p < 0.05$; LAI, injection of local anesthetics; CMI, contrast medium injection; 2′p, 2 min after; RR, blood pressure (Riva Rocci).

Table 6. Statistically significant changes of vital functions in the course of a visceral angiography

Visceral angiography (time →)	↑ LAI	↑ 1 CMI	↑ 2 CMI	↑ 3 CMI	↑ 4 CMI	↑ 5 CMI	↑ 6 CMI	↑ 7 CMI	↑ 8 CMI
Systolic RR	↑	–	–	–	–	–	–	–	–
Diastolic RR	–	–	–	–	↓↓	↓↓	↓	↓↓	↓
Heart rate	–	–	–	–	–	–	–	–	↑
SaO_2	–	–	–	–	–	–	–	–	–
Temperature	–	–	–	–	–	–	–	–	–

See Table 5 for abbreviations.

Table 7. Significant changes of the vital functions in the course of PTA

PTA (time →)	↑ 1 CMI	↑ 2'p First CMI	↑ DL 1	↑ 2 CMI	↑ DL 2	↑ 3 CMI	↑ 2'p Third CMI	↑ 4 CMI	↑ 2'p Fourth CMI	↑ 5 CMI	↑ 6 CMI	↑ 7 CMI	↑ 8 CMI
Systolic RR	–	–	–	↓↓	–	–	↓	↓	–	–	–	–	–
Diastolic RR	–	–	–	–	–	↓	–	↓	↓↓	–	–	–	–
Pulse	–	–	–	–	–	–	–	–	–	–	–	–	↑
SaO_2	↓	↓	↓↓	↓	↓↓	↓↓	↓↓	↓	–	↓↓	↓↓	–	–
Temperature	–	–	–	–	–	–	–	–	–	–	–	–	–

DL, dilatation of a stenosis; for other abbreviations see Table 5.

Table 8. Significant changes of the vital functions in the course of an interventional procedure of the liver

Liver intervention (time →)	↑ LAI	↑ PU1	↑ PU2	↑ 1 CMI	↑ 2 CMI	↑ 3 CMI	↑ 4 CMI	↑ 5 CMI	↑ 6 CMI	↑ 7 CMI	↑ SM1	↑ SM2	↑ SM3	↑ SM4	↑ DL	↑ Stent	↑ Drain
Systolic RR	↑	–	–	–	↑↑	↑	–	–	–	↑↑	↑↑	–	–	–	↑↑	↑↑	↑
Diastolic RR	↑↑	–	–	–	–	–	–	–	–	↑↑	↑	–	–	↑	↑↑	↑↑	↑
Heart rate	↑↑	–	–	–	–	↓↓	↓	–	–	–	↕↕	↕↕	↕↕	–	–	–	–
SaO_2	–	↓↓	↓↓	↓↓	↓↓	↓↓	↓↓	↓↓	↓	–	↓↓	↓↓	↓↓	↓↓	–	↓↓	↓↓
Temperature	–	–	–	↕↕	↑↑	↑↑	↑↑	↑↑	–	–	↑↑	↑↑	↑↑	↑↑	–	–	↑↑

↕↕, The average measurement of data at this point is just as large as the registered preinterventional measurements, and the significance level of the registered intrainterventional variations is $p < 0{,}01$; ↕, the average measurement of data at this point is just as large as the registerd preinterventional measurements, and the significance level of the registered intrainterventional variations is $p < 0{,}05$; LAI, injection of local anesthetic; PU, puncture; SM, manipulations in the region of the biliary system; DL, dilatation in the area of the bile ducts; stent, stent release; drain, installation of a drainage catheter; RR, blood pressure (Riva Rocci); CMI, Contrast medium injection.

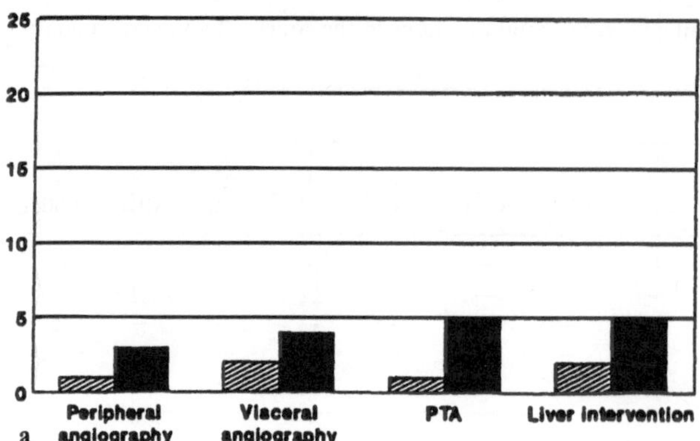

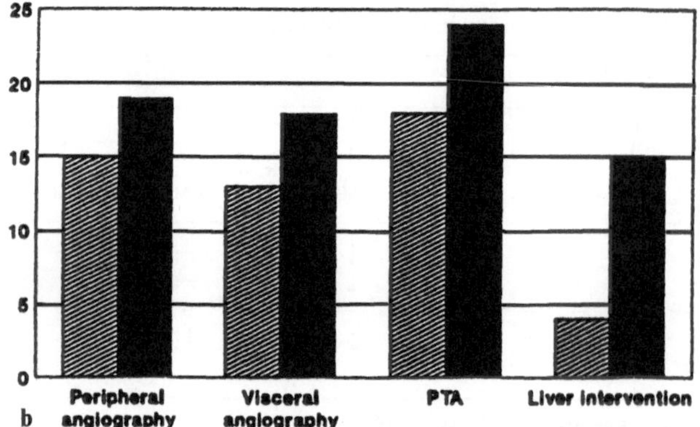

Fig. 1 a, b. Minimax values of systolic blood pressure. **a** Number of patients showing measured values below 100 mmHg. **b** Number of patients showing measured values larger than 160 mmHg. ▨, Before intervention; ■, during intervention

Diastolic Blood Pressure

The results of the statistical calculations of diastolic blood pressure are demonstrated in Tables 5–8. The maximal level observation brought tendencies similar to those of systolic blood pressure. Once again, there was a noticeable crossing over of a large number of patients from preinterventional normotonic values towards the hypertensive group. Moreover, a significant number of patients showed diastolic blood pressure below the tolerance limit (Fig. 2).

Heart Rate

The results of the statistical calculations for heart rate are shown in Tables 5–8. Figure 3 shows the results of the minimax values: All four groups showed patients with pulse rates more than 100/min in the course of the study.

The largest heart rate increase was to be observed in group IV. However, only individual patients showed heart frequencies under 60/min.

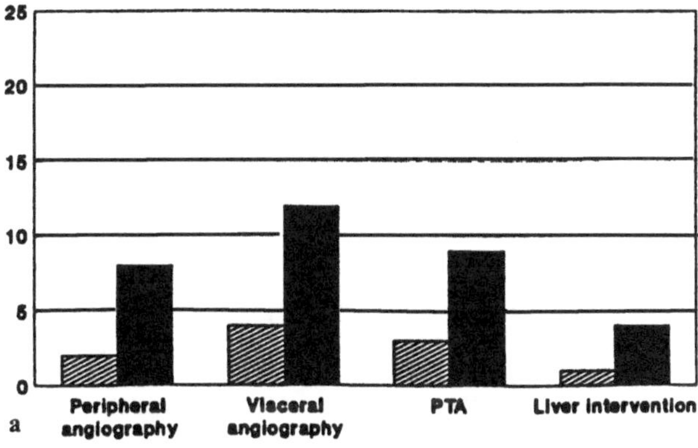

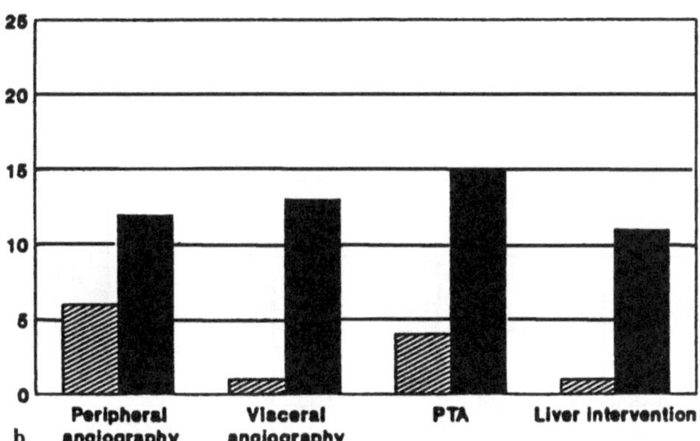

Fig. 2a, b. Minimax values of diastolic blood pressure. **a** Number of patients showing measured values below 60 mmHg. **b** Number of patients showing measured values larger than 95 mmHg. ▨, Before intervention; ■, during intervention

Transcutaneous Oxygen Saturation

Tables 5–8 show the measuring point at which statistically significant variations of the transcutaneous oxygen saturation could be established.

Although patients in group IV were approximately 10 years younger than the other patients, oxygen saturation was often less than 90% during the intervention in this group (Fig. 4). A number of these patients were given 5–15 mg midazolam i.v. or 50 mg promethazine and 50 mg pethidine i.m. to relieve pain. Nevertheless, nine patients showed a decrease in SaO_2 below 90% without previous medication of analgesics or sedatives.

A comparison of the average duration of an procedure with a temporary SaO_2 of less than 90%, with the duration of an intervention where constant saturation levels over 90% were achieved, shows that the procedures with a temporal undersaturation took longer on average. Only within the PTA group did interventions with a permanent SaO_2 greater than 90% take longer (Fig. 5).

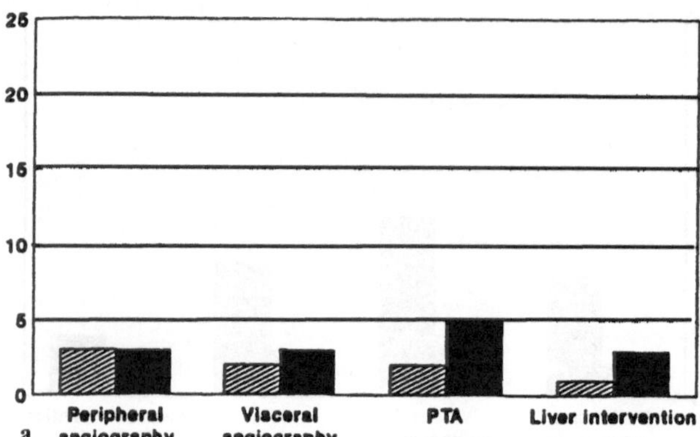

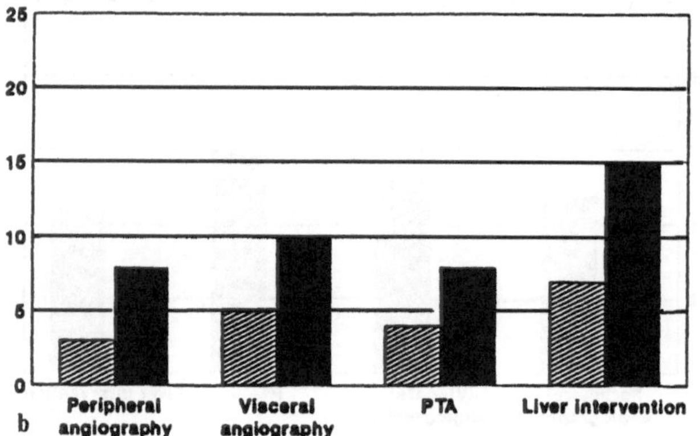

Fig. 3a, b. Minimax values of heart rate. **a** Number of patients showing measured values below 60/min. **b** Number of patients showing measured values larger than 100/min. ▨, Before intervention; ■, during intervention

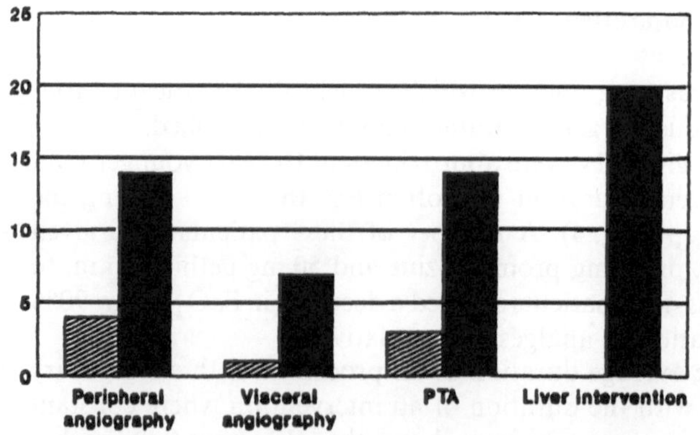

Fig. 4. Minimax values of transcutaneous oxygen saturation (Number of patients showing measured values below 90%). ▨, Before intervention; ■, during intervention

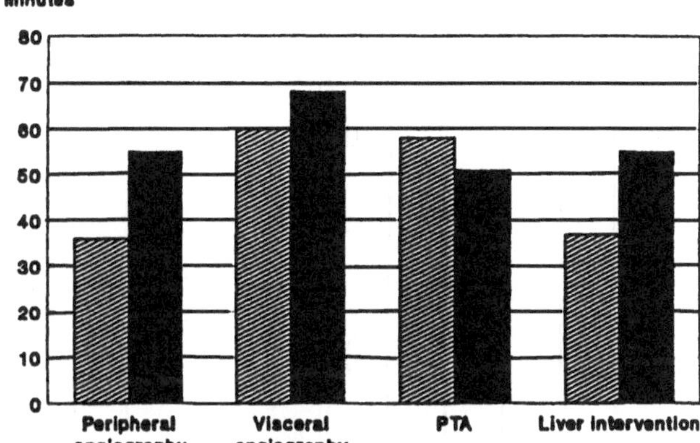

Fig. 5. Duration of the procedure (mean values) and transcutaneous oxygen saturation. ▨, SaO_2 over 90%; ■, SaO_2 below 90%

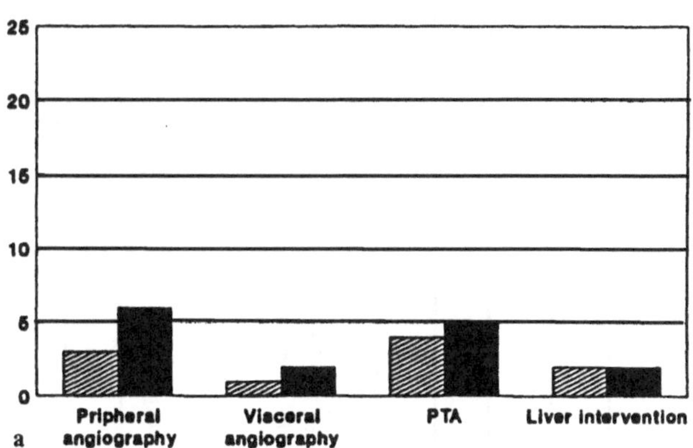

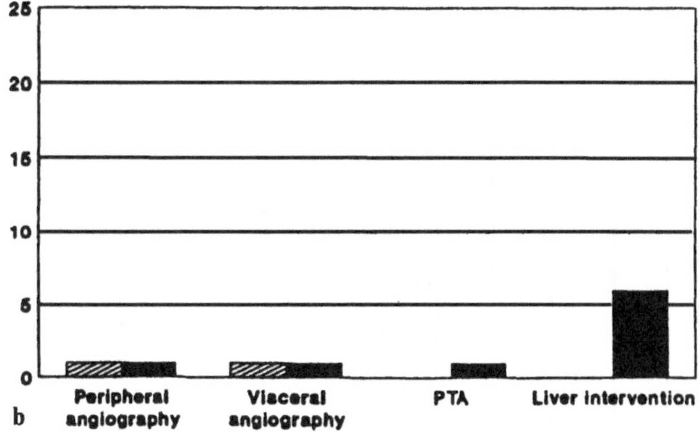

Fig. 6a, b. Minimax values of body temperature. **a** Number of patients showing measured values below 36 °C. **b** Number of patients showing measured values larger than 38 °C. ▨, Before intervention; ■, during intervention

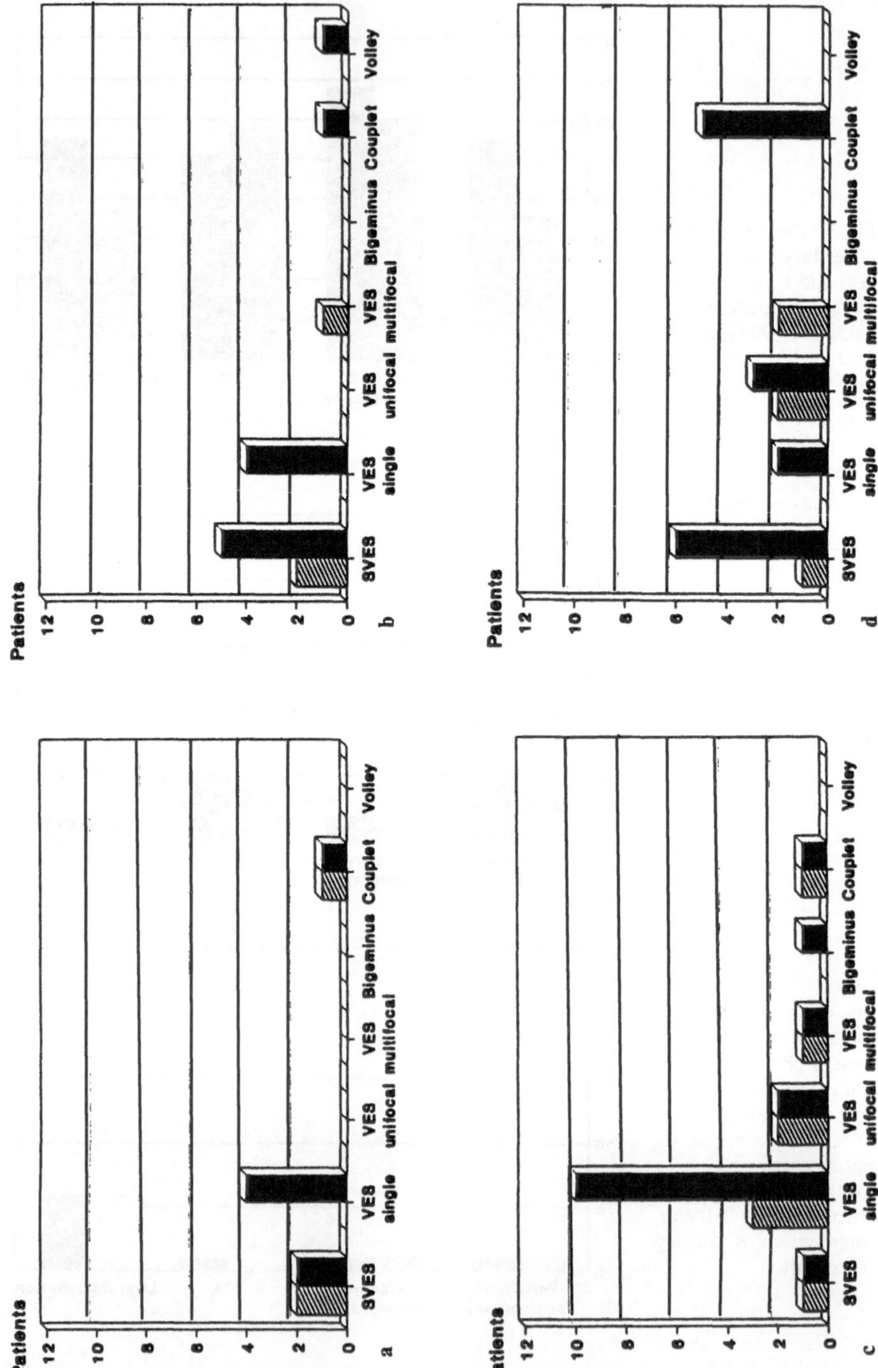

Fig. 7 a–d. Incidence of arrhythmias before and during a procedure. ▨, Before procedure; ■, during procedure

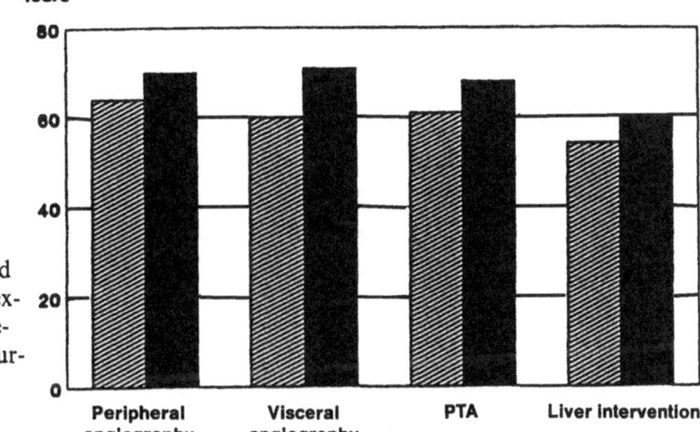

Fig. 8. Extrasystoles and age of patients. ▨, No extrasystoles during procedure; ■, extrasystoles during procedure

Temperature

Statistically significant changes of body temperature could be established only in the course of the interventional procedures in the region of the liver (Fig. 8). Patients of group IV showed temperature levels of over 38 °C more frequently (Fig. 6).

Among the six patients which showed such temperature increases, four received a percutaneous transhepatic cholangiodrainage (PTCD) and two an internal splinting. Three patients had a carcinoma of the pancreatic head, the others bile duct carcinomas (Klatskin tumor).

Electrocardiogram

Figure 7 shows the recorded arrhythmias according to rising complexity and to growing degree of severity. Only the most severe type of arrhythmia occurring during each procedure was listed in this figure.

Peripheral and visceral angiographies more frequently caused a minor rise of uncomplicated arrhythmias. In the PTA group we registered a significant increase of individual ventricular extrasystole (VES).

Significant ECG changes were also registered in the patient group with liver interventions. Parallel to an increase of supraventricular extrasystole (SVES) and uncomplicated VES, the number of patients who showed couplets during the intervention increased significantly. This type of arrhythmia was established in the course of longer procedures. These rhythm abnormalities appeared mostly during exploratory examinations in the region of the hepatoduodenal ligament.

If we compare the average age of the patients who showed no arrhythmias during the examination and the age of those with arrhythmia during the examination we can establish that on average the patients with demonstrable arrhythmic disruption were older (Table 8).

Discussion

A predictor that the growing demands made on IR go hand in hand with a new acceptance of practitioners of this discipline is that recently, adequate patient care and "inpatient management" have obviously gained increasing respect [4, 19, 22, 38]. The results of our study show that impressive changes of vital functions can appear during interventional procedures. Patients who underwent interventional procedures of the liver confirm this finding.

Circulation

To find an adequate explanation for the established changes, we have to point out that the procedures studied took place in two totally different organic systems. While the patients of the first three groups had vascular interventions with considerable amounts of contrast fluid, the patients of group IV had procedures in the area of the bile ducts which can be considered to be "closed systems."

A clarification of the rise in blood pressure during a procedure can be established on the basis of this consideration. In the case of angiographies and PTAs, the additional strain of volume may be the original cause for a systolic pressure rise of over 160 mm Hg and a diastolic pressure rise of over 95 mm Hg in [8]. The increase of the heart rate above 100/min can also be placed in the same context: The additional blood volume which follows the contrast medium injections increases the venous backflow to the heart and consequently the auricular pressure rises. In this way through the Bainbridge reflex it causes a reflectory tachycardia [51].

The given intrainterventional pressure below the lowest tolerance levels can be explained by the histamine release [1, 13, 36] induced by contrast fluid with vasodilation and reduction in blood pressure [7]. This appears all the more evident when significant blood pressure changes, especially during or within the first 2 min after injection of contrast medium, can be observed, whereas hypertonic pressure levels appear somehow later after contrast administration and particularly during the second half of a procedure. Later, the volume of plasma should increase after hyperosmolaric contrast injection, when the circulation system is burdened with a higher dose of contrast fluids during the second half of the procedure.

Because of the small number of kidney interventions (seven patients) involved in the study, we cannot determine accurately the changes of the vital functions which could ultimately come about during a PTA of the renal arteries. This relatively small patient group was assessed together with group III patients showing a dilatation in the extremities. Because in the case of a kidney intervention we are dealing with a visceral organ amply supplied with vegetative fibers, we should expect a higher degree of circulatory disturbances than the results shown here. Hägg et al. [12] already studied a striking increase of plasma renin activity during a renal artery PTA. Even if in our study we were not able to establish a significant alteration in the blood pressure measurements, we recommend monitoring these patients during renal artery PTA.

The reactions of the blood pressure and pulse during a liver intervention can be easily justified by the rise in epinephrine levels and consequent vegetative reactions. This reaction could originally be caused by the strong pain which patients generally feel during such an procedure [40, 43]. Also a release of viscerocardiac reflexes caused by bile leakage and its contact with the peritoneum [41, 47] should be expected. A vagal reaction is the most likely explanation for a drop of blood pressure beneath tolerable levels or a bradycardia [2].

Transcutaneous Oxygen Saturation

As this study shows, not only the circulatory system but also the respiration requires adequate supervision. During the liver interventions a considerable number of patients suffered a decrease of transcutaneous SaO_2 below 90%. Surely, analgesics and sedatives should not be overlooked as a definite risk factor in this context. Intravenous benzodiazepine (midazolam) has a direct depressive effect on the respiratory system. Furthermore, it should not be excluded that the muscular relaxing effect is responsible for a reduced performance of the patients' respiration [15, 46].

In patients who do not need medication during the procedure and still become hypoxic, a vagal reaction has to be considered [2] when the bile ducts and the gall bladder are sufficiently supplied with vagal fibers [16, 17].

The close vicinity of the liver and the lungs might be responsible for an irregular breathing rhythm and cause an additional decrease in respiratory performance. Considering a study from Veyckemans et al. [48] we should exclude the possibility of an inaccurate pulsoximetry reading through the hyperbilirubinemia found in almost all group IV patients.

Individual cases of hypoxic conditions during angiography and PTA have already been observed by other researchers [34]. This hypoxia may have to do with a post dye injection bronchial constriction [39] coupled with the already mentioned histamine release. We should consider further that in arteriography the apnea phase observed during contrast administration could lead to desoxygenation of the blood.

The conclusion that interventions carried under phasal undersaturation lasted longer than those which showed constant over 90% saturation levels can be explained by the fact that longer procedures in general require more contrast medium injections and manipulations in the area of the liver than shorter interventions. The probability of a temporary undersaturation increases through the direct effect of the contrast medium and required apneal phase or through medication given and additional exploratory examinations in the region of the bile duct lifting the vagotonus [2]. In the case of the PTAs, however, a prolonged procedure did not go hand in hand with higher administration of contrast fluid; other measures such as intravascular ultrasound were used in these cases. No additional respiratory methods were used at this stage, so that in this phase the patients, unlike those in the remaining research groups, had more time to improve their respiratory situation.

Temperature

The rise in body temperature and the appearance of septicemia as a possible postoperative complication in the case of liver interventions has been mentioned already [11]. We might add that in individual cases body temperature may rise already during the procedure. The blood vessels and bile ducts of the liver lie closely together within a very confined space, so that communication between the two systems can be established during a puncture or exploratory examination in the course of an intervention. All patients who showed a rise in temperature had cholestasis. An infection of the clogged bile ducts cannot be excluded in these cases [6]. The rise in temperature can be clarified by the bacteremia and the exogenous activation of substances. Like fast-growing tumors, cholestasis per se is able to produce liver cell damage and necrosis even in the absence of cholangitis [27]. This leads to the production of pyrogens by phagocytes, resulting in a rise of body temperature by hypothalamic stimulation. Actually how far a high concentration of endogenous pyrogens, for example, tumor necrosis factor (TNF), sets directly in the blocked bile ducts and is released in the blood stream during an intervention cannot be established at this stage. Nevertheless, the endogenous stimulus of pyrogen release caused by the body's own activities (e.g., necrosis) can be a further reason for intrainterventional temperature changes [7, 33, 42, 44, 45].

The psychological component (such as fear and pain) of the temperature alterations should not be ignored [24, 35].

Some patients had a body temperature of over 38 °C during PTA. Theoretically, instrument contamination could explain a rise in temperature [30] although the fast normalization of the body temperature after the procedure does not support this argument. Another possible cause is a direct effect of the contrast fluid on the hypothalamus [26]. Even used in recommended dosage, contrast fluids are demonstrably capable of overcoming the blood–brain barrier [10] resulting in hypothalamus stimulation.

Electrocardiogram

A different assessment concerning the extrasystoles should be made between groups I–III and group IV. While in the first three groups the characteristics of the injected contrast medium is basically responsible for the arrhythmia, other mechanisms have to be considered for the group with liver interventions.

Klow et al. [23] showed in a study of isolated heart muscle fibers a direct influence of low osmolarity contrast fluid on the myocardium. After the administration there was an increase in resting potential, of repolarization speed and action potential duration, while on the other hand the effective refractory period was decreased. Within this constellation, the probability of arrhythmia increases considerably.

A further factor which can also be responsible for extrasystoles in angiography and PTA is the change in the level of blood calcium after a CF application. The decrease of calcium concentration is the result of general blood dilution effects and the added calcium binding additive (EDTA) in the contrast medium. The direct cell membrane current has also been discussed in this context [18]. It should not be forgotten that ventricular heart rhythm irregularities can occur even under physiological conditions of daily life in healthy individuals [31]. In view of the results from group IV, this aspect should not be overestimated. This group showed complex rhythmical alteration not just once, but constantly in the course of the procedure. What's more, at this point we should mention again that the patient group with the most severe ECG changes were 10 years younger on average than those in the other three groups. Actually one would expect the most stable cardiac condition and correspondingly fewer rhythm disturbances in the younger group. Several studies have already mentioned the complex interwoven relationship between the biliary system, the heart and vagus reactions [9, 21, 29, 32]. That is why unexplainable heart rhythm alterations can be detected during a gallbladder illness or operation. The appearance of a viscerocardiac reflex due to bile leakage has also been discussed in relation to arrhythmia [41, 47].

A further explanation for the arryhthmia could be the changes in levels of blood calcium: The contact between the blood vessels and the biliary system could result in an additional overlapping of bile salts in the blood. A mixture of calcium and these salts [5] could lead to a reduction of the calcium levels and create an extrasystolic condition.

A reduction of SaO_2, observed particularly in group IV, and the following hypoxia can be considered another probable factor responsible for the rhythm alterations [25].

Lown and Verrier stressed that the sympathic rather than the parasympathic section of the autonomous nervous system was responsible for the appearance of ventricular arrhythmias [28]. What's more, the psychological condition of the patient (e.g., fear) and the epinephrine releasing pain are further reasons for the appearance of the extrasystoles.

Obviously, the fact that older patients show extrasystoles during an intervention conforms to the norm in the general population. The tendency towards illnesses leading to arrhythmia (hypertension, coronary heart disease) increases with age [14].

Conclusion

Our study demonstrates that during diagnostic angiography and PTA only mild changes of blood pressure and heart rate take place, while during interventional procedures in the area of the biliary system a decrease of the transcutanous oxygen saturation, an increase of the body temperature and severe arrhythmias should be expected.

These findings indicate that close monitoring of significant vegetative parameters is not necessary during angiography and PTAs, however, must strongly be recommended during interventional procedures of the liver and biliary system.

References

1. Amon EU, Ennis M, Lorenz W, Schnabel M, Schneider C (1990) Histamine release induced by radiographic contrast media. Int Arch Allergy Appl Immunol 92:203–208
2. Andrews EJ (1976) The vagus reaction as a possible cause of severe complications of radiological procedures. Radiology 121:1–4
3. ASGE Publication No. 1022 (1991) Monitoring patients undergoing gastrointestinal endoscopic procedures – guidelines for clinical application. Gastrointest Endosc 37:120–121
4. Barth KH, Matsumoto AH (1991) Patient care in interventional radiology: a perspective. Radiology 178:11–17
5. Baruch E, Lichtenberg D, Barak P, Nir B (1991) Calcium binding to bile salts. Chem Phys Lipids 57(1):17–27
6. Bruch HP, Kern E (1990) Gallenblase und Gallenwege. In: Berchthold R, Hamelmann H, Peiper J (eds) Chirurgie, 2nd edn. Urban and Schwarzenberg, Munich, p 404
7. Dascombe MJ (1985) The pharmacology of fever. Prog Neurobiol 25(4):327–373
8. Dawson P (1989) Cardiovascular effects of contrast agents. Am J Cardiol 64:2E–9E
9. Felderbaum D, Finesilver B (1927) Transient auricular fibrillation in abdominal disease. Am Heart J 2:416–423
10. Goldberg M (1984) Systemic reactions to intravascular contrast media. Anesthesiology 60:46–56
11. Günther RW (1988) Perkutane Gallenwegsdrainage. In: Günter RW, Thelen M (eds) Interventionelle Radiologie. Thieme, Stuttgart, p 363
12. Hägg A, Lörelius LE, Mörlin C, Wide L (1988) Serial measurements of plasma renin activity; aldosterone and cortisol during percutaneous transluminal angioplasty of the renal artery in man. Acta Physiol Scand 134:473–478
13. Herd CM, Robertson AR, Frewin DB, Taylor WB (1988) Adverse reactions during intravenous urography: are these due to histamine release? Br J Radiol 61:5–11
14. Herold G (1990) Kardiologie: Einführung. In: Herold G et al. (eds) Innere Medizin. p 127E and p 118
15. Hoffmann-La Roche (1990) Dormicum. Gut steuerbares Injektionshypnoticum für Anästhesiologie und Intensivmedizin. Hoffmann-La Roche, Basel, p 59
16. Hopton DS (1973) The influence of the vagus nerves on the biliary system. Br J Surg 60:216–218
17. Isaza J, Jones DT, Dragstedt LR, Woodward ER (1971) The effect of vagotomy on motor function of the gallbladder. Surgery 70:616–621
18. Jansen O, Weiss HD, Stolle H, Schallock J (1990) Veränderungen der Plasmahistaminkonzentration und der Blutelektrolytspiegel nach venöser Applikation von nicht-ionischen Kontrastmitteln. Rontgenpraxis 43:104–109
19. Katzen BT, Kaplan JO, Dake MD (1989) Developing an interventional radiology practice in a community hospital: the interventional radiologist as an equal partner in patient care. Radiology 170:955–958
20. Keeffe EB, O'Connor KW (1990) ASGE survey of endoscopic sedation and monitoring practices. Gastrointest Endosc 36:S13–S22

21. Keys JR, Dry TJ, Walters W, Gage RP (1955) Cholecystectomy in patients with coronary heart disease. Proc Staff Meet Mayo Clin 30:587–595
22. Kinnison ML, White RI, Auster M, Hewes R, Mitchell S, Shuman L, Gallacher D (1985) Inpatient admissions for interventional radiology: philosophy of patient management. Radiology 154:349–351
23. Klow NE, Tande PM, Hevroy O, Refsum H (1990) Mechanism of ECG changes and arrhythmogenic properties of low contrast media during coronary arteriography in dog. Cardiovasc Res 24:303–308
24. Kluger MJ, O'Reilly B, Shope TR, Vander AJ (1987) Further evidence that stress hyperthermia is a fever. Physiol Behav 39(6):763–766
25. Kraupp O (1987) Pharmakodynamische Beeinflussung der Rhythmik, Dynamik und Durchblutung des Herzens. In: Forth W, Henschler D, Rummel W (eds) Pharmakologie und Toxikologie, 5th edn. BI Wissenschaftsverlag, Mannheim, p 216
26. Lalli AF (1980) Contrast media reactions: data analysis and hypothesis. Radiology 134:1–12
27. Lang F (1987) Spezielle Pathophysiologie der Leber. In: Lang F (ed) Pathophysiologie Pathobiochemie, 3rd edn. Enke, Stuttgart, p 334
28. Lown B, Verrier RL (1976) Neural activity and ventricular fibrillation. N Engl J Med 294:1165–1170
29. McArthur SW, Wakefield H (1945) Observations on the human electrocardiogram during experimental distention of the gallbladder. J Lab Clin Med 30:349–351
30. McCready RA, Siderys H, Pittmann JN et al. (1991) Septic complications after cardiac catheterization and PTCA. J Vasc Surg 14(2):170–174
31. Meinertz T, Kasper W, Schmitt B, Treese N, Rückel A, Zehender M, Hofmann T, Schuster HP, Pop T (1983) Herzrhythmusstörungen bei Herzgesunden. Dtsch Med Wochenschr 108:527–531
32. Mendelsohn D, Monheit R (1956) Electrocardiographic and blood-pressure changes during and after biliary-tract surgery. N Engl J Med 254:307–313
33. Michie HR, Spriggs DR, Manogue KR et al. (1988) Tumor necrosis factor and endotoxin induce similar metabolic responses in human beings. Surgery 104:280–286
34. Neagley SR, Vought MB, Weidner WA, Zwillich CW (1986) Transient oxygen desaturation following radiographic contrast medium administration. Arch Int Med 146:1094–1097
35. Pechnick RN, Morgan MJ (1987) The role of endogenous opioids in footshock-induced hyperthermia. Pharmacol Biochem Behav 28(1):95–100
36. Pinet A, Corot C, Biot N, Eloy R (1988) Evaluation of histamine release following intravenous injection of ionic and nonionic contrast media. Invest Radiol 23 [Suppl 1]:S174–S177
37. Reuter SR (1991) Medicolegal aspects of intravascular stenting. Semin Intervent Radiol 8(4):311–315
38. Ring EJ, Kerlan RK (1985) Inpatient management: a new role for interventional radiologists. Radiology 154:543
39. Rosenfield AT, Littner MR, Ulreich S et al. (1977) Respiratory effects of excretory urography: preliminary report. Invest Radiol 12:295–298
40. Schmidt RF (1990) Nociception und Schmerz. In: Schmidt RF, Thews G (eds) Physiologie des Menschen, 24th edn. Springer, Berlin Heidelberg New York, p 234
41. Scott HG, Ivy AC (1932) Viscerocardiac reflexes – an experimental study in frogs and dogs. Arch Int Med 49:227–233
42. Sherry B, Cerami A (1988) Cachektin/tumor necrosis factor exerts endocrine, paracrine and autocrine control of inflammatory responses. J Cell Biol 107:1269–1277
43. Silbernagl S, Despopoulos A (1988) Vegetatives Nervensystem. In: Silbernagl, Despopoulos (eds) Taschenatlas der Physiologie, 3rd edn. Thieme, Stuttgart, pp 50–59
44. Starnes HF, Warren RS, Jeevanandem M et al. (1988) Tumor necrosis factor and the acute metabolic response to tissue injury in man. J Clin Invest 82:1321–1325
45. Steinhausen M (1986) Fieber. In: Steinhausen M (ed) Medizinische Physiologie, 1st edn. Bergmann, Munich, p 225

46. Suttmann H, Doenicke A, Bauer M, Loos A, Ebentheuer H, Schneider J (1984) Die Wirkung von Midazolam auf die Atmung. In: Götz E (ed) Midazolam in der Anästhesiologie. International Symposium, Darmstadt, 28–29 October 1983. Editiones Roche, Basel, pp 113–127
47. van Sonnenberg E, Wing VW, Pollard JW, Casola G (1984) Life threatening vagal reactions associated with percutaneous cholecystostomy. Radiology 151:377–380
48. Veyckemans F, Baele P, Guillaume JE, Willems E, Robert A, Clerbaux T (1989) Hpyerbilirubinemia does not interfere with hemoglobin saturation measured by pulse oximetry. Anesthesiology 70:118–122
49. Waltmann AC, Katzen BT, Ring EJ et al. (1988) Society of cardiovascular and interventional radiology: credentials criteria for peripheral, renal, and visceral percutaneous transluminal angioplasty. Radiology 167:452
50. Wilkins RA, Nunnerley HB, Allison DJ, Mason R, Kellet MJ, Cumberland DC, Sandin B (1989) The expansion of interventional radiology. Report of a survey conducted by the Royal College of Radiologists. Clin Radiol 40:457–462
51. Witzleb E (1990) Funktionen des Gefäßsystems. In: Schmidt RF, Thews G (eds) Physiologie des Menschen, 24th edn. Springer, Berlin Heidelberg New York, pp 505–572

Discussion

on the papers by S. KADIR and E. B. KEEFFE

Great interest was shown during the discussion in monitoring guidelines. In this regard, Keeffe pointed to a publication from the American Society for Gastrointestinal Endoscopy, who had published guidelines for clinical application of monitoring in patients undergoing gastrointestinal endoscopic procedures (Gastrointest Endosc 37:120–121, 1991).

In addition, the need for premedication before interventional procedures was discussed. Keeffe reported that, in his experience, gastroenterologists had now come right away from premedication. They had found that personal care of the patient beforehand on the ward in the form of a visit and subsequent accompaniment by a radiological nurse show better anxiolytic effects.

In gastroenterology, sedation is generally nowadays given as conscious sedation with midazolam (2.5–5 mg) or diazepam (5–10 mg), both drugs being titrated over 5–10 minutes. This form of sedation was now used in the majority of all endoscopies, with occasional exceptions for flexible sigmoidoscopies and upper endoscopies. With sedated patients the rules for observation mentioned in his paper must be held to. According to Keeffe, this is also necessary because endoscopies were generally carried out in darkened rooms, which makes direct observation of the patient more difficult. This requirement for a darkened room is, however, now decreasing because of the wider use of video systems, with a corresponding improvement in the possibility for direct observation of patients.

In answer to the question of whether the relatively high rate of apnea during endoscopies with midazolam or diazepam sedation found in a study at Georgetown University might in part have been due to visceral reflexes, Keeffe said that this can not be answered from the data, which had been collected from practitioners in their own practices. There was, however, information about the type of sedatives and their doses: No correlation had been found. Regarding monitoring, it used to be thought that pulse oximetry is only sensible in older patients, whereas now the indication is based more on the presence of risk factors. In vascular interventions, Kadir regarded monitoring by pulse oximetry as necessary in all older unstable patients and for more difficult procedures such as bile duct interventions and embolizations.

While gastroenterological interventions are carried out relatively frequently in outpatients under sedation, this is rather more rare in vascular interventions. In any case, said Kadir, every outpatient who has had sedation must be kept under observation for 4–6 hours, and so a holding area must be included in the basic facilities of any radiology department. Suitable alarm system and, with central observation, monitor systems must be installed.

According to Keeffe, certificates of training regarding competence in first aid procedures and reanimation were increasingly being expected of gastroenterologists. In the United States, 75% of gastroenterologists already possess such certificates. General standards on training did not yet exist, but guidelines on qualification within fellowship programs were being worked on. Some hospitals, however, were already demanding evidence of suitable qualifications in advanced life support when taking on physicians.

Clotting

Pathophysiology of Blood Clotting in Relation to Radiologic Interventions

H.J. HERTFELDER and S. POPOV-CENIĆ

Introduction

Radiologic interventions are associated with a small but nonneglegible risk of thromboembolic complications. In particular, these complications may have fatal consequences when accidental embolic events in cranial or coronary arteries occur. Abnormal activation of the hemostatic system resulting from interventional procedures and its underlying pathomechanisms will be discussed. First, mechanical influences to the vessel wall associated with catheter techniques are shown. Second, the role of the materials and devices used, including the catheters and the various contrast media will be briefly outlined. Finally an anticoagulation regimen for the embolization therapy of intracranial angiomas that has been developed regarding the proposed procoagulant pathomechanisms is presented.

Regulation of Hemostasis

As shown in Fig. 1 the hemostatic system under physiologic conditions exhibits a well-balanced equilibrium between its singular components, i.e., the vasculature, the platelets, the plasmic components of coagulation, and the fibrinolytic system. A shift of balance to one or other side leads to thrombosis or bleeding [2]. For radiologic interventions, alterations in the fibrinolytic

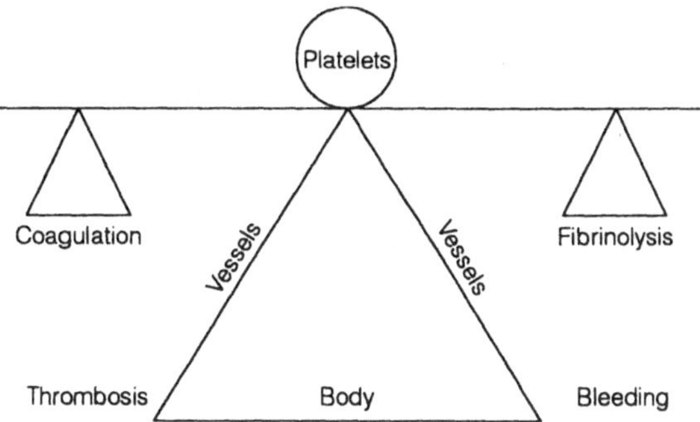

Fig. 1. The balance of hemostasis. The vessels, platelets, coagulation and fibrinolysic proteins, and platelets all cooperate in thrombus formation. (From [2])

system are commonly of minor importance. In contrast, the vessel wall, the platelets, and the plasmic coagulation components play central roles.

Primary manipulations influencing the hemostatic apparatus occur at the vessel wall. Lesions of the endothelial surface and subendothelial structures are induced by the vascular access, the guidewire, and predominantly by contact and manipulations of the catheter tips. Thus intact endothelium, as well as surfaces chronically altered by atherosclerosis may be injured. In both cases the hemostatic system is subsequently activated according to the same principle as outlined in Fig. 2 [5]: Endothelial injury leads to the exposure of structures of the subendothelial matrix, e.g., collagen fibers to the blood stream. The platelets rapidly adhere to collagen. The adhesion is mediated either directly by the collagen receptor of the platelet surface or by the von Willebrand factor (vWF). Binding to collagen induces platelet activation with shape change, aggregation, and release of vasoactive components, e.g., serotonin, and other platelet-activating agents, e.g., ADP, thromboxane A_2 (TXA_2). The interactions between the aggregating platelets are thereby mediated by fibrinogen.

By this way a primary hemostatic plug is formed. The plug resistance against the blood flow at high-shear rates, i.e., in the small arteries, is low. However, it is physiologically stabilized by fibrin formation induced by the activation of the plasmic coagulation enzyme cascade.

The coagulation cascade is simultaneously activated with platelet adhesion in two ways (Fig. 3, [1]): The contact activation or intrinsic pathway is stimulated by the binding of the contact phase proteins (factor XII, prekallikrein, high molecular weight kininogen, and factor XI) to the subendothelium, subsequently inducing the activation of factors IX, X, and II (F IX, F X, and F II, respectively) as shown below.

At the same time the extrinsic pathway is activated by tissue factor, tissue thromboplastin (TTP). TTP, an enzymatically active lipoprotein bound to the cell membrane becomes accessible to the blood stream only upon endothelial cell injury. It converts factor VII (F VII) into its active form (F VII a), then generating active F X a and F II a. The contact phase-dependent activation of F X via F IX a, as well as the extrinsic activation of F X a via F VII a, and the subsequent prothrombin activation into thrombin occur in a highly organized phospholipid-dependent process at the platelet plasma membrane. For optimal activation of the cascade, the activation of the cofactors, factor VIII (F VIII) and factor V (F V), by traces of thrombin is necessary. The activated cofactors (F VIII a and F V a) increase the generation of thrombin (F II a) by several orders of magnitude.

Thrombin plays a multifunctional role in thrombus formation: It converts fibrinogen into fibrin and mediates cross-linking of fibrin by the activation of factor XIII. In particular, thrombin generated at sites of vessel injury promotes further platelet recruitment, i.e., the activation of circulating platelets. Thus, the activation of the coagulation system stimulates the growth of a thrombus by thrombin-induced platelet aggregation and by fibrin stabilization of the thrombus to the secondary hemostatic plug.

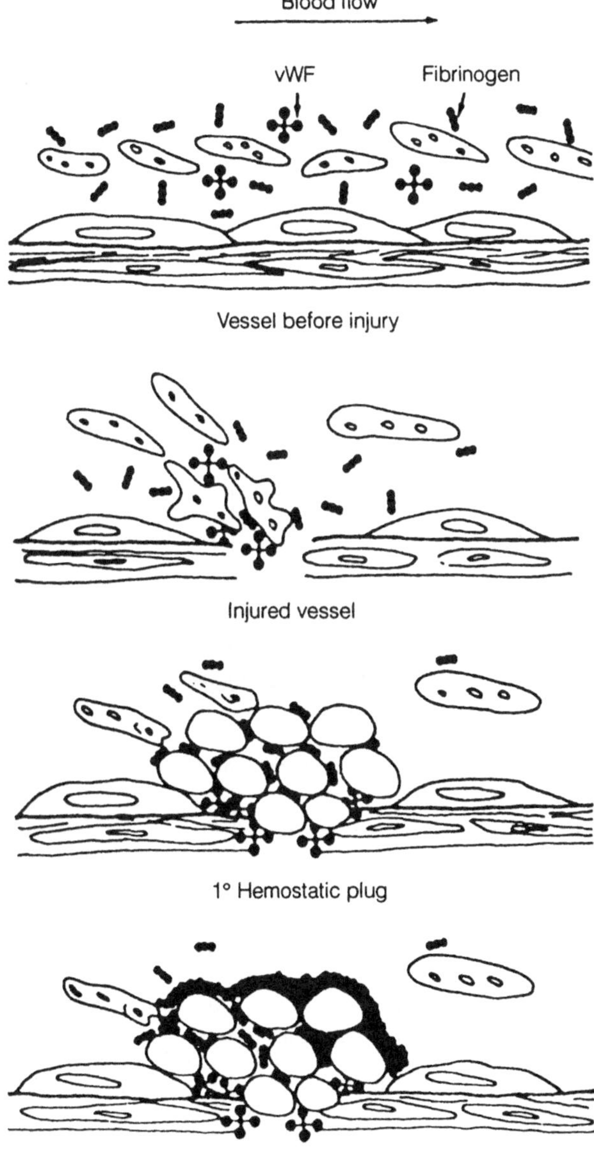

Fig. 2. Adhesive interactions during the formation of a hemostatic plug following vessel injury. (From [5])

The formation of a thrombus is regulated by a variety of inhibitor systems, most of which are associated with the endothelium. The platelet functions are inhibited by prostacyclin (PGI_2), a powerful platelet aggregation inhibitor, released from endothelial cells by epinephrine or thrombin.

The coagulation cascade is also inhibited in at least two endothelium-dependent pathways: (1) The heparin/antithrombin III (AT III) system. The

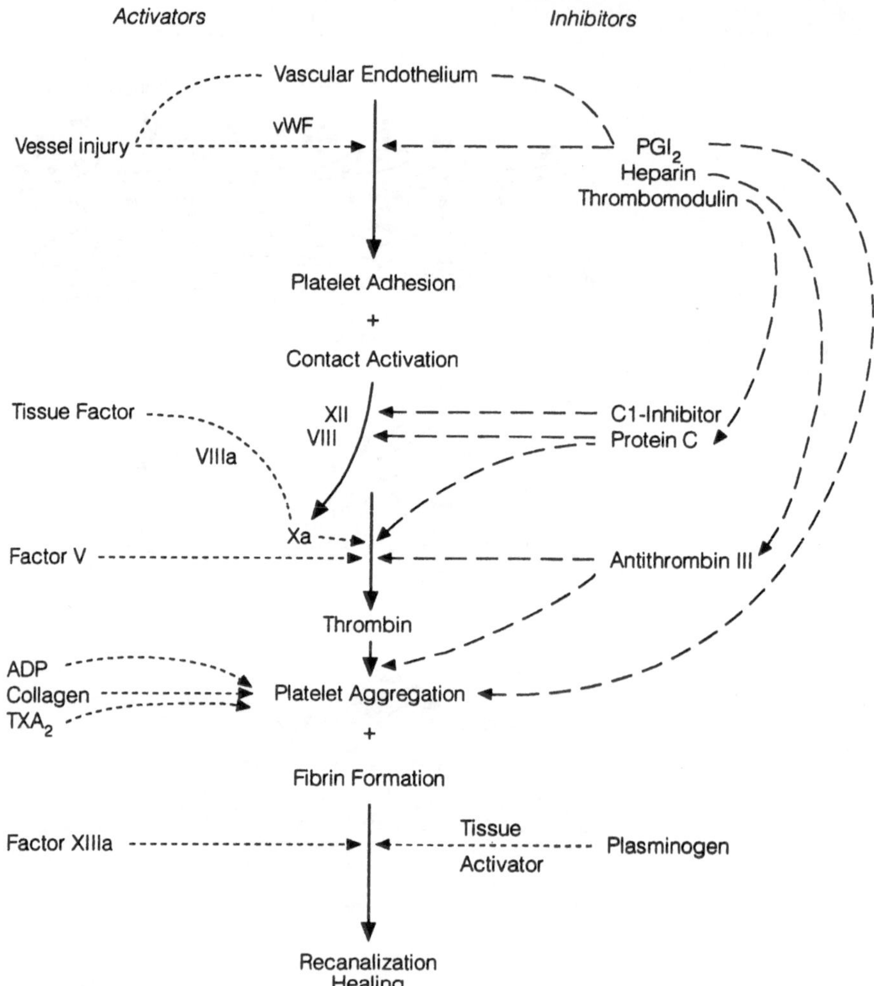

Fig. 3. Overview of hemostasis. The *solid vertical arrows* show cellular and coagulation factor events in the process of hemostasis. Activators and other procoagulants influence hemostasis are noted by the *dotted arrows*. Inhibitory pathways and processes acting to degrade coagulant proteins are indicated by the *dashed arrows*. (From [1], modified by the authors)

intact endothelial surface is coated with heparan sulfate. Heparan sulfate is capable of binding AT III, thereby increasing the affinity of AT III towards the active enzymes (XI a to II a) of the cascade. The enzymes are subsequently inhibited by the formation of inactive complexes with AT III, e.g., the thrombin-AT III complex. (2) Thrombin is bound by thrombomodulin, an endothelial surface-membrane receptor. Thrombomodulin-bound thrombin thereby looses its ability to convert fibrinogen to fibrin. However, it is then able to activate protein C, the central component of the protein C anticoagulant pathway. Activated protein C (APC) proteolytically inactivates F Va and F VIII a, subsequently downregulating the coagulation cascade and inhibiting further thrombin generation. APC also activates fibrinolysis.

However, the size of a developing thrombus is also dependent on its localization at the vessel wall, the size of the injured area, and the hemodynamic conditions in the region of the vascular injury. The hemostatic plugs formed at lesions on the inner surface of large arteries contain only a few layers of platelets, presumably due to the high-shear rates present in those vessels. Nevertheless, microemboli may be released from these lesions leading to the embolization of microcirculation.

Depending on its occlusive effect, once a thrombus has been formed it may alter the hemodynamic conditions by inducing turbulence and promote further thrombus growth. The hemodynamic conditions in a vessel are also influenced by the catheter placed in the vessel. Flow restrictions, in particular at thrombotic lesions, in turn increase the risk of thrombus or embolus formation.

Interaction of Materials with the Hemostatic System

The role of the materials used in radiologic interventions will be discussed only for vascular interventions. The chemical composition and ultrastructural properties of the materials seem to be crucial for hemocompatibility [3]. However, the materials presently used only slightly affect the hemostatic system due to their generally good hemocompatibility. Nevertheless, slight adsorptions of coagulation proteins, e.g., fibrinogen, to the materials seem to be inevitable, thus, platelet adhesion and contact activation of the plasmic cascade can occur.

The effects of the contrast media (CM) on the hemostatic system are still being discussed. It is generally accepted that the CM presently used exhibit more or less anticoagulant properties in vitro [3]. The ionic CM thereby obviously inhibit the coagulation system more than the nonionic CM. The anticoagulant effects are predominantly promoted by the inhibition of (a) fibrin polymerization, (b) the coagulation cascade at a yet unknown level, and (c) the

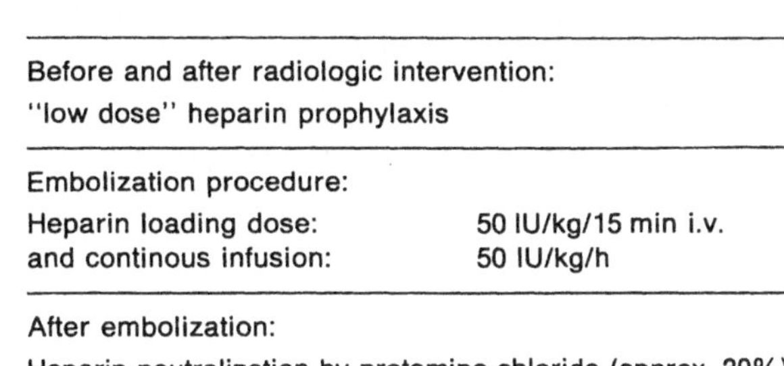

Before and after radiologic intervention:
"low dose" heparin prophylaxis

Embolization procedure:

Heparin loading dose:	50 IU/kg/15 min i.v.
and continous infusion:	50 IU/kg/h

After embolization:
Heparin neutralization by protamine chloride (approx. 30%)

Fig. 4. Anticoagulation regimen developed for embolization therapy of intracranial angiomas

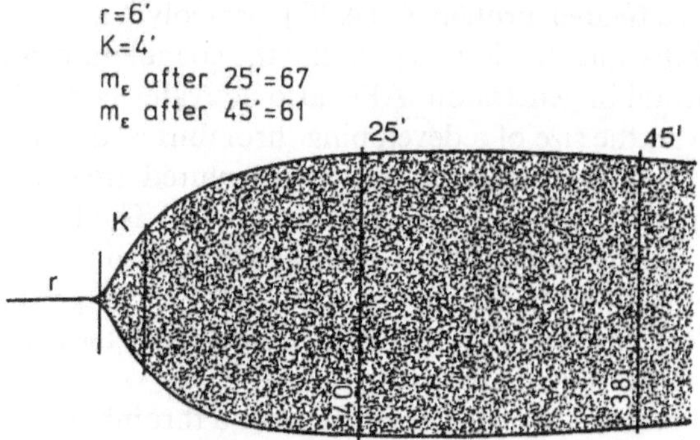

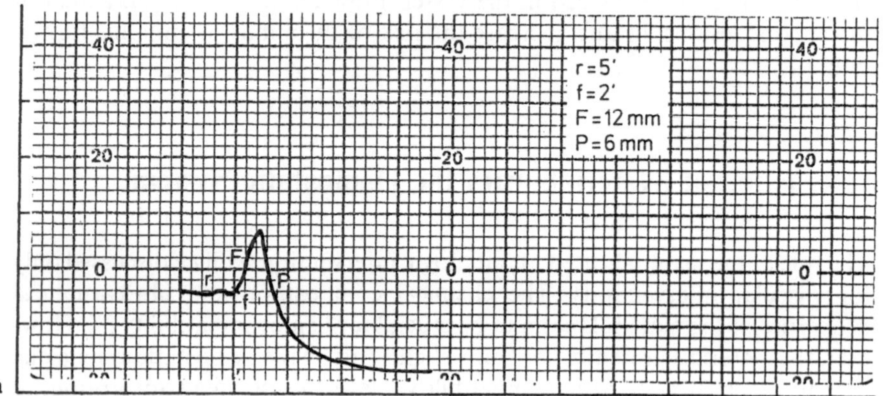

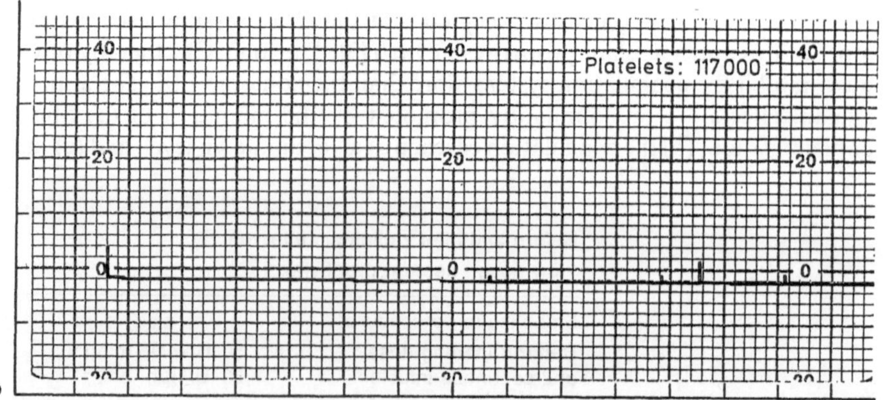

Fig. 5 a–c. Thromboelastograms (*top* in **a** and **c**) and resonance thrombograms of a patient 1 day before (**a**), during (**b**), and 1 day after (**c**) embolization therapy. *r*, reaction time; *K*, clot formation time; m_ε, maximal amplitude; *f*, fibrin formation time; *F*, fibrin leg; *P*, platelet leg

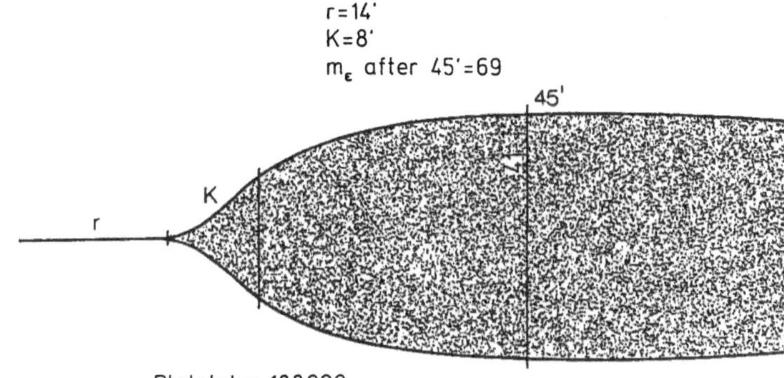

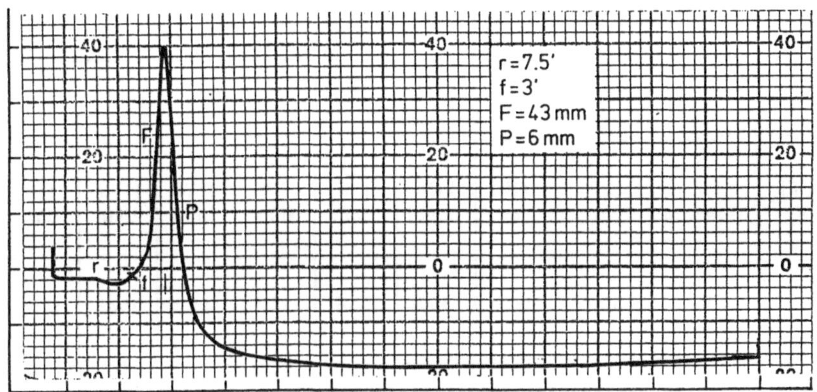

c

platelets [4]. Some rarely occurring thromboembolic complications have been associated with the less anticoagulant properties of the nonionic CM. However, further investigations to examine this issue seem to be necessary [3].

Anticoagulation Therapy in Neuroradiologic Interventions

Regarding the proposed procoagulant alterations in the hemostatic system and in particular the formation of thrombin during interventional procedures, a therapy regimen (Fig. 4) for the application of anticoagulants in neuroradiologic interventions, i.e., for embolizations of intracranial angiomas, has been developed in cooperation with the Department of Neuroradiology of our University Hospital.

All patients receive "low-dose" heparin prophylaxis (3 × 5000 IU/day) beginning on the preinterventional day. Immediately before the intervention, the heparin-loading dose of 50 IU/kg body weight (b.w.) is intravenously admin-

APTT s	PT Quick %	TT s	RT s	FGN mg/dl	F II U/ml	F V U/ml	F VII U/ml	F VIII U/ml	F X U/ml
31,2	82	13.9	18.5	155	1.01	1.25	0.95	0.70	0.65

AT III U/ml	PMG U/ml	α_2-AP U/ml	α_1-AT U/ml	α_2-MG U/ml
1.25	0.81	1.04	1.46	0.75

a

APTT s	PT Quick %	TT s	RT s	FGN mg/dl	F II U/ml	F V U/ml	F VII U/ml	F VIII U/ml	F X U/ml
> 120	43	> 120	19.1	160	1.16	1.08	0.82	0.22	0.98

AT III U/ml	PMG U/ml	α_2- AP U/ml	α_1- AT U/ml	α_2- MG U/ml
1.05	0.79	1.13	1.42	0.71

b

Fig. 6a–d. Plasmic coagulation and fibrinolysis parameters of the same patient 1 day before (**a**), during (**b**), and after (**c**) heparin neutralization, and 1 dy after embolization therapy (**d**). *PT*, prothrombin time; *RT*, reptilase time; *FGN*, fibrinogen; *PMG*, plasminogen; α_2-*AP*, α_2-antiplasmin; α_2-*AT*, α_2-antitrypsin; α_2-*MG*, α_2-macroglobulin

istered within 15 min. The heparin infusion is continued with 50 IU/kg b.w. until the end of the embolization procedure. Thereafter, heparin is partially neutralized by administering approximately 30% protamine chloride (equivalent to 30% of total heparin applied). The reason for this procedure is to obtain a further anticoagulant effect during the first postinterventional hours. Postinterventional "low-dose" heparin prophylaxis is routinely given on the evening after embolization (8 P.M.).

APTT s	PT Quick %	TT s	RT s	FGN mg/dl	F II U/ml	F V U/ml	F VII U/ml	F VIII U/ml	F X U/ml
31.5	97	12.5	18.0	220	1.06	0.95	1.03	0.65	0.88

AT III U/ml	PMG U/ml	α_2-AP U/ml	α_1-AT U/ml	α_2-MG U/ml
1.23	0.90	1.13	1.72	0.85

c

APTT s	PT Quick %	TT s	RT s	FGN mg/dl	F II U/ml	F V U/ml	F VII U/ml	F VIII U/ml	F X U/ml
> 120	56	> 120	18.8	170	1.14	0.95	0.77	0.37	0.60

AT III U/ml	PMG U/ml	α_2-AP U/ml	α_1-AT U/ml	α_2-MG U/ml
1,00	0.77	1.09	1.38	0.71

d

Figures 5 and 6 show a typical example of the course of blood coagulation parameters of a patient undergoing embolization therapy of an intracranial angioma. The thromboelastogram (TEG) and the resonance thrombogram (RTG, Fig. 5a) of the initial preinterventional examination exhibit shortened reaction times (r) indicating a hypercoagulable state. This finding is frequently observed in the patients examined. Apart from a slightly reduced fibrinogen level (Fig. 6a) all plasmic coagulation and fibrinolysis parameters are within their normal ranges. During embolization (Figs. 5b and 6b) an effective anticoagulation is maintained. TEG and RTG show nonclottable samples. Activated partial thromboplastin time (APTT) and thrombin time (TT) are markedly prolonged, prothrombin time (Quick) and F VIII activity are diminished, and all other parameters are not significantly altered. After partial heparin neutralization (Fig. 6c) the samples in TEG and RTG (not shown) are still nonclottable and the APTT and TT are markedly prolonged. Quick and F VIII activity begin to increase again, while no changes are observed in all other parameters. At the postinterventional day (Figs. 5c and 6d) the prolonged r and k in TEG indicate a slight heparin effect. RTG and all plasmic parameters are normalized. This example demonstrates the effectiveness of heparin anticoagulation in the embolization therapy of intracranial angiomas without thromboembolic or bleeding complications.

References

1. Colman RW, Marder VJ, Salzman EW, Hirsh J (1987) Overview of hemostasis. In: Colman RW, Marder VJ, Salzman EW, Hirsh J (eds) Hemostasis and thrombosis. Basic principles and clinical practice. Lippincott, Philadelphia, pp 3–18
2. Corriveau DM (1988) Major elements of hemostasis. In: Corriveau DM, Fritsma GA (eds) Hemostasis and thrombosis in the clinical laboratory. Lippincott, Philadelphia, pp 1–33
3. Dawson P (1991) Contrast agents in clinical angiography. Relevance to thromboembolic phenomena. Front Eur Radiol 8:53–59
4. Gabriel DA (1991) Effects of contrast agents on fibrin structure and platelet surface charge. J Invasive Cardiol 3:31B–40B
5. Hawiger J (1987) Adhesive interactions of blood cells and the vessel wall. In: Colman RW, Marder VJ, Salzman EW, Hirsh J (eds) Hemostasis and thrombosis. Basic principles and clinical practice. Lippincott, Philadelphia, pp 182–209

Use of Anticoagulants and Clotting Agents – Procedures in Patients with Pre-existing Coagulation Disorders

R. F. DONDELINGER

Introduction

The interventional radiologist is faced during daily practice with patients who may show abnormal clotting parameters or a clinically evident bleeding tendency. He must be prepared to recognize such alterations to avoid severe potential complications during or following a diagnostic or a therapeutic invasive percutaneous procedure. An understanding of the basic pathophysiology of coagulation and fibrinolysis is mandatory for the application of specific therapy in the radiology department [1].

Physiologic Homeostasis

Homeostasis results from a dynamic equilibrium between coagulation and fibrinolysis. Simultaneous activity of both systems keeps the blood in a liquid phase and confined within the vascular bed. An excess of coagulation or deficient fibrinolysis leads to intravascular thrombus formation, an excess of fibrinolysis, or deficient coagulation to hemorrhage; the blood breaks through either the normal capillary net or a previously damaged vessel wall.

Coagulation

The Coagulation Cascade

The coagulation process is divided into an intrinsic, an extrinsic, and a common pathway (Fig. 1). The extrinsic pathway is activated in contact with tissue factors such as thromboplastin and involves factor VII (proconvertine), factor X (factor Stuart), and factor V (proaccelerine). The intrinsic pathway is activated by plasma factors such as the prekallikrein-kallikrein system and includes factor XII (factor Hageman), factor XI, factors IX and VIII (antihemophilic factors B and A). Factors X and V are common to both pathways. Coagulation factors are sequentially activated by enzymatic reactions. Inter-

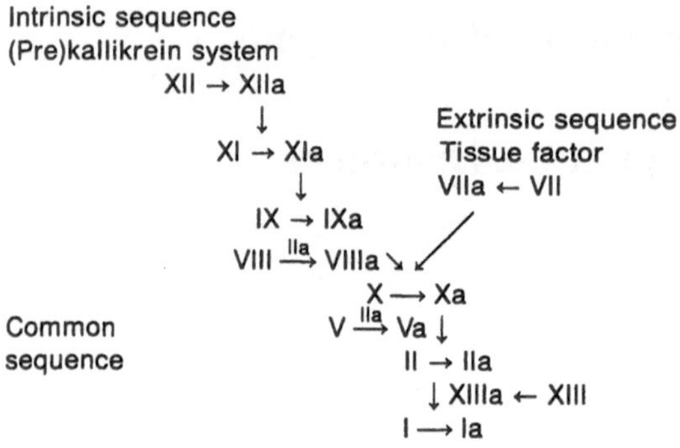

Intrinsic sequence
(Pre)kallikrein system
XII → XIIa
↓
XI → XIa
↓
IX → IXa
VIII $\xrightarrow{IIa}$ VIIIa ↘

Extrinsic sequence
Tissue factor
VIIa ← VII
↙

Common sequence
X → Xa
V $\xrightarrow{IIa}$ Va ↓
II → IIa
↓ XIIIa ← XIII
I → Ia

Fig. 1. Activation sequence of coagulation factors

estingly enough, factor V and factor VIII are not only activated, but they physically disappear during the coagulation cascade. The activation process does not cause a rapid depletion of the other coagulation factors. Various other substances such as phospholipids, calcium, and platelet factor 3 are necessary at different stages of the coagulation sequence. The endpoint of activation of the intrinsic and of the extrinsic pathway is conversion of prothrombin (factor II) into thrombin (factor II a), which in return degrades fibrinogen (factor I) into fibrin (factor I a), which precipitates into crosslink, stable, nonsoluble fibrin polymeres.

Coagulation Tests

The following blood tests explore the process of coagulation and are regularly checked: activated partial thromboplastin time (PTT), prothrombin time (PT), and thrombin clotting time (TCT). PTT (normal 12–15 s) explores the intrinsic pathway, but any anomaly of the common pathway also alters tests which explore the intrinsic sequence. PT (normal 100%) controls the extrinsic pathway. TCT (normal 15–20 s) and dosage of fibrinogen (normal 2–4 g/l) explore the common pathway. Bleeding time (BT; normal 2–4 min) and platelet count (normal 150 000–500 000/ml) explore platelet production and function, and therefore the primary hemostatic ability. More sophisticated radionuclide tests include platelet survival time. The coagulation cascade is far more subtle, but a global overview is helpful for the recognition of a coagulation disorder and for understanding of coagulation tests. Coagulation checks must be systematically ordered before an invasive percutaneous procedure is performed, particularly when no previous medical records are available or when the patient is referred from another institution or is seen on a outpatient basis, whether or not a coagulation disorder is suspected on the grounds of clinical history and examination. Most coagulation factor deficiencies are responsible for repeated clinically significant hemorrhage. Coagulation tests are sensitive not only to a particular coagulation factor, but to a defined portion of the coagulation sequence. They are defined as follows:

- An abnormal PT indicates an anomaly in the extrinsic pathway. When fibrinogen and TCT are normal a defect of factor VII can be present. A selective dosage of factors V, II, VII and X is necessary to identify a congenital deficiency of proaccelerine, prothrombin, proconvertine, or factor Stuart, although these anomalies are rare.
- An abnormal PT and PTT indicates a defect in the common pathway. Presence of coumarin, vitamin K deficiency, or chronic liver disease are frequently identified.
- An abnormal PTT with normal PT and normal TCT indicates a possible defect in the endogenous sequence of factors XII, XI, IX, or VIII. Congenital defects of coagulation factors must be ruled out by specific tests.
- An abnormal PTT and BT reflects von Willebrandt disease, which is defined as a change in normal adhesivity of circulating platelets or afibrinogenemia, disclosed by dosage of fibrinogen.
- An abnormal TCT indicates an anomaly of the common pathway and final phase of coagulation: A structural alteration of fibrinogen (dysfibrinogenemia) can be present or other dysproteinemias, such as myeloma. Fibrinolytic states, diffuse intravascular coagulation, circulating antithrombin, and a deficiency in factor XIII are other possibilities altering TCT. An anomaly of factor XIII, which normally stabilizes fibrin precipitates is responsible for a fragile blood clot, severe bleeding, and a characteristic change in the thromboelastogram. Global coagulation tests may be normal.
- An abnormal BT indicates an anomaly of the primary hemostasis or a qualitative platelet disorder.
- An abnormal BT and an abnormal platelet count defines thrombocytopenia, which can have central causes related to bone marrow deficiency or various peripheral causes.
- When all coagulation factors are normal, but the patient has an obvious bleeding tendency, a defect in factor XII, which initiates the coagulation sequence, must be suspected.
- When all factors of the coagulation sequence are abnormal, diffuse intravascular coagulation is probably present. Liver failure is a common underlying disease, including the particular HELPP syndrome (hemolysis, elevated liver enzymes, and low platelet count) during the postpartum period.

These short guidelines concerning the meaning of coagulation tests should be kept in mind by the interventional radiologist.

Frequent Pathologies Altering Coagulation Tests

A hemostatic defect is often related to a pathological clinical situation, which is either known or occasionally can be revealed by blood tests ordered before an interventional procedure. The most frequent clinical diagnoses responsible for a coagulation disorder include anticoagulation therapy, liver insufficiency of various origin, chronic renal insufficiency, lympho- and myeloproliferative disease, malabsorption syndrome, dysproteinemia, and amyloid and connective tissue disease such as systemic lupus erythematosus.

Correction of Coagulopathy

How can the radiologist correct a coagulation disorder in the radiology department on an emergency basis, either before, during, or after an interventional procedure? Best prevention of complications from a coagulopathy is careful analysis of the patient's history and of available medical records, recognition of chronic underlying diseases, and systematic check of coagulation, particularly in patients with known pathologies such as those mentioned above [12]; however, in an emergency, the following may be useful:

- Perfusion of fresh frozen plasma corrects factors of the coagulation sequence and particularly a deficiency of factor V, XI, XII, XIII.
- Human plasma proteins correct coagulation factors particularly II, VII, X, and IX. Factors V and VIII are not corrected.
- Administration of antihemophilic factor A selectively corrects factor VIII.
- Administration of fibrinogen corrects a- or dysfibrinogenemia.
- Fresh platelet transfusions correct thrombocytopenia.

Heparin Administration During Angiography

One of the most common problems occurs with patients who are on heparin therapy. Many patients with vascular diseases are on efficient heparin therapy; others referred for an interventional procedure may be on prophylactic anticoagulant therapy.

Heparin is an inhomogenous mixture of glycosaminoglycurans. Depending on its molecular structure, heparin components have a variable anticoagulation effect. Heparin acts by accelerating the activity of antithrombin III (AT III) and by neutralizing factors X, XII, XI, and IX of the coagulation sequence. The intravenous or intraarterial injection of heparin has an immediate anticoagulant effect. Therefore heparin is regularly used during angiographic procedures for prevention of clotting around the guidewire or around and inside the catheter or other intravascular devices. The thrombogenic potential of nonionic iodine contrast media largely used in angiographic procedures is emphasized. These contrast agents inhibit thrombin formation in vitro but without clinical significance when heparin is prophylactically used [6, 9, 10].

Potential incompatibility between ioxaglate and papaverine resulting in arterial thrombosis should also be stressed [8]. During peripheral and visceral angiography, 5000 U of heparin are added to 1 l of flushing saline solution and are intermittently injected to rinse the angiographic catheter or the hemostatic valve sheath at the percutaneous puncture point. Before starting a selective supraaortic angiographic procedure, 2000 U of heparin are injected intraarterially. The same amount of heparin is injected when the angiographic catheter remains in a subocclusive position during a selective catheterization. During percutaneous balloon angioplasty or a vascular recanalization procedure, 5000 U of heparin are injected before starting the procedure. A permanent arterial catheter or an injectable guidewire or a hemostatic valve sheath are maintained patent by a systemic or a local intraarterial infusion of 300 to 500 U of heparin/h to prevent pericatheter thrombosis.

Heparin Overdosage

Heparin overdosage resulting in an abnormal PTT and TCT must be recognized by the interventional radiologist. Heparin overdosage can be present in any anticoagulated patient who undergoes an interventional procedure. The interventional radiologist can also inject by error too high a dose of heparin during the procedure. Circulating heparin is removed by the reticuloendothelial system. Half-life of the molecule is variable, depending on the biochemical structure. Some pathological conditions can also alter the half-life of heparin. During pulmonary embolism and deep venous thrombosis the half-life of heparin may be reduced. Immediate therapy of heparin overdosage consists in the injection of protamine sulfate. Reversal is obtained by injection of 1 mg of protamine sulfate per 100 U of heparin.

As an example, let us consider an injection of 5000 U of heparin, which has an estimated half-live of 90 min. At the end of a vascular procedure lasting for 90 min, 2500 U are still circulating and are reversed by the injection of 25 mg of protamine sulfate. The injection should be performed slowly to avoid possible hypotension, bradycardia, or flush. The interventional radiologist should also be aware of the versatile effect of heparin. Anticoagulation can be monitored during interventional procedures lasting for several hours by automatic determination of activated coagulation time which reflects closely PTT [11]. When administration of heparin is ineffective, and AT III deficiency should be ruled out.

Autoimmune Heparin-Induced Thrombocytopenia

Autoimmune heparin-induced thrombocytopenia must be considered in patients who exhibit a progressive decrease of platelet count to 20000 per ml after several days of heparin administration. Platelets aggregate due to a complex mechanism interfering with ADP, epinephrine, and collagen. The clinical result is thrombocytopenia and thrombosis despite heparin administration. Thrombosis can extend into the venous or the arterial system. Acute thrombosis of the abdominal aorta, particularly in the elderly, is a classical clinical presentation. Autoimmune heparin-induced thrombocytopenia seems more frequent than generally accepted. Treatment consists in immediate discontinuation of heparin administration. Systemic or local thrombolytic therapy can reestablish flow in dramatic situations such as thrombosis of the abdominal aorta [4]. Oral anticoagulants must be substituted for heparin therapy.

Oral Anticoagulants

Oral anticoagulants are administered in order to obtain a long-lasting anticoagulation effect. Indications are various, including patients who have undergone cardiovascular surgery, patients with a history of vascular occlusive disease or patients on follow-up after percutaneous transluminal angioplasty (PTA), or a vascular recanalization procedure, after implantation of an inferior vena cava filter or an intraarterial or intravenous stent. Coumarin interferes with the intrahepatic synthesis of the vitamin K-dependent coagulation factors II, VII, IX, and X. Administration of coumarin carries a therapeutic effect after a variable delay of hours or days. The anticoagulation potential of coumarin can be versatile as for heparin, and even a procoagulation effect can be observed. Response of the individual patient to oral anticoagulants is wide and monitored by regular checks of PT.

A therapeutic anticoagulant range is obtained when PT is 1.5 to 2 times the normal value. This corresponds to a reduction of coagulation factors by 90%. Reversal of the oral anticoagulant effect is obtained by intravenous injection of 10 mg of vitamin K. The biological response is obtained several hours or days after injection. The anticoagulant effect of coumarin can also be neutralized by the administration of 2 to 4 units of fresh frozen plasma. It should be reminded that in patients with liver insufficiency, vitamin K is ineffective and human plasma proteins must be given.

Circulating Platelets

Platelets are complicated cell structures which have important physiological properties. The adhesive property is one of the most prominent and is balanced by the antiplatelet agent prostacyclin (PGI 2). The aggregation property of platelets is promoted by fibrinogen, calcium, ADP, thromboxane A_2, β-thromboglobulin, and other factors. Platelets have also a vasoconstrictive property through the activation of the arachidonic acid pathway resulting in thromboxane A_2 and thromboxane B_2. Platelets have a coagulation promotion property by the absorption of prothrombin and of coagulation factors X and V. They are also responsible of activation of factor XI. Within the platelets, granules are produced and released through the platelet membrane. α-Granules contain several platelet factors, thromboglobulin, and coagulation factors VIII and V. The amine storage granules release serotonin, ADP, and calcium. Another group of granules are lysosomial vesicles.

Thrombocytopenia

A low platelet count reflects thrombocytopenia. Patients with a platelet count of 50000/ml are at risk of hemorrhage. Patients with a platelet count of 20000/ml will definitely experience spontaneous bleeding or at the vascular puncture site after removal of an angiographic catheter. On the other hand, patients with chronic thrombocytopenia may compensate by an increased platelet function. Occasionally, they may show no hemorrhagic complication during a percutaneous interventional procedure, while their platelet count is as low as 5000/ml. Acute viral infections or other conditions may be responsible for a low platelet count, which rapidly normalizes again. Patients with chronic thrombocytopenia have often previously received multiple platelet transfusions over years and in return they have produced antiplatelet antibodies. Chronic thrombocytopenia is therefore difficult to treat. Chronic thrombocytopenia and particularly immune thrombocytopenic purpura (von Werlhoff disease) is classically treated by steroids and immunoglobulins. We have found that partial splenic embolization results in normalization of platelet count for 2–5 years and persists even after the splenic parenchyma has grown again to the preexisting size of spleen before embolization [3]. Thrombocytosis (over 500000/ml) favors thrombosis and can be present in various conditions, including in the early phase after splenectomy or splenic arterial embolization or in oncological patients.

Platelet Aggregation

Aspirin

The aggregation property of platelets favoring thrombosis is classically reduced by the administration of aspirin. Aspirin is widely given in patients following PTA. Aspirin inhibits the synthesis of prostacyclin (PGI 2). Carrying an antiaggregation and a vasodilation effect, the intake of aspirin creates an irreversible acetylation of cyclooxygenase which blocks the arachidonic acid pathway. Platelet aggregability and α-granule release of platelets is reduced, but adherence and granule release from adherent platelets is not affected. Even long-term intake of aspirin will usually not result in severe clinical bleeding. A single dose varying from 150 to 1500 mg has a platelet-inhibiting effect for about 2 weeks. Patients taking aspirin have a bleeding time up to 15 min. The antiplatelet effect is obtained with low doses of heparin less than 500 mg/day, whereas a higher dose will have an aggregation effect. Activity of aspirin is reversed 3 to 10 days after therapy is discontinued.

Dipyridamole

Dipyridamole is another common oral antiplatelet drug. Dipyridamole acts as a phosphodiesterase inhibitor and prevents breakdown of cyclic AMP. Usual dose is 50 to 75 mg per day. The drug reduces adhesion and aggregation of platelets, platelet granule release and also inhibits change in platelet shape [7].

Diffuse Intravascular Coagulation

Acute diffuse intravascular coagulation is readily diagnosed by typical clinical features associating thrombosis and bleeding. Symptomatic treatment is heparin. Definitive treatment is aetiological. Minimal and chronic diffuse intravascular coagulation may be encountered in oncological patients, including bronchogenic non-small-cell cancer, small-cell lung cancer and aneurysm of the abdominal aorta. Patients show slightly or moderately elevated fibrinolytic split products. Chronic and minimal intravascular coagulation does not require specific treatment.

Fibrinolysis

Fibrinolytic Sequence

Endogenous fibrinolysis is a complex process by which the precipitated fibrin polymeres are fragmented into soluble fibrinolytic split products (FSP). The steps of fibrinolysis are summarized in Fig. 2. Circulating plasminogen or plasminogen which is entrapped in the clot is activated into plasmin by a plasminogen activator (PA). Plasmin acts by degrading fibrin and fibrinogen into fibrin split products. Current plasmin inhibitors are α_2-antiplasmin, α_2-macroglobulin and AT III. Depending on their molecular weight, FSP may show an anticoagulant heparin-like effect. The level of FSP is measured in the plasma; their presence confirms ongoing fibrinolysis. In vivo thrombolysis also liberates platelets or red cells immobilized in the thrombus. Endogenous physiological fibrinolysis results from activation by urokinase and tissue type PA.

Plasminogen Activators

Therapeutic fibrinolysis is performed by either systemic or local administration of an endogenous or exogenous PA. Streptokinase (SK) is a first genera-

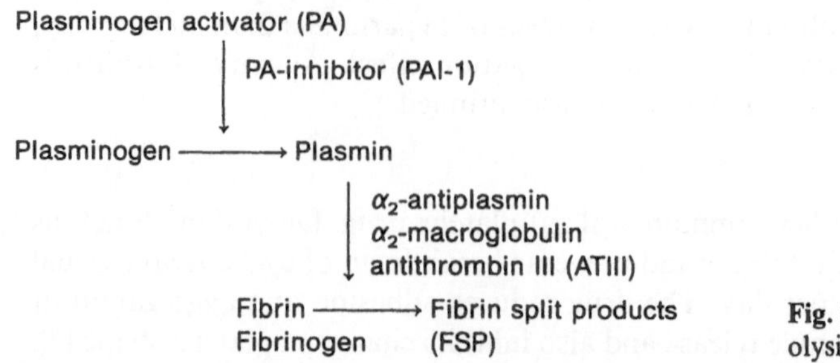

Fig. 2. Sequence of fibrinolysis

tion PA derived from β-hemolytic streptococci. Therefore SK is antigenic and may be responsible for pyretic reactions in 5%–10% of patients. A loading dose of 250000 U neutralizes circulating SK antibodies when present. SK acts on plasminogen after formation of an intermediate SK activator complex, which is bound in an isostoichiometric ratio to plasminogen. SK has a low fibrinolytic/fibrinogenolytic ratio. Clearance half-life is about 25 min.

Urokinase (UK) is also a first generation PA and is produced from human fetal renal cell cultures. It has no antigenic property and activates plasminogen directly, without formation of an intermediate activator complex. UK has a high fibrinolytic/fibrinogenolytic ratio. UK is about 20 times more expensive than SK for a given treatment by local infusion. Clearance half-life is about 12 min.

Recombinant tissue plasminogen activator (rtPA) is a second generation PA and is produced by recombinant DNA techniques from human melanoma cells. The molecule is available either as double chain or as a single chain configuration. rtPA activates plasminogen selectively in the presence of fibrin. Clearance half-life is about 2–7 min. The drug is expensive and clot specific, giving a limited systemic fibrinolytic effect during local infusion.

SK bound to the intermediate activator complex (Anistreplase) is available as an inactive acylated plasminogen activator complex (APSAC), which is reactivated following spontaneous deacylation in the plasma in the presence of physiological pH values.

Saruplase or recombinant unglycosylated single chain urokinase-type plasminogen activator (scu-PA) or prourokinase is activated into UK by hydrolysis of one peptide bond.

A great deal of research was undertaken trying to combine various PA into synergistic combinations, and by creating hybrid and chimeric molecules, but without proven clinical advantage [2]. Clinical trials which compare SK and rtPA on a large scale gave similar results. It must be remembered that up to 15% of the population are resistant to any exogenous PA.

Indications

Interventional radiologists use local fibrinolytic or thrombolytic infusion for treatment of acute or subacute ischemia of lower limb arteries, hand and finger arteries, renal, hepatic and superior mesenteric arteries, pulmonary, cerebral and coronary arteries, occluded arterial grafts, dialysis shunts, central vein thrombosis, etc.

Dose Regimens

Local infusion protocols differ greatly and can be divided into aggressive high dose infusions given over a short time period and soft protocols using reduced doses over longer time periods.

For UK, described dose regimens vary from 20000 to 100000 U/h or 10000 U/min. For SK, dose regimens vary from 5000 to 30000 U/h or 3000 U every 2–3 min. For rtPA, dose varies from 0.02 to 0.05 mg/kg per hour.

Low dose heparin (300–500 units/h) is maintained either systemically or locally and keeps the infusion catheter or the injectable guide wire clean from thrombi.

Complications

The basic idea of local thrombolysis is to achieve dissolution of thrombus without a general fibrinolytic effect. However, after a 24-h infusion, a systemic effect is almost always present and the patient is at risk for complications.

The most feared complications are:
- Hemorrhage at the puncture point or at remote sites (retroperitoneal or cerebral bleeding)
- Distal emboli which can impair arterial ischemia during thrombolysis
- Thrombosis around the infusion system and secondary embolization.

Severe complications are observed in 18%–50% of cases of local thrombolysis when using SK and in 5%–16% of cases when using UK [5].

Contraindications

The best prevention of complications is strict observation of contraindications. Absolute contraindications are active bleeding, cerebral vascular episode, brain tumor, and uncontrolled coagulopathy. Major relative contraindications include a recent history of bleeding, recent surgery or postpartum, deep organ or vessel puncture, and major trauma. Minor relative contraindications include ulcerative colitis, gastric ulcerations, active tuberculosis, necrotic tumor, severe arterial hypertension, hepatic or renal insufficiency, bacterial endocarditis, partially thrombosed aortic aneurysm, cardiac thrombi, etc.

Reversal of Thrombolysis

Local thrombolytic infusion is monitored by clinical observation of the ischemic limb, by repeated coagulation tests, and repeated arteriography. A low fibrinogen level before starting PA infusion (1.5 g/l) or a rapid decrease of fibrinogen during the first 6 h of treatment (0.8 g/l) is a good predictor of hemorrhagic complications, but such a complication can occur while coagulation tests are normal or before they are altered.

A hyperfibrinolytic state is treated by the following measures:
- Stop thrombolytic infusion
- Perfusion of aprotinin 500000 U in 10 min followed by 20000 U over 4 h
- Injection of 10 mg/kg of tranexamic acid
- Replenish coagulation factors by fresh frozen plasma, but fresh plasminogen brought in excess can be reactivated by circulating PA
- Platelets transfusions
- Perfusion of fibrinogen concentrate
- α_2-Antiplasmin or other PA inhibitory may be available in the future(?)

Fibrinolytic therapy must be followed by heparin, because of depletion of the stock of plasminogen, exposing the patient to the risk of thrombus formation, as endogenous fibrinolysis is deficient.

References

1. Bookstein JJ, Moser KM, Hougie C (1982) Coagulative interventions during angiography. Cardiovasc Intervent Radiol 5:46–56
2. Collen D, Gold HK (1989) Fibrin specific thrombolytic agents and new approach to coronary fibrinolysis. In: Julian D, Kubler W, Norris RM, Swan HJC, Collen D, Verstraete M (eds) Thrombolysis in cardiovascular disease. Dekker, Basel, pp 45–47
3. Dondelinger RF, Kurdziel JC (1990) Splenic embolization. In: Dondelinger RF, Rossi P, Kurdziel JC, Wallace S (eds) Interventional radiology. Thieme, Stuttgart, pp 502–512
4. Goffette P, Kurdziel JC, Dondelinger RF (1989) Local urokinase infusion for total occlusion of the lower abdominal aorta. Eur J Radiol 9:121–124
5. Goffette P, Kurdziel JC, Dondelinger RF (1991) Local arterial thrombolytic infusion. Therapeutic effects and complications. Acta Radiol 32:305–310
6. Mamon JF, Hoppensteadt D, Fareed J, Moncada R (1991) Biochemical evidence for a relative lack of inhibition of thrombin formation by nonionic contrast media. Radiology 179:399–402
7. Murray PD, Garnic JD, Bettmann MA (1982) Pharmacology of angioplasty and intravascular thrombolysis. AJR 139:795–803
8. Pilla TJ, Beshany SE, Shields JB (1986) Incompatibility of hexabrix and papaverine. AJR 146:1300–1301
9. Rasuli P, McLeish WA, Hammond DI (1989) Anticoagulant effects of contrast materials: in vitro study of iohexol, ioxaglate and diatrizoate. AJR 152:309–311
10. Robertson HJ (1987) Blood clot formation in angiographic syringes containing nonionic contrast media. Radiology 163:621–622
11. Scott JA, Berenstein A, Blumenthal D (1986) Use of the activated coagulation time as a measure of anticoagulation during interventional procedures. Radiology 158:849–850
12. Silverman SG, Mueller PR, Pfister RC (1990) Hemostatic evaluation before abdominal interventions. AJR 154:233–238

Discussion

on the papers by H. J. HERTFELDER and R. F. DONDELINGER

Rudofsky proposed that coagulation as it concerned interventions be discussed considered separately for the time periods before, during and after the procedure. The first question was which clotting parameters shall be checked before PTA and which ranges of values seem to be acceptable as baseline criteria. Hertfelder pointed out that this evaluation is also dependent on the type of procedure. Dondelinger said he always requires details on Quick's test, thrombocytes, and bleeding time. According to the hematology literature, the risk of significant bleeding occurring rise at a Quick of less than 60% and a thrombocyte count of under 50000. The measurement of the bleeding time is not standardized, so the normal values vary. In outpatients, observation of the bleeding from the skin incision, which is always necessary, gives a good indication of the functions of the coagulation system according to Dondelinger, especially before biopsies. Dondelinger, too, thought that the acceptable range of values depend on the type of procedure. In any nonurgent procedure when there is no primary disease that makes stopping anticoagulation seem risky, a Quick of at least 40% was expected as a starting condition.

Gross-Fengels gave two practical examples of decision-making situations. Shall an anticoagulated patient with a Quick of between 30% and 40% undergo a necessary vascular dilatation using a reduced dose of heparin, or shall the Quick first be raised so that the full dose of heparin, usually 5000 U, can be given during the intervention? If the Quick was reduced for other reasons, e.g., liver disease, Rudofsky thought that further investigation are necessary first, while Hertfelder recommended checks of factors 2, 7, and 10 and of antithrombin 3 and 4.

Walter pointed out the difference described in the older laparoscopic literature between the liver bleeding time and the percutaneously measured bleeding time. This can be important in the context of liver biopsies. Here, a check of the coagulation status was recommended in all patients with existing liver parenchyma diseases.

The second theoretical case concerned a patient with a coumarin-induced Quick of 25% who is scheduled only for diagnostic angiography. Here, the question concerned the possibility of minimizing the risk of bleeding by using thinner catheters. In Dondelinger's view, this is not sufficient; in such cases he preferres to lift the anticoagulation until a Quick of over 40% is reached, as long as this is not associated with a severe risk of, for instance, embolization from a heart valve.

In the further discussion Rudofsky drew attention to the question of checking coagulation parameters during and after the intervention. Studies by Hertfelder and coworkers had shown that heparinization with 5000 U represented sufficient anticoagulation during the whole time taken for an intervention, as the half-life of heparin is of the same order as the mean duration of a vascular intervention. Dondinger said that this means that the blood heparin concentration is about 2500 U at the time of removal of the catheter and cannulation system. In patients with an intact clotting system this represents an acceptable value regarding the benefit-risk balance between thrombosis and bleeding. Checking the coagulation system during and after the intervention seems unnecessary in such patients.

The situation shall be judged differently in patients with preexisting coagulation disorders, particularly with preexisting coumarin therapy or long-term heparinization. Hertfelder pointed out that even with "low-dose" heparinization, the tissue pools are partly full of heparin, and so the fall in the blood concentration of additionally administered heparin is significantly slowed. Checking the clotting time and also the PTT concentration before removing the cannula seems to be indicated in such cases.

With local lytic therapy, a systemic effect can often be seen, the systemic effects of the lysis depending on both the dose as well as the length of the lytic therapy. Long-term lyses thus produces systemic lysis as well as the local lytic effect. In lyses of the order of up to 4 h, systemic effects are first seen at doses of over 500 000 IU urokinase.

In response to a question from Radü about the indications for adjuvant medication with rtPA or urokinase in carotid artery dilatation, as recommended by a Japanese study group, Rudofsky said he thought this was not indicated, because the risk of peripheral embolization is increased by giving lytic substances and furthermore the risk of hemorrhage into a brain infarct after embolization rises. This risk is also feared with ulcerated carotid stenoses in the context of local and systemic lytic therapy. The general indications and the high risks of dilatation of carotid stenoses were not discussed further.

Concomitant Drug Therapy During Radiologic Interventions

Drug Therapy During Venous Interventions and Vena Cava Filter Procedures

C.L. Zollikofer, F. Antonucci, G. Stuckmann, and P. Mattias

Introduction

In principle, drug therapy in venous intervention and vena cava filter implantation consists, as in arterial intervention, of the administration of local anesthesia and the prevention or treatment of perioperative thrombosis, and of sedation and analgesia as requested.

Further adjunctive drug therapy may be needed for hypo-hypertension, vaso-vagal reaction etc., the treatment of venous spasms, and the prevention of postinterventional thrombosis, restenosis and intimal hyperplasia following recanalization, percutaneous transluminal angioplasty (PTA) and stenting of veins.

General Principles for Venous Interventions

Routine Practices

Intravenous Line. Before starting any interventional radiologic procedure we install a peripheral (central) venous line for sufficient hydration of the fasting patient and for immediate and easy access to administer drugs and/or volume as needed.

Technical Monitoring. Regular blood pressure measurements (5 to 15-min intervals) and registration of oxygen saturation using a finger oscillometer are done routinely.

Local Anesthesia. For the interventional access to the venous system mepivacaine or lidocaine (Scandicain, Xylocaine) are used. For an inguinofemoral or internal jugular approach 10 ml is usually sufficient. Only a few milliliters are needed for peripheral access, such as in hemodialysis fistulas.

Periinterventional Antithrombotic Regimen. The main antithrombotic drug used in venous intervention is heparin. In contrast to arterial interventions, no platelet inhibitors are usually used since their effect on the venous side is disputable. For recanalization and dilatation of venous obstructions, as well as for foreign body removal and vena cava filter placements, we use 5000 IU heparin i.v. starting after the placement of the hemostatic-introducing sheath into the access vein. For prolonged interventions of more than 2-h duration, approximately 2000 IU heparin per hour of procedure is added. Unless contraindicated, heparin infusion at 800–1000 IU per hour is maintained for 72 h in all implant procedures, such as filters and stents.

Special Indications

Sedatives and Analgesics. Sedatives and analgesics are not used routinely by us. If increased pain is anticipated or the patient is restless, premedication with 5 mg midazolam (Dormicum) and 1 mg per 10 kg body weight nicomorphine (Vilan) is given i.m. 20 min before the procedure (normal coagulation parameters!).

If needed nicomorphine and/or midazolam are given in fractions of 2 mg i.v. during the procedure. Retrograde amnesia from midazolam is a desirable side effect. However, particularly in elderly patients with cerebral arteriosclerosis, midazolam may provoke paradoxic reactions or cause severe sedation in doses as low as 1 mg i.v.

ECG Monitoring. ECG monitoring is performed in patients at risk or in patients where guidewires and catheters have to be manipulated through the heart.

Hyper/Hypotension. Hypertensive patients should have their medication as usual on the day of intervention. If necessary our preferred hypertensive drug is nifedipine (Adalat), 10 mg sublingually.

In our experience perioperative hypotension rarely occurs in venous interventions. Treatment is with 5 mg ephedrine i.v. in cases of peripheral vasodilation or with a rapid infusion of saline or gelatine solution (Physiogel) in cases of vasodilation and/or volume loss. Atropine is the drug of choice for vasovagal reactions.

Spasmolytic Drugs. Venous spasms may be induced by the selective catheterization of small caliber veins, such as in hemodialysis fistulas or spermatic veins. Our preferred spasmolytic drug is nitroglycerin given intravascularly in doses of 0.1–0.2 mg. Alternatively lidocaine is used.

Adjunctive Drug Therapy for Specific Procedures

Percutaneous Transluminal Angioplasty and Stenting in the Venous System

Percutaneous Transluminal Angioplasty

Usually no further drug treatments apart from those described under general principles are needed for percutaneous transluminal angioplasty (PTA) of veins. The most important intraoperative drug is heparin for the prophylaxis of thrombosis. Heparinization is usually discontinued at the end of the procedure unless thrombolysis had to be performed, e.g., for an acutely occluded hemodialysis shunt.

Stenting in the Venous System

Since PTA of venous stenoses generally shows a high recurrence rate and because of a primarily high resistence or tendency to recoil, endovascular stenting has been advocated for the following indications:

a) Palliative treatment of tumor compression of the vena cava and large central veins
b) Nontumorous external compression of the vena cava, such as in Budd-Chiari syndrome or mediastinitis
c) Postoperative strictures in large native veins
d) Postthrombotic stenoses of large veins, the venous spur (May-Thurner syndrome), or congenital webs
e) Stenoses of the venous outflow tract including brachiocephalic veins in chronic hemodialysis fistulas

For all these indications our concomitant drug therapy consists of the intraoperative administration of 5000 IU heparin. Heparinization is continued for 72 h and patients are transferred to oral anticoagulation with coumarin. A similar protocol is used by other authors [1–3]. If oral anticoagulation is contraindicated, we use a platelet inhibitor, 250 mg aspirin daily. We do not use preoperative treatment with platelet inhibitors.

In cases which need the recanalization of a partially or totally occluded vein or following acute occlusion, local thrombolysis is performed with fibrinolytic agents such as urokinase, clot aspiration, and/or PTA. For fibrinolysis of large veins, such as the innominate and vena cava, prolonged regional clot lysis may be necessary, necessitating close monitoring of coagulation parameters (partial thromboplastin time, fibrinogen levels).

Role of Postoperative Anticoagulation and/or Platelet Inhibitors in PTA and Stenting

Generally vascular stents are embedded into the vascular wall by intimal overgrowth and endothelialization. Initially, however, the stent becomes covered by a certain amount of thrombus formation. According to animal experiments by Nöldge et al. and Palmaz et al. [4, 5], this amount of laminal-thrombus formation eventually determines the thickness of the intimal layer that will be present later. A restricted or turbulent arterial flow caused increased thrombus deposition with consequently thicker fibromuscular intimal reaction. Furthermore, for a given stent surface thrombus formation was relatively constant. This caused a thicker thrombus layer for a given stent in a small-diameter vessel as compared to a larger diameter vessel. Theoretically therefore platelet inhibitors and anticoagulation with coumarine until endothelialization of the stented surface is complete should minimize the risk of thrombotic occlusions and increased intimal hyperplasia. This could be proven in animal experiments, where a combination of heparin, aspirin, dipyridamole, and low-molecular dextran was most effective [6].

Whether the same theory also applies to veins is not known for certain. In our own experiments, stents implanted in popliteal and iliac veins remained patent over a period of 6 and 12 months, respectively, with various amounts of intimal thickening. The dogs were given 125 mg aspirin daily for a period of 30 days postoperation. The intimal layers measured 70–500 μm in the completely patent popliteal veins and 30–1000 μm in the iliac veins. Two out of seven femoropopliteal veins showed signs of previous thrombosis with recanalization. However, in human patients intimal overgrowth and endothelialization of the stents vary a lot more than in animals, where all stents were covered by a neoendothelium after 5–12 weeks in veins and after 4–6 weeks in arteries.

In human iliac-artery stents, we have found bare areas of metal surface after 18 months. Similarly, endothelialization in stented venous tumor stenoses seems definitely delayed and may even be partially absent after 1.5 years. Radiation therapy and/or corticoid or chemotherapy may be a possible explanation [7]. In our experience the amount of intimal reaction in benign stenoses may also vary considerably without any good explanation. Therefore, we propose long-term oral anticoagulation with coumarine for at least 6 months for venous stenting, particularly for tumor stenosis, since tumor invasion probably causes a deteriorated endothelial surface with an increased risk of acute occlusion, as was shown in one of our patients with malignant stenosis. In cases where oral anticoagulation was contraindicated (bleeding of tumor etc.), platelet inhibitors (aspirin) were given. However, as stated previously, there is no solid scientific basis for this and it was done primarily to ease our conscience.

Stenting of the Venous Outflow Tract in Hemodialysis Shunts

This procedure is mainly complicated by severe intimal hyperplasia and the occurrence of new lesions. Probably the increased arterialized flow with consequent turbulence in the hemodialysis shunts is the main factor responsible. However, acute thrombosis is comparatively rare in our experience. In most cases our patients were anticoagulated for 3–6 months. Platelet inhibitors were given only in two patients in whom coumarin had to be discontinued early after stenting. There was no positive effect with regard to intimal reaction. Apart from the pain medication as described under general principles, we use perivenous infiltration of the stenotic vein segment before dilatation and stenting because dilatation of these usually very fibrotic stenoses can be very painful. Perivenous infiltration with local anesthetics is most helpful.

Vena Cava Filters

To our knowledge no adjunctive therapy is usually given apart from intraoperative heparinization with 5000 IU heparin. Since contraindications of oral anticoagulation are one of the main indications of vena cava filters, usually no further anticoagulant therapy is given. However, some investigators suggest short-term anticoagulation for 10–14 days to prevent acute caval thrombosis [Günther, personal communication, University of Aachen/Germany].

Percutaneous Foreign Body Retrieval

Apart from the intraoperative prophylaxis of thrombosis with 5000 IU heparin no further drugs are generally necessary.

Conclusions

In addition to local anesthesia and intraoperative heparinization, further drugs are only rarely needed in venous interventions. An intravenous line and blood-pressure recording are routine for all interventions.

Postoperative anticoagulation for at least 6 months is strongly recommended after venous stent procedures.

References

1. Rösch J, Uchida BT, Hall LD, Antonovic R, Ivancev K, Petersen BD (1992) Gianturco expandable stents in the treatment of superior vena caval syndrome. CVIR Vol 15, No 5, 1992
2. Olcott EW, Ring EJ, Robert JP, Ascher NL, Lake JR, Gordon RL (1990) Percutaneous transhepatic portal vein angioplasty and stent placement after liver transplantation: early experience. JVIR 1:17–22
3. Walker HS, Rholl KS, Register TE, von Breda A (1990) Percutaneous placement of hepatic vein stent in the treatment of Budd-Chiari syndrome. JVIR 1:23–27
4. Noeldge G, Richter GM, Siegestetter V, Garcia O, Palmaz JC (1988) Tierexperimentelle Untersuchungen über den Einfluß der Flußrestriktion auf die Thrombogenität des Palmaz Stentes mittels 111-Indium-markierter Thrombozyten. ROFO 152:264–270
5. Palmaz JC, Tio FO, Schatz RA, Alvarado R, Rees C, Garcia O (1988) Early endothelialization of balloon-expandable stents: experimental observations. J Intervent Radiol 3:119–124
6. Palmaz JC, Garcia O, Kopp DT, Tio FO, Ciaravino V, Schatz RA, Rees C, Alvarado R, Lancaster JL, Borchert RD (1989) Balloon-expandable intraarterial stents: effect of antithrombotic medication on thrombus formation. In: Zeitler E, Seyfert W (eds) Pros and cons in PTA and auxiliary methods. Springer, Berlin Heidelberg New York, pp 170–178
7. Hoepp LM, Elbadawi A, Cohn M, Dachelet R, Peterson C, De Weese JA (1979) Steroids and immunosuppression. Effect on anastomotic intimal hyperplasia in femoral arterial Dacron bypass grafts. Arch Surg 114:273–276

Adjunctive Medication, Therapy, and Special Monitoring in Embolization Procedures

W. GROSS-FENGELS, R. FISCHBACH, M. KUHN, P. SIEMENS, and K. LACKNER

Adjunctive Medication in Embolization Procedures

Transcatheter arterial embolizations are established and effective interventional procedures [1, 2, 20, 22, 25, 27, 31, 35, 38, 39, 42, 45]. Compared to other interventional methods, e.g., angioplasties, these procedures are often more complex. They are frequently associated with side effects and have a higher complication rate [11, 12, 16, 33, 40]. The various aspects of adjunctive medical treatment, further accompanying therapies, and the importance of special patient monitoring are discussed. The measures presented have the following aims:

1. Subjective complaints of the patient relating to the intervention are to be reduced in order to improve acceptance of the procedure
2. Specific reactions associated with the embolization procedure, such as paroxysmal hypertension and sudden hormonal discharge, have to be controlled
3. Overall safety and effectiveness of the intervention must be increased

Transcatheter arterial embolization procedures may be efficacious in several different pathologies: malignant tumors, vascular malformations, varicoceles, and hemorrhage – spontaneous, traumatic, or iatrogenic (Fig. 1). Sometimes embolization of entire organs, e.g., renal artery embolization in end-stage renal insufficiency, is performed.

Technical details and adjunctive medications vary considerably depending on the anatomical target area. Embolization procedures are feasible in the following organs and systems: CNS, liver, kidney, spleen, bronchial arteries, pulmonary arteries, pelvis, the upper or lower limbs, and the gastrointestinal tract.

It has to be understood that transcatheter arterial embolizations are relatively time-consuming procedures and often large doses of contrast media are necessary.

Sudden, uncontrolled movements during the critical phase of an intervention due to pain or patient distress may result in catheter dislocation and subsequent incorrect embolization. Pain and agitation of the patient may lead to early termination of the intervention. Complementary medical therapy and patient monitoring in hepatic artery chemoembolization are described in detail in the following. Recommendations for other locations are presented also.

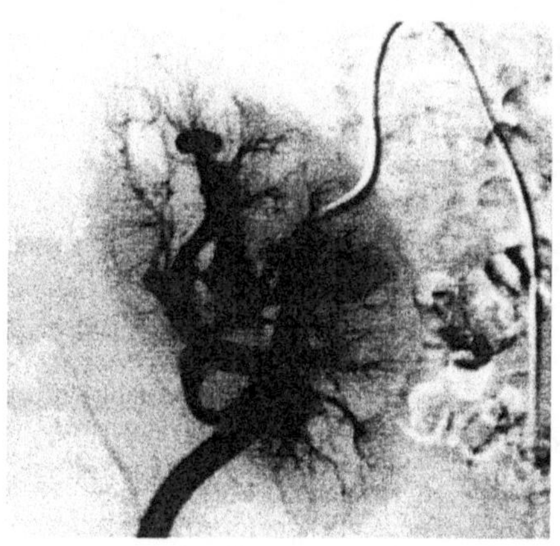
a

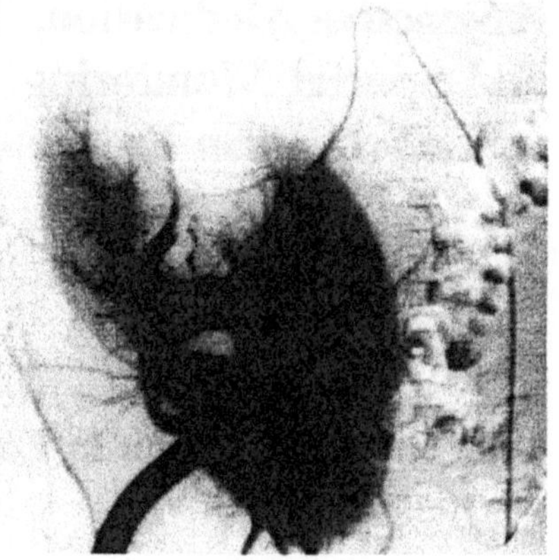
b

Fig. 1 a, b. Two weeks after diagnostic puncture of a kidney transplant for suspected transplant rejection severe bleeding occurred necessitating repeated blood transfusions and tamponade of the bladder due to blood clots. **a** Intraarterial digital subtraction angiography (IA-DSA) before embolization: false aneurysm with arteriovenous (AV) fistula in the cranial portion of the transplant. **b** IA-DSA after embolization: complete occlusion of the aneurysm and the AV fistula; small infarct distally to the occluded artery. The bleeding was interrupted immediately, no further tamponade occurred and the transplant could be preserved

Embolization–Chemoembolization of the Liver

Several studies were able to demonstrate a prolongation of the survival time compared to untreated controls. Preoperative chemoembolization may facilitate resection of hypervascular tumors or may even make an operative therapy feasible due to a significant reduction in tumor volume. Furthermore, embolization procedures are valuable in life-threatening tumor hemorrhages. Several contraindications to hepatic artery chemoembolization have to be recognized and these are summarized in Table 1. The risk of inducing severe side effects or complications correlates with the tumor volume. Several anatomic variations have to be considered and redistribution of the nutritive liver supply, as observed in liver cirrhosis, must be regarded. Fatal courses after chemoembolization of the liver have been described. Our review of the literature yielded a 4% in-hospital mortality [1, 8, 9, 14, 43].

Medication and Materials for Chemoembolization of the Liver

The injection of embolization materials into the celiac artery has to be avoided. Coaxial catheter systems usually allow a more distal catheter placement in the proper hepatic artery or in segmental branches [4, 10, 18, 26, 28, 34]. The

Table 1. Chemoembolization of the liver – contraindications (modified from [18])

Contraindications	
Karnofsky index	≤ 50
Severe hepatic dysfunction:	
Bilirubin	> 2.5 mg
Cholinesterase	< 1000 IU
Prothrombin time (Quick)	< 50%
Partial thromboplastin time	> 1.5 × control
Severe renal dysfunction:	
Creatinine	> 2.5 mg/dl
Myelodepression:	
White blood cells	< 2000
Platelets	< 100 000
Portal vein occlusion	
Surgical resection feasible	
Untreated extrahepatic TU manifestation	
Acute infection	
Severe ascites	

TU, Tumor.

intended level of occlusion governs the selection of suitable embolization materials. Occlusion of the proper hepatic artery in its proximal segment, e.g., using Gianturco-Anderson-Wallace coils, seems to be indicated only in otherwise uncontrollable hemorrhages. The capillary or precapillary level should be occluded for the best results. Tables 2 and 3 list embolization materials and chemotherapeutic agents that are in use for the treatment of hepatocellular carcinoma or secondary liver neoplasms.

Monitoring

Occlusion of the hepatic artery causes serious changes in the perfusion of the liver and hepatic metabolism. In the healthy individual nutritive blood supply to the liver is derived mainly from the portal system and only to a lesser extent from the hepatic artery [6]. In portal hypertension or portal-vein obstruction secondary to tumor expansion, the normal blood-supply pattern may change significantly. This means that hepatic-artery occlusion can lead to extensive liver necrosis resulting in hepatic coma. Thus laboratory parameters have to be followed closely. Table 4 presents details about patient monitoring. It has to be stressed that in addition to liver-function disturbance, renal function can be impaired leading even to hepatorenal syndrome with dialysis-dependent renal insufficiency. Moreover, a sudden release of tumor-specific hormones in endocrine-active processes can cause dramatic situations (see below).

Table 2. Materials for chemoembolization of the liver – treatment of hepatocellular carcinoma [from 5–9, 18–20, 24, 34, 36, 37, 41, 46]

Materials	Amount	Reference
5-Fluorouracil	1 g	Junyuan [24]
Mitomycin C	10 mg	
Gelfoam particles	*	
Mitomycin C	10 mg	Takayasu [46]
Doxorubicin (Adriamycin)	20–40 mg	
Gelfoam particles	*	
Mitomycin C	*	Carrasco [7]
Doxorubicin (Adriamycin)	*	Chuang [8]
Floxuridine (FUDR)	*	
Ivalon 250–590 μm	*	
Cisplatin	1.5–2 mg/kg b.w.	Sasaki [41]
Lipiodol	10 ml	
Gelfoam particles	*	
Epirubicin	40–60 mg	Bokemeyer [5],
Cisplatin	24–36 mg	Grote [19]
Lipiodol	4–6 ml	
Doxorubicin (Adriamycin)	40–100 mg	Nakamura [34]
Lipiodol	5–20 ml	
Doxorubicin (Adriamycin)	20–50 mg/m^2	Hashimoto [20]
Lipiodol	5–10 ml	
Gelfoam particles	*	
Doxorubicin (Adriamycin)	20–60 mg and/or	Ohishi [37]
Mitomycin C	10–20 mg	
Lipiodol	*	
Cisplatin	50 mg	
Gelfoam particles	*	
Epirubicin	40–60 mg	Gross-Fengels [17]
Ivalon 250–590 μm	*	
Ethibloc	0.2–1 ml	

b.w., body-weight; *, no specification possible or made by the authors.

Complications, Side Effects, and Special Monitoring

The type and incidence of side effects and specific requirements for monitoring hepatic embolization procedures can be taken from Tables 5 and 6. Most of the patients will experience moderate or severe abdominal pain, necessitating adequate pain relief in the subacute phase (see below). Often the cystic artery cannot be identified in selective hepatic artery angiography. A partial occlusion of this vessel cannot be avoided in all cases. If collateralization is good no significant sequelae will develop, but especially after upper abdominal surgery, e.g., gastrectomy, such collaterals are occluded and there is a high risk of postembolization cholecystitis. Some groups therefore recommend cholecystectomy before performing hepatic artery chemoembolization. Several in-

Table 3. Materials for chemoembolization of the liver – treatment of metastases [from 8, 13, 14, 18, 25, 31, 38]

Materials	Amount	Reference
Mitomycin C	*	Chuang [8]
Floxuridine (FUDR)	*	
Ivalon 250–590 μm	*	
Mitomycin C microencapsulated	10–30 mg	Kato [25]
Mitomycin C	10–15 mg/m^2	Patt [38]
Floxuridine (FUDR)	100 mg/m^2	
Gelfoam particles or GAW coils	*	
Fluorouracil microspheres	30 mg/kg b.w.	Pfeifer [39]
Mitomycin C	ca. 25 mg	Daniels [13]
Cisplatin	ca. 75 mg	
Collagen	ca. 7.5 ml	
Cisplatin	150 mg	Mavligit [31]
Ivalon 150 μm	15 ml	(metas. occ. mal. melanoma)
Mitomycin C	20 mg	Gross-Fengels [18]
Ivalon 250–590 μm	*	
Ethibloc	0.2–1 ml	

GAW, Gianturco-Anderson-Wallace; b.w., body weight; *, no specification possible or made by the authors.

Table 4. Chemoembolization of the liver – monitoring of laboratory parameters

Parameters	Changes
SGPT (ALT)	→ 10-fold ↑
SGOT (AST)	→ 10-fold ↑
GLDH	→ 10-fold ↑
LDH-5	→ 5-fold ↑
Cholinesterase	↓
Albumin	↓
Partial thromboplastin time	Prolongation
Prothrombin time (Quick)	↓
Alkaline phosphatase	→ 3-fold ↑
Bilirubin	→ 3-fold ↑
Creatinine	↑
Na, K, Mg, Ca	↑↓
Uric acid	↑↑↑
Amylase	↑
White blood count	→18000 ↑
CEA[a]	↑ → ↓↓ (within 1 week)
Alpha-fetoprotein[a]	↑ → ↓↓ (within 1 week)

[a] Depending on tumor type.

Table 5. Chemoembolization of the liver – acute side effects and complications

Side effects/complications	Incidence (%)	Monitoring
Pain	53–95	Clinical
Systemic hypertension	10	Blood pressure control
Nausea, vomiting	40–64	Clinical, laboratory electrolytes
Fever, chills	16–55	Clinical, temperature control
Gallbladder infarction	2	Ultrasound, CT
Dyspnea	5	Oximetry
Acute renal failure	3	Lab.: creatinine, Na, K
Renal or mesenteric embolism	1	Clinical, angiography
Carcinoid syndrome	–	Clinical, laboratory serotonin
Hemorrhage (puncture site)	15	Clinical, laboratory Hb

Table 6. Chemoembolization of the liver – subacute side effects and complications

Side effects/complications	Incidence (%)	Monitoring
Abscess	5	CT, ultrasound
Sepsis	3	Blood cultures
Tumor necrosis	–	CT, laboratory: LDH
Tumor rupture	–	Clinical, CT
Cholecystitis	10	Ultrasound
Pancreatitis	2	Ultrasound, CT, laboratory: amylase
Subileus	4–13	Abdominal plain film, ultrasound
Transient liver dysfunction	10–18	Laboratory: albumin, prothrombin time, SGOT, SGPT, bilirubin
Leukocytosis	75	Blood count
Anemia (<8 g/dl)	–	Blood count
Thrombopenia (<50000)	–	Blood count
Leukopenia (<3000)	–	Blood count
Potassium ↑, ↓	–	Laboratory: K
Hyperuricemia	–	Laboratory: uric acid
Oliguria	6	Urine volume
Hepatorenal syndrome	5–10	Laboratory: creatinine, K, Na
Metabolic acidosis	–	Blood gases, pH
DIC	1–2	Laboratory: fibrinogen, platelets
Ascites	21	Ultrasound
Pleuritis, pleural effusion	6	Ultrasound, chest X-ray
GI ulcera, gastritis	6	Endoscopy, hemoccult test

vestigators stress the risk of hemorrhage from the puncture site secondary to the impaired systemic coagulation in reduced liver function. Hemorrhage may also occur secondary to paroxysmal systemic hypertension, indicating the need for close blood-pressure controls.

In the first weeks after chemoembolization, liver abscess formation or tumor necrosis in the embolized region may be observed (Fig. 2). Sterile conditions are particularly important in embolization procedures, as is prophylactic periinterventional antimicrobial therapy. The risk of tumor necrosis or rupture of the tumor into the peritoneal cavity is increased if attempted surgical liver resection was not possible due to tumor size. These patients need even closer follow-ups in the early post-interventional stage (1–7 days).

The necrosis of hepatic parenchyma after embolization can cause hyperuricemia and a massive shift in serum electrolytes. Disseminated intravascular coagulation, constituting a vital threat, can result from circulating tumor cells or cell fragmentation. We lost one (1.9%) of our 53 patients to such a complication. Disseminated pulmonary microembolism resulted in respiratory insufficiency. Furthermore blood pH-shifts are possible and can cause severe acidosis. Laboratory checks (Table 4) are necessary, especially in prolonged or complicated cases. Sonographically detectable ascites may be a symptom of progressive liver dysfunction. After a hepatic embolization procedure, we also recommend a chest X-ray before the patient is discharged to rule out pleural effusion. Plain abdominal radiography may show a paralytic subileus (Fig. 3).

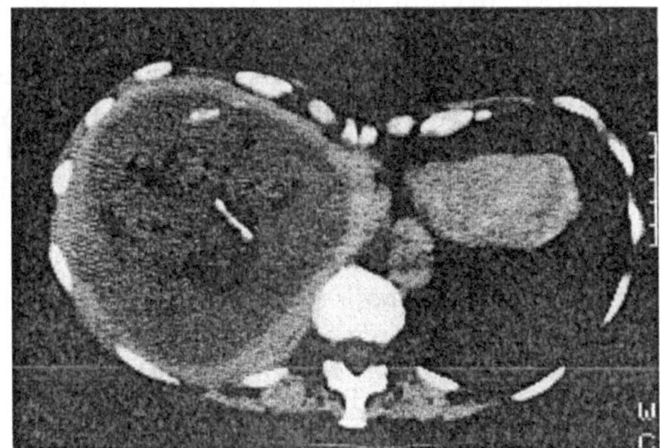

Fig. 2. Four weeks after chemoembolization of a hepatocellular carcinoma. Computed tomography: gas formation within the necrotic tumor, no clinical signs of abscess formation

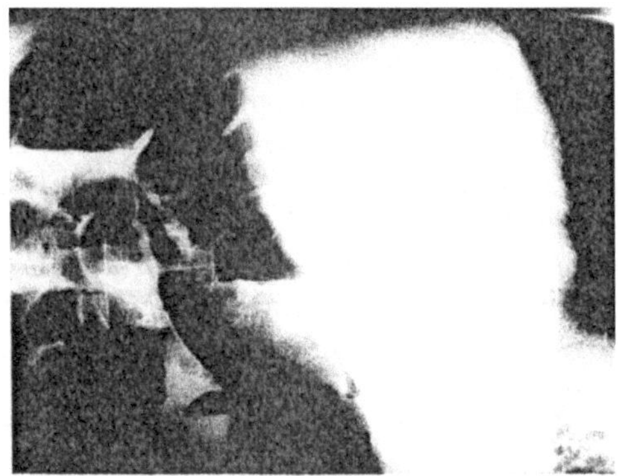

Fig. 3. Two days after chemoembolization of liver metastases from colorectal carcinoma. Plain abdominal radiography: paralytic subileus which resolved under symptomatic therapy

Adjunctive Medication

We perform embolization only in inpatients. Hospital admission is at the latest on the day before the intervention. No solid foods or milk products are allowed after midnight. Clear liquids like tea or water are allowed up to 2 h before the intervention. As with other interventions the patients should take their regular medication in the morning of the procedure. We believe that an adjunctive medical treatment is mandatory in hepatic artery embolization [17]. Protocols, special medications, and dosages are listed in Table 7.

An i.v. line is required for all interventions. Intramuscular administration of adjunctive drugs is not recommended. The onset of specific drug effects cannot be controlled exactly and the risk of producing hematomas is high since coagulation is usually reduced. In almost all medication administered, dosages have to be adapted to the individual liver function, this means usually that dosages have to be reduced. Furthermore, a disturbed liver function will prolong the effects of the drugs given.

Positive effects of sufficient hydration before embolization are well known. According to Daniels et al. [13, 14, 44] prophylactic antibiotic medication should also be given. Their experimental studies have demonstrated a reduced risk of hepatic necrosis with antimicrobial therapy. Antibiotics with a known nephrotoxicity, as for example gentamycin, are not recommended, since they may augment the nephrotoxic effect of chemoembolization.

Almost every patient undergoing chemoembolization needs some form of analgetic treatment. The intraarterial administration of local anesthetics before injecting the embolization material has proved to be of value. Sedation is done routinely in our patients. A short-acting benzodiazepine (e.g., midazolam in a solution of 1 mg midazolam/ml) is used. If opioid analgesics, e.g., pethidine, are given, synergistic effects with midazolam can occur. Acute respiratory insufficiency and apnea have been reported. Thus specific antagonists like flumazenil (Anexate) should be at hand. The sedative effects of midazolam may also be augmented if chlorprothixene is given simultaneously. The deep sedation produced requires specific preparations and may necessitate consultating an anesthesiologist.

We routinely use low-dose anticoagulation in hepatic embolizations (e.g., 5000–7500 IU heparin i.a.). Heparinization prevents thrombus formation in the coaxial catheter system. On the other hand occlusion of the hepatic artery should be achieved by the administered embolization material (e.g., Ivalon, Gelfoam) and not by the formation of lysable thrombi, since hepatic artery thrombosis would yield an uncontrollable type of arterial occlusion.

If chemoperfusion of the portal venous system is done in addition to hepatic artery embolization, adequate pain relief is of even greater importance. Postintervention fever can be relieved and the total dosage of analgesics needed may be reduced by antiphlogistic drugs.

A computed tomography (CT)-guided blockade of the celiac plexus can be indicated for pain relief. We perform this procedure if severe pain exists before

Table 7. Chemoembolization of the liver – adjunctive medication and supportive therapy

	Medication	Dosage
Hospital admission:		≥ Day before the procedure, nothing p.o. after midnight
Night sedation:		
Flunitrazepam	Rohypnol	0.5–1 tablet or
Nitrazepam	Mogadan	0.5–1 tablet
Morning of the intervention:		
Regular medication	as usual	
i.v. line		∅ 1.2–1.4 mm
Prehydration:		
0.9% NaCl solution/ Ringer solution		500–1000 ml/2 h
Antibiotics:		
Cefazolin	Gramaxin	2 g/day i.v. and
Metronidazole	Clont	1.5 g/day i.v.
avoid gentamycin		
Angiography suite:		
Analgesics:		
Pethidine-HCl	Dolantin	0.5 (0.25) mg/kg body weight i.v. at intervals ≥ 30 min
Lidocaine-HCl-1%	Xylocain	≤ 100 mg = 10 ml i.a.
Sedation:		
Midazolam	Dormicum	2 mg + 1.5 mg etc., i.v. 3 ml + 12 ml 0.9% NaCl = 15 ml solution 1 ml = 1 mg or
Chlorprothixene	Truxal	25 mg i.v. 1 ml + 4 ml 0.9% NaCl = 5 ml solution 1 ml = 10 mg
Anticoagulation:		
Heparin-Na	Liquemin	100 IU/kg body weight i.a.
On the ward:		
I.v. hydration		2 l/day for 2 days
Antibiotics		5 days
Analgesics:		As needed
Morphine		10 mg + 5 mg etc.
Pethidine-HCl	Dolantin	0.5 (0.25) mg/kg body weight i.v.
Antiphlogistics:		5 days
Paracetamol	Ben-u-ron	3 × 500 mg p.o. or
Indomethacin	Amuno	3 × 25 mg p.o.

the embolization or if the tumor or lymphnode metastasis involve mesenteric structures. Another indication is seen in persistent severe pain on the fifth day after embolization. Other groups use high peridural anesthesia or inhalational anesthetics depending on the different embolization techniques employed. Table 4 and 8 give details on further side effects and complications resulting from liver embolization.

Table 8. Chemoembolization of the liver – therapy of side effects and complications

Side effect/complication	Therapy	Drugs	Dosage
Subileus	Nasogastric tube with suction Nothing per os Infusions		
Hyponatriemia, Hepatorenal syndrome	Replacement of Na, K Corticosteroids	Na, K Hydrocortisone	As needed i.v. 0.5–1 g/day i.v.
Nausea	Triflupromazine-HCl Dimenhydrinate Ondansetron-HCl Metoclopramide-HCl	Psyquil Vomex Zofran Paspertin	5 mg i.v. 65 mg i.v. 10 mg i.v. 10 mg i.v.
Liver abscess	Percutaneous drainage		
Bleeding	Hydroxyethyl starch (Transfusions: informed consent !!!)	HAES-st. 6%	0.5–1 l/day i.v.
Hyperuricemia	Fluids Allopurinol Benzbromarone and Allopurinol	 Zyloric Uricovac c.	2 l/day 300 mg p.o. 40+200 mg p.o.
Systemic hypertension	Nifedipine Dihydralazine Clonidine	Adalat Nepresol in combination with Catapresan	10 mg s.l. 25 mg i.v. 0.15 mg i.v.

Table 9. Chemoembolization of the liver – antagonizing endocrine-active tumors (modified from [42, 43])

Substance	"Blocking agent"
Gastrin	Somatostatin H_2-receptor blockers Proton pump inhibitors
Serotonin	Somatostatin Methysergide Cyproheptadine
Insulin	Glucose Diazoxide Somatostatin
Histamine	Chlorpromazine Cyproheptadine Diphenhydramine
Kinins	Aprotinin β-Blockers Chlorpromazine Phenoxybenzamine
Substance P	α-Mimetics

In spite of local administration, the chemotherapeutic agents will produce some systemic effects. These effects are less marked than in systemic chemotherapy, nevertheless potential side effects of the substances used should be accounted for. Depending on the drug used effects include myelodepression, leukocytopenia, thrombocytopenia, cardiac arrhythmia, cardiomyopathy (Adriamycin), renal dysfunction, nausea, vomiting, and neurotoxicity. Nephrotoxic effects have to be considered especially with the use of cisplatin. Diuresis should be enforced by the administration of sufficient fluids and manitol, and the substitution of sodium. Several chemotherapeutic agents are inactivated by heparin, thus heparin and chemotherapeutic drugs should not be mixed.

In the embolization of endocrine active tumors [30, 32], life-threatening side effects have to be expected and sophisticated monitoring is imperative. Certain hormone-specific effects can be counteracted by the use of specific "blocking agents" (Table 9). Postinterventional monitoring in the intensive care unit has to be considered in such cases.

Special Aspects of the Embolization of Other Areas

Depending on the anatomic site, varying complications are associated with embolization procedures. Some important aspects are summarized in Table 10.

Embolization of *pelvic tumors* may cause myoglobinuria secondary to necrosis of muscle tissue. Sufficient fluids have to be provided to enforce diuresis. The value of steroids in the therapy of paralysis of the extremities due to damage to the vasa nervorum has not been documented in controlled studies, but a trial seems to be warranted.

Embolization of the spleen should be done under periinterventional antibiotic coverage according to Dondelinger et al. [15]. Partial occlusion of the splenic-arterial vessels can produce a secondary thrombosis of the splenic vein. Thus temporary heparinization is suggested in such cases. Changes in the immune system with the risk of infections have to be considered. The incidence of secondary malignomas seems to be increased after radiation of the spleen or operative intervention. Incomplete *renal embolization* can induce hypertensive crisis. Thus antihypertensive substances should be at hand and close monitoring of blood pressure is mandatory. If pain relief is not sufficient with i.v. analgesics, peridural anesthesia should be discussed. The function of the contralateral kidney has to be maintained. Careful embolization without reflux, reduced contrast load, and fluid balance is necessary.

The high rate of preexisting and often asymptomatic cerebral infarcts has to be kept in mind when performing an embolization of *pulmonary arteriovenous fistulas* [2, 21]. Before the embolization a cranial CT scan should be done for legal reasons. If a cerebrovascular accident occurs in spite of preventive measures, cerebral microcirculation can be improved by the administration of hydroxyethyl starch.

Table 10. Embolization of other areas – special aspects depending on embolization type [from 3, 15, 23, 29]

Anatomic site	Complication	Treatment
Pelvic tumor	Myoglobinuria	Improve diuresis, hemodialysis if needed
	Paralysis of the extremities	Corticosteroids!?
Spleen	Systemic infection	Antibiotics indispensable vaccination
	Pancreatitis	Nothing p.o.
	Gastrointestinal ulcer	H_2 blockers, antacids
	Splenic vein thrombosis	Heparin
Kidney	Systemic hypertension	Nifedipine, nitrates
	Pain	Peridural anesthesia
	Compromising function of contralateral kidney	Avoid reflux. Provide fluids (> 2 l/day) esp. if CheE is performed, reduced contrast load
	Sepsis	Antibiotics if nephrectomy does not follow
	Chills	Pethidine (Dolantin) i.v.
Bronchial artery	Oesophageal bronchial fistula	Nothing p.o.
	Ischemic myelitis	Avoid reflux, corticosteroids!?
Pulmonary AV malformation	Embolic stroke	Improve microcirculation, e.g., with hydroxyethyl starch (HAES-st. 6%) Obtain cranial CT *before* intervention

In conclusion, embolization procedures are highly effective but are associated with significant side effects and complications. Adjunctive medication and proper monitoring will increase the safety and acceptance of these interventions.

References

1. Allison DJ, Jordan H, Hennessy O (1985) Therapeutic embolization of the hepatic artery; a review of 75 procedures. Lancet 1 (8429):595–599
2. Barth C, White RI, Kaufman S, Terry P, Roland J-M (1982) Embolotherapy of pulmonary arteriovenous malformations with detachable balloons. Radiology 142:599–606
3. Basche S, Leisering W, Kachel R (1988) Die Bedeutung der Embolisationstherapie für die Prognose des Nierenzellkarzinoms. In: Schneider GH, Vogler E (eds) Digitale bildgebende Verfahren. Springer, Berlin Heidelberg New York
4. Bechtel W, Wright KC, Wallace S, Mosier B et al. (1986) An experimental evaluation of microcapsules for arterial chemoembolization. Radiology 161:601–604
5. Bokemeyer B, Grote R, Schmoll E, Freise J, Schmoll HJ, Galanski M, Schüler A, Schmidt FW (1986) Chemoembolisation hepatocellulärer Karzinome mit Lipiodol, Epirubicin and Cisplatin. Dtsch Med Wochenschr 114:128–132
6. Breedis C, Young G (1954) Blood supply of neoplasms in the liver. Am J Pathol 30:969–986

7. Carrasco C, Soo CS, Chuang VP, Wallace S (1983) Transcatheter management of hepatic neoplasms. Appl Radiol 12:47–48, 50, 52–54
8. Chuang VP, Wallace S (1983) Interventional approaches to hepatic tumor treatment. Semin Roentgenol 18:127–135
9. Chuang VP, Wallace S (1981) Hepatic artery embolization in the treatment of hepatic neoplasms. Radiology 140:51–58
10. Clouse ME, Lee RGL, Duszlak EJ, Lokich JJ et al. (1983) Peripheral hepatic artery embolization for primary and secondary hepatic neoplasms. Radiology 147:407–411
11. Coldwell D, Roth H, Mortimer J, Press O, Nance D, Harley J, Goldman M (1988) Alternation in liver function tests after hepatic arterial embolization. Proc Annu Meet Am Soc Clin Oncol 7:A422
12. Coldwell DM, Hottenstein DW, Ricci JA, Wengert PA (1985) Emphysematous cholecystitis as a complication of hepatic arterial embolization. Cardiovasc Intervent Radiol 8:36–38
13. Daniels JR, Sternlicht M, Daniels AM (1988) Collagen chemoembolization: pharmacokinetics and tissue tolerance of cisplatin in liver and kidney. Cancer Res 48:2446–2450
14. Daniels JR, Sternlicht M, Daniels AM (1989) Collagen for embolization: therapeutic embolization of primary and metastatic cancer in liver. Publication Regional Therapeutics, Santa Monica
15. Dondelinger RF, Kurdziel JC (1990) Embolization of the spleen. In: Dondelinger RF, Rossi P, Kurdziel JC, Wallace S (eds) Interventional radiology. Thieme, Stuttgart
16. Doppman JL, Girton M, Vermess M (1982) The risk of hepatic artery embolization in the presence of obstructive jaundice. Radiology 143:37–43
17. Gross-Fengels W (1989) Medikamentöse Zusatztherapie bei radiologischen Interventionen. In: Friedmann G, Steinbrich W, Gross-Fengels W (eds) Angioplastie, Embolisation, Punktion, Drainagen – Interventionelle Methoden der Radiologie. Schnetztor, Konstanz
18. Gross-Fengels W, Friedmann G, Kuhn M, Huber R, Dommaschk J, Neufang KFR (1991) Techniken, Ergebnisse und Risiken der Chemoembolisation von malignen Lebertumoren. Aktuel Radiol 1:97–104
19. Grote R, Schmol E, Rosenthal H, Bokemeier B (1989) Chemoembolisation hepatozellulärer Karzinome. Fortschr Rontgenstr 151:15–22
20. Hashimoto N, Kawai S, Mikuriya S et al. (1989) Effects of transcatheter arterial chemoembolization with oral chemotherapy on hepatic neoplasms. Cancer Chemother Pharmacol 23:21–25
21. Hewes RC, Auster M, White RI (1985) Cerebral embolism – first manifestation of pulmonary arteriovenous malformation in patients with hereditary hemorrhagic telangiectasia. Cardiovasc Intervent Radiol 8:151–155
22. Hirai K, Kawazoe Y, Yamashita K, Aoki Y, Fujimoto T, Sakai T, Majima Y, Abe M, Tanikawa K (1989) Arterial chemotherapy and transcatheter arterial embolization therapy for non-resectable hepatocellular carcinoma. Cancer Chemother Pharmacol 23:S37–S41
23. Jaschke W, Hoevels J, Schulz V (1989) Die Behandlung von Hämoptysen durch Embolisation thorakaler Arterien mit Ethibloc. Fortschr Rontgenstr 150:536–542
24. Junyuan G, Zhicheng H, Pengcheng L, Daoyu H (1987) Intraarterielle Chemotherapie und Embolisierung der Arteria hepatica bei primären Lebercarcinomen. Rontgenpraxis 40:211–214
25. Kato T, Nemoto R, Mori H, Takahashi M et al. (1981) Arterial chemoembolization with mitomycin C microcapsules in the treatment of primary or secondary carcinoma of the kidney, liver, bone and intrapelvic organs. Cancer 48:674–680
26. Kaufmann G, Richter G (1988) Embolisationsmaterialien: In: Günther R, Thelen M (eds) Interventionelle Radiologie. Thieme, Stuttgart
27. Kim T, Chuang V, Ricketts R, Zaatari G, Atkinson G, Andrews HG, Ball T, Ragab AH (1986) Improved surgical resectability of childhood hepatic malignancies by primary transcatheter embolization. Proc Am Soc Clin Oncol 5:203

28. Kubota H, Nimura Y, Hayakawa N, Shionoya S (1989) Hepatic transcatheter arterial embolization with gastroduodenal artery-blocking by finger compression. Radiology 170:562–563
29. Löhr E, Schmit-Neuerburg P, Heckemann R (1985) Embolisations-Therapie von primären Weichteiltumoren und metastatischen Raumforderungen im Beckenbereich. Radiologe 25:359–363
30. Martensson H, Nobin A, Bengmark S, Lunderquist A, Owman T, Sanden G (1984) Embolization of the liver in the management of metastatic carcinoid tumors. J Surg Oncol 27:152–158
31. Mavligit G, Charnsangavej C, Carrasco H, Patt Y, Benjamin R, Wallace S (1988) Regression of ocular melanoma metastatic to the liver after hepatic arterial chemoembolization with cisplatin and polyvinyl sponge. JAMA 260:974–976
32. Mitty HA, Warner RRP, Newman LH, Train JS et al. (1985) Control of carcinoid syndrome with hepatic artery embolization. Radiology 155:623–626
33. Nagasue N, Galizia G, Kohno H, Chang Y, Hayashi T, Yamanoi A, Nakamura T, Yukaya H (1989) Adverse effects of preoperative hepatic chemoembolization for resectable hepatocellular carcinoma: a retrospective comparison of 138 liver resections. Surgery 158:81–86
34. Nakamura H, Hashimoto T, Oi H, Sawada S (1988) Iodized oil in the portal vein after arterial embolization. Radiology 167:415–417
35. Nakao N, Miura K, Takahashi H, Ohnishi M et al. (1986) Hepatocellular carcinoma: combined hepatic, arterial, and portal venous embolization. Radiology 161:303–307
36. Ohishi H, Uchida H, Yoshimura H, Ohue S et al. (1985) Hepatocellular carcinoma detected by iodized oil. Radiology 154:25–29
37. Ohishi H, Yoshimura H, Uchida H, Sakaguchi H, Yoshioka T, Ohue S, Matsui T, Takaya A, Tsujii T (1989) Transcatheter arterial embolization using iodized oil (lipiodol) mixed with an anticancer drug for the treatment of hepatocellular carcinoma. Cancer Chemother Pharmacol 23:33–36
38. Patt YZ, Chuang VP, Wallace S, Hersh EM et al. (1981) The palliative role of hepatic arterial infusion and arterial occlusion in colorectal carcinoma metastatic to the liver. Lancet 349–350
39. Pfeifer KJ, Eibl-Eibesfeldt B, Huber RM, Kenn RW, Mangel E, Mayr B (1988) Mikroembolisation von Lebermetastasen. In: Schneider GH, Vogler E (eds) Digitale bildgebende Verfahren. Springer, Berlin Heidelberg New York
40. Powell-Tuck J, McIvor J, Reynolds KW, Murray-Lyon IM (1984) Prediction of early death after therapeutic hepatic arterial embolization. Br Med J (Clin Res) 288:1257–1259
41. Sasaki Y, Imaoka S, Kasugai H et al. (1987) A new approach to chemoembolization therapy for hepatoma using ethiodized oil, cisplatin, and gelatine sponge. Cancer 60:1194–1203
42. Schild H (1988) Embolisation der Leber. In: Günther R, Thelen M (eds) Interventionelle Radiologie. Thieme, Stuttgart
43. Schultheis KH (1985) Embolisation–Chemoembolisation. Beitr Onkol 21:201–228
44. Sternlicht M, Sales S, Daniels JR, Daniels A (1989) Renal cisplatin chemoembolization with angiostat, gelfoam, and ethiodol in the rabbit: renal platinum distributions. Radiology 170:1073–1075
45. Suzuki K, Kono N, Ono A, Osuga Y, Kiyokawa H, Mineo I, Matsuda Y, Miyoshi S, Kawata S, Minami Y et al. (1988) Transcatheter arterial chemo-embolization for humoral hypercalcemia of hepatocellular carcinoma. Gastroenterol Jpn 23:29–36
46. Takayasu K, Moriyama N, Muramatsu Y, Suzuki M, Ishikawa T, Ushio K, Matsue H, Sasagawa M, Yamada T (1984) Splenic infarction, a complication of transcatheter hepatic arterial embolization for liver malignancies. Radiology 151:371–375

Drug Therapy, Monitoring, and Function Testing in Neuroradiologic Interventions

A. Laurent, Y. P. Gobin, F. Launay, A. Aymard, A. Casasco, A. L. Bailly, E. Houdart, and J. J. Merland

Introduction

In the Department of Interventional Neuroradiology at Lariboisière Hospital, we take care of malformative or tumoral disorders of the central nervous system, and of the head and neck: cerebral arteriovenous malformations (AVMs, [5, 13, 15, 22, 23]) and medullary AVMs [4, 10, 20, 21], intracranial aneurysms [1, 2, 9], superficial AVMs of the face or limbs [7, 26], and hypervascularized tumors [3, 8].

In most cases therapeutic interventions are performed through arterial routes, at other times through venous access, and by direct puncture in the case of superficial AVMs and some tumors. The interventions consist mainly of embolizations. Various materials are used: acrylic glue, alcohol, calibrated microspheres, noncalibrated particles (absorbable or not), balloons, pasty mixture (Ethibloc). In some cases the therapeutic intervention consists of a vascular recanalization, obtained by an infusion of drugs (fibrinolysis), or by an angioplasty.

In neuroradiologic interventions we have three imperatives. Firstly, the anesthesia must allow a neuroradiologic examination of the patient at any time. Secondly, three complications have to be prevented and treated if necessary: thromboembolism because of the risk of ischemic stroke, infection because of the risk of bacterial graft on implants, and spasm because it reduces the guidability of catheters and can cause ischemic strokes. Thirdly, we need provocative tests of the brain functions to predict (and avoid) secondary complications; these tests are a modified Wada test, a hypotension test, and a Xylocaine and a coloring test.

Premedication, Anesthesia, and Monitoring in Neuroradiologic Interventions

Premedication

An anxiolytic premedication is given systematically before each catheterization: 2 mg/kg per os hydroxyzine (Atarax). An antiallergic premedication is essential if the patient has an allergic history (asthma, urticaria or eczematous reactions, allergic reactions to drugs or iodine). This premedication consists in giving the patient 10 mg prednisolone (Solupred) in the morning and 100 mg hydroxyzine (Atarax) in the evening for 3 consecutive days. To be efficient, corticoids have to be started at least 18 h before an iodine injection.

Anesthesia

The anesthesia must guarantee the safety of the intervention and the comfort of the patient [14]. The first condition of safety is the complete immobility of the patient during the catheterization and the angiographic controls. The anesthesia has to obtain this immobility combined with the possibility of carrying out a clinical neurologic evaluation at any time. This neurologic surveillance requires good collaboration between the neuroradiologist and the anesthetist to evaluate neurologic signs, according to the localization of the intervention. Hemodynamic monitoring is done with an automatic tensiometer, an electrocardioscope, and a finger-pulse oximeter.

The patient has to be comfortably positioned on the radiologic table, particularly as neuroradiologic interventions are often long (1–3 h). Neuroradiologic interventions are usually not very painful, except the arterial punctures which requires a good local anesthesia. Patient anxiety is the rule in interventional procedures and may increase with each intervention if they are repeated. This justifies an anxiolytic premedication as a preparation to anesthesia.

Drugs and Doses

The anesthetic protocol we generally perform is a diazanalgesia which combines a benzodiazepin, midazolam (Hypnovel), given in a continuous infusion with a pump or in repeated injections (2–5 mg/h) and an analgesic drug, Fentanyl or alfentanyl (Rapifen) that we inject i. v. and discontinuously. In our opinion, midazolam is well adapted to neuroradiologic interventions as it has few side effects, induces no pain at the injection site, and has an amnesic effect, which is useful if interventions are repeated. With this diazanalgesia, the patient is relaxed and motionless. At any given moment it is possible to neutralize these drugs with their specific antagonists: midazolam is neutralized by flumazenil (Anexate) and fentanyl and midazolam by naloxone (Narcan). These antagonist drugs wake the patient and allow his neurologic examination. In most cases the analgesia is slight and we do not need the antagonist drugs to perform neurologic examination.

Anesthesia of Children

For children older than 8 years, we use a neuroleptanalgesic, sometimes associated with anesthetic halogen gas (halothane) or ketamine injection (Ketalar) during the painful punctures. For younger children we perform in most cases a general anesthesia with intubation and assisted ventilation.

Anesthesia During Diagnostic Angiographies

The monitoring is the same as for interventions. The anesthetic consists of low doses of midazolam associated in some cases with central analgesics (fentanyl, alfentanyl).

Anesthesia for Superficial Vascular Malformations and Osteoplasties

Interventional procedures for superficial vascular malformations are commonly short but painful because they imply multiple and iterative punctures and injections of irritating agents (alcoholic mixtures). We associate the diazanalgesia with either halogen gas or nitrogen protoxide. If it is possible, we also use propofol (Diprivan), which is injected i. v., discontinuously or continuouly (pump).

Specialized Monitoring

Neuroradiologic interventions require specific monitoring: a clinical neurologic follow-up, which is made possible by the diazanalgesia, monitoring machines or systems which can be associated with neuroradiologic maneuvers, cerebral blood flow measurements with ^{133}Xenon [17] transcranial Doppler [12], and evoked potentials of the brain stem or the spinal cord.

Prevention of Infections

Infections are prevented by the observance of classic asepsis rules in all cases and by prophylactic antibiotic treatment in some cases. Asepsis is guaranteed by means of various protections (surgical masks and clothing, sterile gloves, sterile wrapping of the radioprotective shields and gears), by respecting sterile conditions during the manipulation of "small materials" for catheterization (catheters, guides, Luer locks, cockstops, introducers, needles, etc.), and by a strict local asepsis all around the vascular access zone: shaving, cutaneous disinfection (antiseptic solutions), and adhesive sterile drapes.

Antibiotic Therapy for Interventions Done by Arterial Catheterization

Severe and symptomatic septic complications rarely occur during arterial interventional procedures [24]. Thus, we do not routinely use antibiotic prophylaxis for neuroradiologic interventions. We use it only in patients with cardiac valvular diseases. In these cases the antibiotic consists of a combination of a β-lactam (oxacillin: Bristopen) and an aminoside (gentamycin: Gentalline). The first i. v. injection is given at the beginning of the anesthesia. Treatment is carried on i. v. for 48 h.

Antibiotic Therapy for Venous Catheterization

We administer antibiotics in all cases. We use two types of antibiotic therapy according to the site of intervention:

- For trunk and upper limb venous interventions, we use a single i.v. injection of 30 mg/kg β-lactam (oxacillin: Bristopen) at the beginning of the anesthesia. This treatment is aimed at gram-positive bacteria, such as staphylococcus.
- For interventions done through femoral veins, we use a broad-spectrum antibiotic aimed at gram-positive and gram-negative bacteria, because of the nearby anogenital area. It consists of a single i.v. injection at the beginning of anesthesia and of a combination of antibiotics (Augmentin): amoxicillin (200 mg) and clavulanic acid (2 g).

Antibiotic Therapy for Bone Cementoplasties

We use the same antibiotic therapy as for femoral vein catheterization.

Prevention of Thromboembolism During Neurocervicofacial Radiologic Interventions

Thromboembolic complications are prevented by some precautions in catheter use in all cases, combined with anticoagulant drugs in selected procedures.

Precautions in Catheter Use

Routine precautions relative to catheter thrombogenicity [19] are very useful: repeated rinsing of the catheters (especially after the use of a guidewire), continuous rinsing of "dead spaces" (between a coaxial external catheter and a microcatheter, and between a guidewire and a catheter) with a saline perfusion under pressure, and washing and rinsing of materials with heparinized saline solution.

Anticoagulant Protocol

Indications

Anticoagulant drugs are given to prevent thromboembolism which complicates some interventional neuroradiologic procedures, such as temporary or definitive clampage of brain afferent arteries, endosaccular-selective treatment of arterial intracranial aneurysms, and embolization of brain AVMs. During the embolization of high-flow AVMs, the risk of thromboembolic complications is low because of the apparent low viscosity of the blood and the preferential flow to the AVM. In these AVMs, anticoagulant drugs are not necessary. In low- or medium-flow AVMs we use heparin which can be neutralized immediately if bleeding occurs. Anticoagulants are sometimes used after the embolization of some medullary vascular malformations (medullary AVM, meningeal fistulas with perimedullar drainage, extramedullary arteriovenous fistulas with perimedullary drainage) if they have a giant venous component, and if a total occlusion has been obtained. Then a risk of spinal compression by an acute venous thrombosis, which has to be prevented by anticoagulant drugs exists.

Moreover, as a general rule, anticoagulants are used if microcatheterization of cerebral vessels is prolonged over 30 min.

Drugs and Doses

When anesthesia is started (induction) we give an i.v. injection of 250 mg aspirin (Aspegic) except in high-flow AVMs. After the vascular access has been installed, we begin heparin therapy consisting of an initial i.v. bolus of 1000 U followed by a continuous i.v. infusion (pump) at the rate of 30 U/kg per hour. We used to give 3000 U bolus, but we have observed in many cases that anticoagulation was then too strong (partial thromboplastin time, PTT, four- to five times upper control). This may be explained by interaction between heparin and iodinated contrast media [6].

Biological Follow-up

Biological monitoring is started after the first hour of anticoagulant therapy. Heparin doses are subsequently modified to obtain a patient's PTT of between two- and three times upper control. Thirty minutes before the end of the session, a final PTT control is done. It allows the calculation of the protamine-sulfate dose that is necessary to obtain a satisfactory hemostasis at the access site by manual compression of the punctured artery.

In case of hemorrhage, heparin is neutralized by an i.v. injection of an equivalent protamine-sulfate dose.

Aspirin (Aspegic)

Interest

The antiaggregation effect of aspirin adds to the effect of heparin. It can be neutralized by platelet transfusion only.

Indications

We combine aspirin with heparin in some cases with a high risk of thromboembolism, e.g., (a) procedure-related risks: clampage of brain vessels, selective occlusion of intracranial aneurysms, and (b) patient-related risks: red blood cell hyperaggregability, which can be due to infectious or inflammatory diseases, some blood diseases, or to contrast media [25] , and hypercoagulability related to protein C deficiency (personal history of repeated thrombophlebitis). As no biologic test detecting red blood cell hyperaggregability is readily available, we consider a high level of fibrinogen or an acceleration of the sedimentation rate as risk factors. "Plasmatic dilution" may be justified if such abnormalities exist. This dilution of plasmatic proteins, which are responsible for aggregation mechanisms, is obtained by an i.v. infusion of macromolecular or isotonic fluids.

Doses

We use an i.v. bolus of 500 mg aspirin at the beginning of the intervention.

Fibrinolytics

Introduction

Fibrinolysis techniques are used more and more often in neuroradiologic interventions for cerebral thromboembolic accidents, whether or not they are iatrogenic. The main difficulty is still the imperative necessity to perform the fibrinolysis within a short time after the accident: 6 h in the region of the carotid artery and 6–24 h in the vertebrobasilar region. Contraindications to fibrinolysis are the other difficulties, i.e., general contraindications (coagulation disorders, evolutive peptic ulcer, recent surgical intervention, arterial hypertension, age over 75 years), and neurologic contraindications (ischemia associated with hypodensity on CT scan or brain edema – both increase the risk of bleeding in the ischemic region). On the other hand, thromboembolism may occur during angiography-guided neuroradiologic interventions. Thus, a fibrinolysis may be indicated and performed through a superselective catheter.

The fibrinolysis protocol is the same in both the iatrogenic and non-iatrogenic groups.

Procedure

The therapeutic procedure is carried out in several steps: angiographic diagnosis of the cerebral arterial occlusion, installation of a microcatheter in the thrombus, discontinuation and neutralization of anticoagulant drugs, and infusion of fibrinolytic agents.

Drugs and Doses

Three drugs can be used: (1) urokinase, (2) streptokinase, and (3) recombinant tissue plasminogen activator (rTPA). Two of them are used in our department: urokinase (Urokinase) and rTPA (Actlyse).

Urokinase

Urokinase is now the most often used fibrinolytic agent. Its advantages are a short half-life, no immunoallergic reaction, and a lower risk of bleeding than streptokinase. Its disadvantage remains its high cost.

We use urokinase as follows: initial bolus (100000 U) directly injected into the thrombus, angiographic control, then discontinuous injections up to a usual total dose of 400000 U. In some cases it is useful to raise the dose up to 900000 U (the maximum dose allowed) within 90 min even if no changes in the fibrinogen level occur. The effectiveness of thrombolysis is judged by the angiographic controls and the transcranial Doppler. Biologic control of coagulation is done at regular intervals (prothrombin time, PTT, thrombin time, fibrinogen level, fibrin degradation products, and platelet counts).

After fibrinolysis, and if the fibrinogen level is over 1 g/l, heparin is given if a lesion remains which could be responsible for cerebral embolism: ulcerated carotid plaque, cardiac rhythmic disorder. A CT scan is done routinely after the fibrinolysis to verify if any bleeding, ischemia, or edema has occurred. The CT scan frequently reveals hemorrhagic petechiae in basal ganglia after fibrinolysis of the MCA, without any clinical symptoms (according to J. Theron's experience).

rTPA

rTPA has a short half-life (6 min). It is used as follows: repeated bolus of 1 mg (total dose 20–50 mg) for 1.5 –2 h.

Preventive and Curative Treatment of Arterial Spasm

Interest

Calcium channel-blockers have been known for years to be active in experimental spasm in animals [11]. They are used mainly in neuroradiologic interventions to relieve the arterial spasm which occurs during catheterization. They are used either preventively (i.v. injection) or curatively (intraarterial injection). It is difficult to estimate the rate of spasm occurring during catheterization. Spasm is rarely localized nor very tight. Most frequently the spasm is diffuse, slight, asymptomatic, but it reduces the catheter's guidability and access to the lesion. Calcium channel-blockers are used in some cases to facilitate a catheterization which could be difficult because of tortuosities, stenoses, narrowed arteries, bifurcations etc.

In 1987 we designed a study to verify if nimodipine (Nimotop) could facilitate catheterization and embolization of brain AVMs [16]. Nimodipine was given i.v. at a rate of 5–10 ml/h (0.25–0.50 mg/kg per minute, 1–2 mg/h for 60 kg) to patients with AVMs who were undergoing endovascular treatment. In group A patients received nimodipine 12–24 h before the beginning of the catheterization, group B patients received nimodipine at the beginning or during the catheterization, and the control group patients received no nimodipine. Efficiency was judged on several criteria: number of acrylic glue injections during the intervention, time between the beginning of the procedure and the first acrylic glue injection, and mean duration of the embolization procedure. The results of the study are summarized in Table 1. In short, this study showed that nimodipine can facilitate the catheterization and emboliza-

Table 1. Effects of nimodipine (Nimotop) on the catheterization and embolization of arteriovenous malformations

	Acrylic glue injections (number/procedure)	Delay before first acrylic glue injection (h)	Mean duration of embolization procedure (h)
Nimodipine 12–24 h before catheterization 5–10 ml/h ($n = 13$)	1.9	2.0	2.9 (t test: $p = 0.0029$)[a]
Nimodipine at the beginning of or during the catheterization 5–10 ml/h ($n = 9$)	1.1	2.3	3.3 (t test: $p = 0.0573$)[a]
Control ($n = 25$)	1.4	1.7	4.1

[a] t test: comparison with control group.

tion of cerebral AVMs. The mean duration of embolization procedures is significantly shortened ($p=0.0029$) if drug infusion is begun 12–24 h before the procedure, but not significantly if the infusion starts with the procedure ($p=0.0573$). This can be explained by the time required to obtain a stable plasmatic level of the drug, which is about 8 h with a nimodipine infusion at 2 mg/h.

Protocol for Preventive Treatment by i.v. Nimodipine Infusion (Pump)

The infusion is started at 6 A.M. (at least 3 h before the beginning of catheterization). The pump infusion is set at 5 ml/h (0.25 mg/kg per minute, 1 mg/h for 60 kg) and connected to a saline base infusion. The nimodipine dosage is increased at the beginning of the procedure (generally up to 10 ml/h) to obtain a decrease in the patient's systolic blood pressure (around 20–30 mmHg), which shows that a good efficacy-impregnation has been obtained.

Protocol for Curative Treatment of the Spasm, with i.a.-Nimodipine

Nimodipine (2 ml) is diluted in 10 ml saline. This solution is then injected directly into the artery through the catheter in bolus of 1–2 ml. If necessary, one or two other bolus are injected while controlling the blood pressure.

Function Tests

Tests with Barbiturates as Anesthetic Drugs

In the Wada test of speech lateralization [28], the drug used was amobarbital, an anesthetic drug [28]. It was injected directly into the common carotid artery. It could also be used in other cerebral arteries to test various neurologic functions related to different vascular territories.

Other areas commonly examined in INR include the rolandic artery, pre- and postcentral artery, callosal artery, anterior choroidal artery, lenticulostriatal artery, thalamo-perforating artery, Heubner artery, calcarine artery, transmesencephalic artery, cerebellar and postero-inferior cerebellar artery, and radiculomedullar artery.

Indications

This functional test is used in case an AVM is located in a functional area. The afferents to the AVM may vascularize part of the normal adjacent parenchyma. If a deficit occurs after the selective injection of the barbiturate into the

AVM afferent, embolization becomes contraindicated. The catheter has to be pushed ahead in the artery, over normal branch issues, towards the nidus of the AVM, in a segment of the artery that gives no afferent to the normal brain.

Drugs and Doses

We use methohexital (Brietal), a barbiturate which acts quickly and shortly. When injected hyperselectively, it induces a transient neurologic deficit. Its half-life is 3.9 h ± 2 h. The drug is used in a 1% solution (dilution of 500 mg drug powder in 50 ml saline or glucose).

Technique

After the catheter has been pushed into the artery in a position that allows embolization, methohexital is injected into the microcatheter (2 mg for a middle cerebral artery, 5 mg for a carotid artery), and the patient immediately undergoes a neurologic examination. This examination has to be quick and focussed only on the neurologic function related to the functional area under examination. Exhaustive examinations are not possible because of the short symptomatic period of methohexital (1–2 min).

We have frequently observed that a methohexital test can be negative at the first injection but becomes positive after embolization. If a single afferent vascularizes both the AVM and the normal brain, the drug may be aspirated by the AVM at the first injection, but after a flow reduction in the AVM, the drug may go to the AVM and the normal branch. Such cases explain the skepticism of some operators who talk about "false negative". In fact false negatives do not exist if repeated injections are done.

Methohexital injection can modify EEG data, brain stem-evoked potentials, and spinal-evoked potentials. This underlines its usefulness in neuroradiologic interventions.

Hypotension Test for Carotid Clampages

Interest

The hypotension test consists of inducing a reduction in the systolic blood pressure (around 40–50 mmHg) after a carotid clampage has been well-tolerated clinically and angiographically (supplementary vessel supply, flow). This is in order to increase an potential arterial insufficiency which then becomes symptomatic. Some carotid clampages with endovascular balloons are clinically well tolerated during the immediate follow-up: this invites the detaching of the balloon. In the following hours or days, a neurologic deficit may occur. This could not have been predicted from the clinical and angiographic data previously obtained during the intervention. We have observed such cases of delayed deficits [17], some of which have been related to arterial hypotension.

Technique

After 15 min of clampage, we induce arterial hypotension with a calcium channel blocker, nicardipin (Loxen). Nimodipin is diluted in 5% glucose and injected i.v. at a rate of 1 mg/min until a 40–50 mmHg reduction in the systolic blood pressure occurs. This hypotension is prolonged for 10 min. Examination can detect neurologic deficits or abnormalities. This helps to decide if the balloon can be detached or not.

After this, the drug is discontinued. The blood pressure quickly returns to normal in most cases, simply by increasing the saline infusion rate. In some cases, however, it is necessary to infuse macromolecular fluids for 1 or 2 h.

The information given by the hypotension test is immediately available. It can be compared with the data from ^{133}Xenon cerebral blood flow [17] or transcranial Doppler.

Monitoring

This test is done under permanent monitoring of blood pressure, pulse, ECG, and arterial oxygen saturation.

Xylocaine Test

Interest

The test consists of selectively injecting an anesthetic drug into a catheterized afferent to a lesion to verify if this branch also vascularizes a nerve (by vasa nervorum). We use it before the embolization of vessels that also vascularize peripheral nerves if the embolic material can occlude vessels of the nervous elements. This risk is high with fluid emboli (alcohol, acrylic glues) and with very small particles (under 100 μm in diameter). It is low with bigger particles since a revascularization via the surrounding vessels is possible from below the occlusion.

Indications

These are shown by branches of the external carotid artery which participate in cranial nerve vascularization, inferior gluteal artery (sciatic nerve), sacral arteries etc.

Drugs and Doses

Xylocaine (Lidocaine) is injected selectively through the catheter in the position for embolization. According to the diameter and flow of the arterial pedicle 1–3 ml of a 1% solution is injected (e.g., 1 ml in ascending pharyngeal artery, 3 ml in inferior gluteal artery).

Color Test

Interest

Injected selectively into an artery, the coloring allows a visual delimitation of the cutaneous territory which is vascularized by this artery. It allows the identification of the cutaneous zone one wishes to embolize. In cases of arterial chemotherapy for chest cancers with a cutaneous extension, the color test is useful to verify if the cutaneous extension depends on the internal mammary artery and/or the external mammary artery. It is useful to administer chemotherapy through a single implanted catheter. If the color test shows that the external mammary artery also participates in the tumoral vascularization, one can embolize it proximally to increase the internal mammary artery territory in which a microcatheter is then left. The test also allows the identification of a cutaneous zone one does not want to embolize because of the risk of necrosis (especially with fluid emboli and particles under 100 μm diameter).

Coloring and Doses

We use two colorings: patent blue (Guerbet laboratory) or methylene blue (Pharmacie Centrale des Hôpitaux): 1 cc diluted in saline (1 vol/10 vol). We quickly inject 1, 2, or 5 cc of the solution. Skin coloring often occurs quickly and lasts for a short time.

Indication

These are superficial vascular malformations, tumors with cutaneous extension, or tumors vascularized by an artery which also vacularizes a cutaneous zone etc.

Drug Therapies After Neuroradiologic Interventions

Drug Therapy After the Embolization of Brain AVMs with Acrylic Glue

Acrylic glue is commonly used in the embolization of AVMs. It induces an edema which involves the embolized vascular structures and adjacent tissues [18, 27]. The toxic effect of acrylic glue appears within the hours following the embolization and persists for some days or weeks, depending on the volume of acrylic glue injected. In cerebral AVMs, toxic effects induce various symptoms: deficit, epileptic seizure, headache.

Drugs and Doses

Since 1986 we have verified many times that this edema responds very well to steroids, that antiepileptic drugs can avoid epileptic seizures, and that analgesic drugs are rarely useful. For this reason we routinely administer methylprednisolone (Solumedrol) and clonazepam (Rivotril) after acrylic glue embolization [15, 22]. Corticotherapy is short enough not to induce any drug dependence. Car driving and physical activities are forbidden for 1 week after embolization.

Protocol

Methylprednisolone is started at the moment of the acrylic glue injection: 80 mg i.v. first, followed by 20 mg i.v. every 6 h for 24 h. It is interrupted on the second day or, in case of headaches, replaced by oral methylprednisolone for 2–3 days. 3 mg clonazepam orally (at three intervals) for 3 days is also used. It is automatically prescribed, even in cases of preexistent antiepileptic treatment.

Drug Therapy After Embolization of Superficial Vascular Malformation

Interest

In the case of superficial vascular malformation, a painful inflammatory edema occurs after embolization with Ethibloc or alcohol. This edema can be avoided if antiinflammatory drugs are given routinely.

Drugs and Doses

Antiinflammatory indomethacin (Indocia) (50–100 mg) or one 400 mg morniflumate (Nifluril) suppository is administered in the evenings for a few days. Analgesics used are paracetamol (Doliprane), rectally or orally.

References

1. Aymard A, Merland JJ, Rufenacht D, Reizine D, Guimaraens L (1987) Endovascular treatment of aneurysms of the terminal vertebral artery. J Neuroradiol 14:1–9
2. Aymard A, Gobin AP, Hodes JE, Bien S, Rufenacht D, Reizine D, George B, Merland JJ (1991) Endovascular occlusion of vertebral arteries in the treatment of unclippable vertebrobasilar aneurysms. J Neurosurg 74:393–398
3. Beaujeux R, Laurent A, Hodes JE, Wassef M, Merland JJ (1991) Calibrated sphere embolization of craniofacial tumors and AVMS. Neuroradiology 33 [Suppl]:562–564
4. Biondi A, Merland JJ, Reizine D, Aymard A, Hodes JE, Lecoz P, Rey A (1991) Embolization with particles in thoracic intramedullary arteriovenous malformations: long-term angiographic and clinical results. Radiology 177:651–658
5. Casasco A, Lylyk P, Hodes JE, Kohan G, Aymard A, Merland JJ (1991) Percutaneous transvenous catheterization and embolization of vein of Galen aneurysms. Neurosurgery 28:260–266
6. Eloy R, Corot C, Belville J (1991) Contrast media for angiography: physicochemical properties, pharmacokinetics and biocompatibility. Clin Mater 7:87–197
7. Enjolras O, Riche MC (1991) Hemangiomes immatures et malformations vasculaires superficielles – Les grands atlas médicaux. MEDSI/McGraw-Hill, Paris
8. Garcia-Cervigon E, Bien S, Rufenacht D, Thurel C, Reizine D, Tran Ba Huy P, Merland JJ (1988) Pre-operative embolization of naso-pharyngeal angiofibromas. Report of 58 cases. Neuroradiology 30:556–560
9. George B, Aymard A, Gobin PY, Merland JJ, Mourier KL, Cophignon J (1990) Traitement endovasculaire des anévrysmes intracraniens. Intérêt et perspective d'après une série de 92 cas. Neurochirurgie 36:273–278
10. Gueguen B, Merland JJ, Riche MC, Rey A (1987) Vascular malformations of the spinal cord: intrathecal perimedullary arteriovenous fistulas fed by medullary arteries. Neurology 37(6):969–979
11. Handa J, Yoneda R, Koyoma T (1975) Experimental cerebral vasospasm in cats: modification by a new synthetic vasodilatator YC-93. Surg Neurol 3:195–199
12. Harders A, Bien S, Eggert HR, Laborde G, Merland JJ, Rufenacht D (1989) Haemodynamic changes in arteriovenous malformations induced by superselective embolisation: transcranial Doppler evaluation. Neurol Res 10:239–245
13. Hodes JE, Aymard A, Casasco A, Rufenacht D, Reizine D, Merland JJ (1991) Embolization of arteriovenous malformations of the temporal lobe via the anterior choroidal artery. AJNR 12:775–780
14. Launay F, Sankowska A, Reinmund M (1990) Anesthésie pour anévrysmes intracraniens traités par voie endovasculaire: 31 cas. Agressologie 31(5):268–270
15. Laurent A, Merland JJ, Rufenacht D, Guimaraens L, Assouline E (1985) Treatment of supra-tentorial AVMs by IBC embolization, with a new technique, neurologic follow-up. Proceedings of the XIIIth Congress of the European Society of Neurology, Amsterdam 11–15 Sept 1985 (ed. J. Volk). Excerpta Medica, Amsterdam–New York, pp 315–318
16. Laurent A, Rufenacht D, Cervigon E, Merland JJ (1987) Cathéterisme et embolisation des malformations artérioveineuses cérébrales: intérêt des inhibiteurs calciques. Press Med 16:10
17. Laurent A, Weitzner I, Luft A, Merland JJ (1988) Significance of pre-operative cerebral blood-flow measurements in endovascular occlusion of the internal carotid and middle cerebral arteries. Radiology 175 [Suppl] (RSNA) 121
18. Laurent A, Wassef M, Drouet L, Ignaud G, Merland JJ (1989) Etude histologique de plusieurs matériaux d'embolisation et d'un nouveau type de matériel sphérique et adhésif. ITBM 3(10):357–366
19. Laurent A, Eloy R, Merland JJ (1991) Thrombogenicity of arterial catheters depends on catheter type, not base material. Neuroradiology 33 [Suppl]:560–561
20. Merland JJ, Reizine D (1990) Embolization techniques in the spinal cord. In: Dondelinger RF, Rossi P, Kurdziel J-C, Wallace S (eds) Interventional radiology. Thieme, Stuttgart, pp 433–443

21. Merland JJ, Assouline E, Rufenacht D, Guimaraens L, Laurent A (1986) Dural spinal arteriovenous fistulae draining into medullary veins. Clinical and radiological results of treatment (embolization and surgery) in 56 cases. Proceedings of the XIIIth Congress of the European Society of Neurology, Amsterdam 11–15 Sept 1985 (ed. J. Volk). Excerpta Medica, Amsterdam–New York, pp 283–290
22. Merland JJ, Rufenacht D, Laurent A, Guimaraens L (1986) Endovascular treatment with isobutyl cyanoacrylate in patients with arteriovenous malformations of the brain. Indications, results and complications. – XIIIth symposium Neuroradiologicum Stockholm. Acta Radiol Suppl 369:621–622
23. Merland JJ, Aymard A, Gobin YP, Laurent A, Rufenacht D, Garcia-Cervigon E, Guimaraens L (1990) Endovascular therapy of cerebral AVMs: technique and results in 125 patients. Radiology 177 [Suppl]:94
24. Meyer P, Reizine D, Aymard A, Guerin JM, Marciano S, Habib Y (1988) Septic complications in interventional angiography: evaluation of risk and preventive measures, preliminary studies. J Intervent Radiol 3:73–75
25. Monnier L, Laurent A, Othmane A, Dufaux J, Mills P, Moyse D, Merland JJ (1991) Produits de contraste et microcirculation: étude de l'agrégation et de la déformation erythrocytaires. Rev Imag Med 3:237–242
26. Mourao GS, Hodes JE, Gobin YP, Casasco A, Aymard A, Merland JJ (1991) Curative treatment of scalp arteriovenous fistulas by direct puncture and embolization with absolute alcohol. Report of three cases. J Neurosurg 75:634–637
27. Vinters H, Galil KA, Lundie MJ, Kaufmann JCE (1985) The histotoxicity of cyanoacrylates. A selective review. Neuroradiology 27:279–291
28. Wada J, Rasmussen T (1960) Intracarotid injection of Amytal for the lateralization of cerebral speech dominance: experimental and clinical observations. J Neurosurg 17:266–282

Drug Therapy in Computed-Tomography-Guided Interventional Procedures

A. JACOB and W. STEINBRICH

Introduction

The number and variety of computer tomography (CT)-guided interventions has risen considerably over the past years. CT interventions can be divided into two main groups relating to their intention, namely, diagnostic and therapeutc. These in turn can be subdivided following technical, morphologic, and functional aspects.

Diagnostic Interventions

Diagnostic interventions include biopsies, the aspiration of tissue and fluids, temporary neural blocks, and percutaneous application and imaging of contrast medium, e.g., for arthrography or pancreaticography.

Therapeutic Interventions

Therapeutic interventions include:

a) The removal of pathological fluid collections with or without sclerosis of the containing cavity by aspiration or drainage of (pseudo-) cysts and abscesses.
b) The temporary or definitive blocking of neural structures for tumor or degenerative pain relief and neurovascular dysregulations (hyperhydrosis, Raynaud phenomenon etc.).
c) The curative or palliative intralesional therapy of benign and malignant primary and secondary tumor with alcohol, chemotherapeutics, other substances, hyperthermic or kryothermic probes, and mechanical devices such as drills.
d) Diverse procedures such as vertebroplasty with acrylate compounds in metastatic or osteoporotic vertebral compression, CT-guided stabilization of fractures of the pelvic girdle, and the aspiration of inferior vena cava (IVC) thrombi.

These procedures are generally less invasive, more to-the-point, and bear less morbidity and mortality than their surgical or medical counterparts. They are characterized by a very good ratio of effort to effect, at least as far as the strain on the patient is concerned.

Nevertheless a certain amount of preparation for patient, technicians, interventionist, and other involved persons before, during, and after an intervention is indispensable in order to make it a success and not to lose the assumed benefit [1–5].

The different therapeutic entities and monitoring methods will only be discussed briefly because they have already been extensively put forth. Instead some applications for different CT-guided interventions will be proposed. Therefore the title of this contribution could also have read "Patient Care in Interventional CT".

Adjunctive Medication and Monitoring

Goals

When discussing adjunctive medication one first has to define the desired effects or goals. These are patient comfort and increased patient satisfaction through sedation and amnesia, anxiolysis, analgesia, immobilisation, and the prevention of nausea and vomiting, and patient safety through the monitoring of circulation, respiration, electrolytes, blood clotting, and other vital parameters. Another important aspect of patient safety is the ability to handle side effects and complications of technically necessary (e.g., contrast media), or actually effective drugs (e.g., alcohol), or prophylactic antibiosis in contaminated or "dirty" procedures.

Patient Comfort

One of the main purposes of providing comfort is to let the patient experience the procedure in the same way as the interventionist: as an elegant, minimally invasive measure replacing a cumbersome, potentially dangerous and lengthy operation with significant procedural risk and postprocedural morbidity.

There is no reason why the patient should look back on the intervention as a nightmare he would never let happen again. On the contrary, he should spread the news of an unexpectedly harmless manipulation done in a friendly environment by friendly and competent people, who even cared to look after him later.

An inherent drawback of CT examinations is the akward positioning. Comfort, immobilization, and lastly success rate can be greatly enhanced by an effort to achieve stable and minimally uncomfortable positioning.

Sedation

Sedation allows the patient to see the ongoing procedure from a distance. It reduces the natural anxiety and excitement. The first and mostly sufficient step of anxiolysis is the preprocedure visit. This has been documented several times. Furthermore in CT-guided interventions the active cooperation of the patient is usually vital. So the positive effects of sedation must be carefully weighed against the need for a cooperative patient. In our opinion, sedation is only needed in cases of very long or painful procedures or overly anxious patients.

A benzodiazepine, whose elimination half-life should be tailored to the length of the procedure, is the drug of choice in this situation. It also provides an anterograde amnesia of differing length.

Dosage must take into consideration age, weight, former drug abuse, and others [2].

Analgesia/Anesthesia
The best possible analgesia is avoidance of pain through appropriate techniques and strategies. Vogelzang and associates point this out in the case of hepatobiliary interventions, where they propose choosing the left hepatic access wherever possible [6, 7]. Another beautiful example is the transrectal approach to pelvic abscesses, which can be done without any medicaton at all, as shown by Gazelle et al. [8]. Unfortunately this does not apply to all situations.

Different kinds of pain are encountered during different procedures: the "fast", sharp, superficial pain while traversing a layer of tissue susceptible to pain, which is mainly mediated by the myelinated A fibers, and the "slow", deep visceral pain provoked, e.g., by stretching (dilating) tissue for large-bore catheters or by taking bone biopsies, conducted by unmyelinated C fibers.

The first one is efficiently handled with local anesthetics, the second can be treated with centrally acting analgesics, namely opioids, if need be together with a short-acting sedative [9–11].

The use of nitrous oxide instead of i.v. narcotics has been proposed several times [12, 13]. This is a safe, well-known, short-acting, and easily reversible analgetic, which cannot produce anesthesia unless given in toxic concentration above 80% of inhaled volume [14].

Another successful technique is regional anesthesia through regional blocks like intercostal, pleural, or celiac plexus blocks, which may itself be done by interventional radiologic techniques [15–18].

General anesthesia is only necessary in selected cases, especially in children, in patients with a disturbance of consciousness, and on demand. It is always done by an anesthetic crew and is certainly beyond the scope of this paper. After all it may be the easiest way to go for the radiologist.

Patient Safety

The term comprises all measures which reduce risk and enhance safety before, during, and after an intervention.

General Considerations in CT Interventions
Preprocedural Evaluation. An important element of preprocedural evaluation is getting in contact with the patient and assessing and possibly correcting risk

Table 1. Patient care for CT interventions: preprocedural evaluation

Action	Person responsible
Check radiologic equipment	Interventionist
Check interventional material	Interventionist
Check anesthetic equipment	Anesthetist/nurse/interventionist
Check indication/alternatives	Interdisciplinary consultation
Preprocedure visit	Interventionist
Review medical chart	Interventionist
Take history	Interventionist
Do short physical examination	Interventionist
identify high risk	Interventionist
Cancel or delay procedure	Interventionist
Correct medical problems	Referring clinician/anesthetist
Explain procedure	Interventionist
Reassure patient	Interventionist
Establish relationship	Interventionist
Obtain informed consent	Interventionist
adjust medication	Interventionist
adjust diet	Interventionist
Order patient preparation	Interventionist
Inform surgeon/anesthetist/ICU about planned procedure	Interventionist
Premedication on call	ward
Premedication on site	Anesthetist/nurse/interventionist

ICU, intensive care unit.

factors [1, 19]. A partial list of standard preprocedural evaluation is given in Table 1, as outlined by the literature, and from our own experience.

Lyons, in a recent review on *Anesthesia and Sedation in Interventional Radiology* states: "State of the art practices in radiological techniques are rarely supported by state of the art practices in sedation" [4]. He continues in saying that "anesthetic support for *all* sessions requiring sedation is not a realistic option," and concludes that the radiologist must be able to identify patients at high risk.

For that purpose he proposes a small check list (Table 2) with simple questions about the patient's medical history. If any question is answered with "yes," continuous monitoring with appropriate devices for oxygen saturation, heart rate and rhythm, and blood pressure is recommended (Table 3).

An interesting discussion about the prophylactic use of antibiotics was recently generated by an article by Spies et al. [20–22]. All authors agree that a manifest infection should obviously be treated with antibiotics, if possible specifically targeted to the infecting organism(s). The question of the prophylactic use of antibiotics remains open.

Spies proposes to classify interventional procedures into four categories, following the American National Academy of Science/National Research Council classification of surgical wounds:

- *Clean*, if there is no entry into the gastrointestinal, biliary, respiratory, or genitourinary tracts, if there is no break in technique and no inflammation is encountered.
- *Clean-contaminated*, if there is entry into the gastrointestinal or respiratory tracts without spillage and into noninfected biliary or genitourinary tracts, and if there are at best minor breaks in technique.
- *Contaminated*, if there is entry into the gastrointestinal or respiratory tracts with spillage and into colonized – which means the presence of microorganisms without host response – biliary, or genitourinary tracts and if there are major breaks in technique.
- *Dirty*, if there is entry into clinically infected biliary or genitourinary tracts or if pus or a perforated viscus is encountered.

  Based on that classification he assigns attributes to different radiologic interventions and recommends the prophylactic use of antibiotics dependent upon the expected spectrum of organisms.

A typical example of a "clean" procedure, where no prophylaxis is indicated, are biopsies of solid tumors without entry into any of the above-mentioned tracts. A frequent example of a "dirty" procedure is the drainage of an abdominal abscess.

Table 2. Patient care for CT interventions: checklist for identifying high risk (from [4])

Question	Yes	No
Is patient over 60 years or under 15 years?		
Does patient weigh more than 100 kg?		
Is there a history of reaction to contrast media?		
Is there any degree of		
liver failure?		
renal failure?		
respiratory failure?		
heart failure?		
Has the patient had a myocardial infarction or stroke in the past 6 months?		
Is the patient less then conscious or alert?		
Does the patient take sedative or analgesic drugs?		
Is the procedure complex?		

Table 3. Patient care for CT interventions: recommendations for monitoring (from [4])

All patients	Special facilities
Conscious level	Conscious level
Color	Oxygen saturation (pulse oxymeter)
Pulse	Heart rate & rhythm (continuous ECG)
Blood pressure	Blood pressure (automatic oscillotonometer)

Additionally he recommends an "endocarditis prophylaxis" in patients with corresponding risk factors like prosthetic cardiac valves.

There is an apparent lack of randomized, blind studies in this field.

Intraprocedural Care and Monitoring. There are a number of possible side effects and complications associated with an interventional radiologic procedure.

Side effects may stem from the mechanical manipulation itself, like a minor pneumothorax, or from the administration of drugs, like respiratory depression from narcotics. They occur in a certain percentage of procedures and can partly be avoided, but must be anticipated, monitored, and eventually treated appropriately.

The frequency of *complications* like the inadvertent puncture of a vessel with major bleeding or a severe anaphylactic reaction to contrast media can be kept to a minimum with proper techniques and careful history taking. The key to early detection of a possible side effect or complication is careful monitoring of the patient's vital functions. As already mentioned above and as Hurlbert puts it, "pulse oximetry, ECG, and automated blood-pressure monitoring (should) become the norm on every patient in the interventional radiology suite" [2]. These devices need to be observed, however, to be of use [23].

If a patient requires anesthesia, the facilities to conduct a general anesthesia must be at hand [5].

A crucial point in patient safety is the close cooperation with the referring specialities and an interested anesthesist. Indication, intention, and accomplishment of the process should be clear to all involved.

Withers and coworkers quote: "At the University of California, San Diego, we have found that with an interventional radiology-anesthesia team, complex procedures more often are successful and patients are remarkably more compliant and content" [5].

Interventional technicians and radiologists should periodically be trained in cardiopulmonary resuscitation.

Table 4 lists the necessary actions and precautions during the procedure.

Postprocedural Care. Postprocedural care begins with the surveillance of the patient in the recovery area, which ideally is the surgical recovery room. Factors to consider are catheter care in drainage procedures, clinical follow-up, or the review of histologic results. A list is given in Table 5.

Quality Assurance. A very important issue is the quality and appropriateness of interventional procedures. This implies the recording of all relevant procedural data, including intent and outcome, and their periodical analysis. Peer reviewers could participate in the analysis.

If too low a success rate or too high a complication rate is detected, careful review of current techniques must follow and corrections be made. This process should be documented to be understandable on later occasions. It will eventually lead to empirically based standards of interventional techniques.

Table 4. Patient care for CT interventions: intraprocedure care and monitoring

Action	Person responsible
Reassure patient	Interventionist
Briefly reassess patient	Interventionist
Use sterile techniques	Interventionist
Proceed quickly	Interventionist
Do least manipulation possible	Interventionist
Consider multiple small interventions	Interventionist
Administer medication	Anesthetist/nurse/interventionist
Monitor respiration	Anesthetist/nurse/interventionist
Monitor heart rate and rhythm	Anesthetist/nurse/interventionist
Monitor blood pressure	Anesthetist/nurse/interventionist
Monitor oxygen saturation	Anesthetist/nurse/interventionist
Correct disorders, if needed	Anesthetist/nurse/interventionist

Table 5. Patient care for CT interventions: postprocedural monitoring and care

Action	Person responsible
Monitor patient in recovery room	Interventionist/nurse/anesthetist
Keep verbal contact	Interventionist/nurse/anesthetist
Reassure patient	Interventionist/nurse/anesthetist
Monitor respiration	Interventionist/nurse/anesthetist
Monitor heart rate and rhythm	Interventionist/nurse/anesthetist
Monitor blood pressure	Interventionist/nurse/anesthetist
Monitor peripheral blood saturation	Interventionist/nurse/anesthetist
Dismiss patient from recovery room	Interventionist
Give written advice for:	Interventionist
Further monitoring, if any	Interventionist
Patient care and medication	Interventionist
Catheter care	Interventionist
Control exams	Interventionist
Further referrals to radiology suite	Interventionist
Postprocedure visits	Interventionist
Write comprehensive report	Interventionist
Assess complications	Interventionist
Obtain results (histology...)	Interventionist
Record results, complications, etc.	Interventionist
Do clinical follow-up	Interventionist
Develop standards	Interventionist
Do quality control	Interventionist
Educate residents	Interventionist

Obviously the progress can be accelerated if the data from several institutions or whole countrys are combined. Consequently there are attempts to this aim, e.g., from the American National Heart, Lung, and Blood Institute or from the Society of Cardiovascular and Interventional Radiology (SCVIR, [24]). Participation in such programs has to be encouraged.

A second point to be made is the presence of a core team of interventionists doing the procedures and training the young interventional doctors and technicians. A lot of credit can be lost if interventions are done incompetently by untrained personnel. A formal training program should therefore be set up. The SCVIR committee on fellowship training has devised preliminary guidelines for such a program.

Specific Considerations in CT Interventions

CT interventions do not differ fundamentally from other imaging-guided procedures as far as adjunctive medication and monitoring is concerned. Only the guidance itself is different and mostly more precise. Thus CT imaging could be

Table 6. Patient care for CT-interventions: interventional CT-guided procedures

	Fine needle aspiration/ biopsy	Large catheter drainage/ dilatation	Neural block, neurolysis	Intralesional tumor therapy
Preprocedural care				
Diet adjustment	NPO 4 h	NPO 8–12 h	NPO 4 h	NPO 8–12 h
Medication adjustment	Anticoagulation, aspirin, antidiabetics, diuretics			
Intraprocedural care				
Contrast media	If needed for guidance			
Drugs/devices for therapy	None	Antibiotics as tested	Alcohol for lysis	Alcohol, chemotherapy, drills
Antibiotic prophylaxis, no infection	No	In biliary/genitourinary pro.	No	Yes
Antibiotic prophylaxis, infection suspected	No	Yes	Cancel	Yes (cancel)
Analgesia -	Local anesthetic	Local/regional anesthetic	Local/regional anesthetic	Local/regional anesthesia
Sedation	None/benzodiazepine	Benzodiazepine +i.v. narcotics	Benzodiazepine +i.v. narcotics	Benzodiazepine +i.v. narcotics
Antagonists	Flumazenil	Flumazenil, naloxon		
Anesthetic team	No	Rarely	No	Rarely
Monitored functions	Respiration, blood pressure		+ Heart rate/rhythm, O_2 saturation	
Complications	Bleeding, infection, tract seeding	Bleeding, infection	Bleeding, infection, hypotension	Bleeding, infection
Alternatives	Open biopsy	Open drainage	Surgical lysis	Diverse
Postprocedural care				
Recovery area	1–4 h	4 h/inpatient	4 h/inpatient	4 h/inpatient
Monitored functions	Respiration, blood pressure		+ Heart rate/rhythm, O_2 saturation	
Follow-up	Obtain results, organize catheter care etc.			

Table 7. Patient care for CT interventions: organ-, region-, or disease-related problems

	Problem	Diagnosis	Prevention/action
Biliary/genitourinary	Pain control	n/a	Pleural/intercostal/ celiac plexus block, epidural anesthetic
Celiac block, sympathectomy	Hypotension	Monitoring	I.v. fluid administration
Hydatid cyst aspiration	Anaphylaxis	Monitoring	Prophylaxis [25], treatment
Liver abscess	Spillage	CT imaging	Transhepatic puncture
Liver hemangioma	Bleeding	Imaging, monitoring	Transhepatic puncture
Thorax	Pneumothorax	expiration view	Drainage rarely needed

n/a, not applicable.

viewed as part of the intraprocedural monitoring because it helps detect and avoid possible complications through misplaced needles and catheters. A guideline about possible approaches to CT interventions is given in Table 6.

Special considerations for certain procedures are summarized in Table 7.

Conclusion

CT interventions like other radiologic interventions are highly sophisticated, minimally invasive procedures, which can often replace major surgery. If the full benefit for the patient both objectively and subjectively is to be achieved, a number of supportive precautions and actions have to be taken. Some aspects of adjunctive medication and monitoring in interventional CT have been discussed.

The well-being of the patient and not just technical aspects should always be at the center of the effort undertaken. This will also decide upon the future of interventional radiology, which is underlined by Barth, when he says: "Commitment to patient care will be the best guarantee for the continued existence of interventional radiology among other clinical specialties" [1].

References

1. Barth KH, Matsumoto A-H (1991) Patient care in interventional radiology: a perspective. Radiology 178:11–17
2. Hurlbert BJ, Landers DF (1987) Sedation and analgesia for interventional radiologic procedures in adults. Semin Intervent Radiol 4(3):151–160
3. Lind LJ, Mushlin PS (1987) Sedation, analgesia, and anesthesia for radiologic procedures. Cardiovasc Intervent 10:247–253
4. Lyons G (1989) Anaesthesia and sedation in interventional radiology. J Intervent Radiol 4(3):109–112
5. Withers CE, Scheller MS, Van Sonnenberg E (1988) Anesthesia for interventional radiologic procedures. Semin Intervent Radiol 5(2):125–131
6. Vogelzang RL, Nemcek AA Jr (1988) Towards painless percutaneous biliary procedures: new strategies and alternatives. J Intervent Radiol 3(3):131–134
7. Vogelzang RL (1988) Pain control for percutaneous biliary procedures. Semin Intervent Radiol 5(3):207–212
8. Gazelle GS, Haaga JR, Stellato TA, Gauderer MW, Plecha DT (1991) Pelvic abscesses: CT-guided transrectal drainage. Radiology 181:49–51
9. Miller DL, Wall RT (1987) Fentanyl and diazepam for analgesia and sedation during radiologic special procedures. Radiology 162:195–198
10. Ayre-Smith G (1987) Fentanyl and diazepam for analgesia and sedation during radiologic special procedures (letter). Radiology 164:285
11. Redmond PL, Kumpe DA (1987) Fentanyl and diazepam for analgesia and sedation during radiologic special procedures (letter). Radiology 164:284
12. Braun SD, Miller GA Jr, Ford KK et al. (1985) Nitrous oxide: effective analgesic for vascular and interventional procedures. Am J Roentgenol 85(1):377–379
13. Katzen BT, Edwards KC (1983) Nitrous-oxide analgesia for interventional radiologic procedures. Am J Roentgenol 140:145–148
14. Larsen R (1987) Anästhesie, 2nd edn. Urban and Schwarzenberg, Munich, pp 152–154
15. Rosenblatt M, Robalino J, Bergman A et al. (1989) Pleural block: technique for regional anaesthesia during percutaneous hepatobiliary drainage. Radiology 172:279–280
16. Lieberman RP, Lieberman SL, Cuka DJ, Lund GB (1988) Celiac plexus and splanchnic nerve block. A review. Semin Intervent Radiol 5(3):213–222
17. Lieberman RP, Nance PN, Cuka DJ (1988) Anterior approach to celiac plexus block during interventional biliary procedures. Radiology 167(2):562–564
18. Whiteman MS, Rosenberg H, Haskin PH, Teplick SK (1986) Celiac plexus block for interventional radiology. Radiology 161:836–838
19. Lasser EC, Berry CC, Talner LB, Santini LC, Lang EK, Gerber FH, Stolbe B (1987) Pretreatment with corticosteroids to alleviate reactions to intravenous contrast material. N Engl J Med 317:845–849
20. Spies JB, Rosen RJ, Lebowitz AS (1988) Antibiotic prophylaxis in vascular and interventional radiology: a rational approach. Radiology 166(2):381–387
21. Hunter DW, Simmons RL, Hulbert JC (1988) Antibiotics for radiologic interventional procedures (editorial). Radiology 166:572–573
22. Van Waes PF, Simoons Smit IM (1988) Use of antibiotics in interventional radiologic procedures: an important lesson still to be learned (editorial). Radiology 166:570–571
23. Eichhorn JH, Cooper JB, Cullen DJ et al. (1986) Standards for patient monitoring during anaesthesia at Harvard Medical School. J Am Med Assoc 256:1017–1020
24. Cascade PN, Kastan DJ (1990) Monitoring and evaluating the quality and appropriateness of angiographic/interventional radiologic procedures. Radiology 174(3):926–928
25. Gargouri M, Ben Amor N, Ben Chehida F, Hammou A, Gharbi HA et al. (1990) Percutaneous treatment of hydatid cysts (Echinococcus granulosus). Cardiovasc Intervent 13(3):169–173

Discussion

on the papers by C. L. ZOLLIKOFER, W. GROSS-FENGELS, J. J. MERLAND, and A. JACOB

Due to the limited time available, only the paper by Zollikofer was discussed in this session. An interesting question here concerned the necessity for anticoagulation after using caval filters. The general view was that this is not needed for nitinol or titanium filters, while for Günther filters anticoagulation for a further 10 days was recommended.

As an incidental comment, Roeren pointed out that anticoagulation is also not necessary after transjugular insertion of a stent into the liver to create a portosystemic shunt, because this method was only used to treat patients in Chaild's B or C liver cirrhosis. These patients generally have coagulation disorders. Furthermore, the stent was quickly endothelialized, so only aspirin therapy for a few weeks to prevent thrombocyte aggregation seem necessary.

Contrast Media

The Pathophysiology of Contrast Media Use

P. Aspelin

Introduction

The ideal contrast medium should only influence X-rays and not have any effect on the living tissues. Unfortunately, this is impossible and all contrast media have side effects.

The use of contrast media in interventional radiology is increasing. In many instances, the amount of contrast medium used is larger than in diagnostic radiology. Also the length of the procedure exceeds that in diagnostic studies many times. This makes the choice of contrast medium of great importance and a knowledge of what is happening to the organs is of high interest.

In the following presentation my intention is to describe some of the important physiologic events that happen when a contrast medium is injected into the blood stream and circulation. The presentation will be in the same order as the contrast media reach the body. I will, thus, start with in vitro, in syringes if blood is mixed with contrast media and will continue to the vessel endothelium, how the blood components are influenced and in special instances the coagulation of blood, how renal and general toxicity of different contrast media affect the choice of medium.

Four different types of contrast media will be discussed: ionic monomeric (IM), ionic dimeric (ID), nonionic monomeric (NIM), and nonionic dimeric (NID) contrast media. I will try to do a personal "ranking" of the advantages and disadvantages of these four contrast media.

In Vitro Investigations

If blood is withdrawn into syringes which contain contrast medium, an in vitro reaction of blood/contrast medium may occur. One event that has been seen, especially with a nonionic contrast medium, is an increased red-cell aggregation within the syringes [3, 25]. This can be observed either as conglomerates, "clumps" of red blood cells, or red-blood-cell aggregates, which due to gravity "descend" in the syringes. These aggregates can be mistaken for blood clots [28] and before injection, the syringes should be shaken, which will easily disperse these aggregates. Several experimental investigations have shown that this in vitro increased red-cell aggregation has very little, if any, in vivo significance. These aggregates disperse when they come in isosalinic solutions, e.g., "plasma", thus when injected into the patients circulation. Also these aggregates are shear dependent and most of the aggregates will have been dispersed already by the high shear rates that are created in the syringes and catheters through which this mixture is injected [3, 26]. Also another phenomenon can be seen when syringes with a contrast medium–blood mixture are shaken. A complete transparent material that simulates hemolysis can occur. Despite the macroscopic appearance, however, there is no detectable hemolysis, and intact red cells are easily separated from contrast medium by centrifugation [3].

It can be clearly shown that increased in vitro red-cell aggregation occurs more with NIM than with IM or ID contrast media. The transparent solution that simulates hemolysis might appear with all contrast media. A real hemolysis can occur only when a high ratio of high-osmotic (IM) contrast medium is mixed with blood.

Viscosity

One factor that might be of importance in choosing a contrast medium is the viscosity of the contrast medium. When injected through small catheters, the viscosity of the contrast medium is of importance. The viscosity of a contrast medium is proportional to the size of the contrast-medium molecule, and the contrast medium with the lowest viscosity is the ionic monomer followed by ID, NIM, and NID. The contrast medium viscosity is reduced by heating.

In Vitro Coagulation

Firstly, it must be said that in vitro there is no definite proof that any contrast medium is procoagulant [5, 6, 21, 22, 32]. However, it is quite obvious, that the ionic monomers are more anticoagulant than ionic dimers which are more anticoagulant than nonionic contrast media. Glass syringes are more surface activating than plastic syringes, which might be procoagulant, and therefore plastic syringes are to be preferred [9].

However, one must stress that blood which stands undisturbed for a long time may coagulate and even if contrast media have anticoagulant properties, blood should never be left undisturbed in the syringes, and an angiographic technique that reduces the possibility of a mixture of blood and contrast media in syringes and catheters is to be preferred.

In Vivo Investigations

Endothelium

The first "organ" that contrast media come in contact with after the in vitro period is blood and the endothelium. Several investigations have shown that contrast media interact with the endothelium and that different contrast media affect the endothelium in different regards [12, 17, 23, 35]. There is a correlation between morphologic changes in the vessels and an increase in vascular permeability. Also a disruption in the endothelium is predisposing for thrombus formation in vivo. There is also a clear correlation between endothelial damage and the time during which the endothelium is exposed to the contrast medium.

It has been shown that not only the hyperosmolality but also the chemotoxicity of a contrast medium affects the endothelium. The hyperosmolality induces cell shrinkage and expansion of the intracellular clefts with destruction of the cells. Several of these effects are reversible. However, a comparison with sodium chloride shows that sodium chloride in concentrations equiosmolar with IM contrast media have an injurious effect similar to that of nonionic contrast media. This indicates that the chemotoxicity of a contrast medium also plays an important role in causing endothelial damage. Thus, studies on endothelium both experimentally and in the human umbilical cord have shown that the nonionic contrast media induce less changes than the IM or ID contrast media. This has especially been shown in the blood-brain barrier, which might be regarded as a specific mode of change in endothelial cells where the non-ionic contrast media show less destruction of the blood-brain barrier than the ionic contrast media [15].

Contrast Media–Blood Component Interactions

This is an extensive subject and will not be reviewed in detail. Most of these studies have, however, been performed in vitro.

Red Blood Cells

The red blood cells are influenced by contrast media. They can be influenced either by the chemotoxicity, osmolality, or ion imbalance of the contrast medium. High-osmotic contrast media induce shrinkage and crenation of the red blood cells and in high concentration stiff, rigidified "dessicocytes," and even hemolysis may occur. Even low-osmotic contrast media, both ID and NID, induce crenation of the red blood cells even in isoosmotic solution. This indicates that there is also a chemotoxic effect on the red-blood-cell membrane from contrast media. Of most importance, especially in vivo and in the microcirculation, is probably the shrinkage and rigidification of the red blood cells. This reduces the ability of the red blood cells to form a rouleaux and red-cell aggregation, which strongly influence red-blood-cell rheology and blood viscosity [2].

Whole-Blood Viscosity

It is now generally accepted that the non-Newtonian viscous characteristics of blood are the consequence of at least two different mechanisms related to the red cell, red-cell aggregation and red-cell deformation. At low shear rates, there is a rise in whole-blood viscosity, which increases with a decreasing shear rate. This increase in whole-blood viscosity has been shown to be due to a reversible aggregation of red cells. At high shear rates, the blood viscosity decreases with increasing shear rate due to disaggregation and red-cell deformation. An important determinant of red-blood-cell viscosity is the hematocrit and all these three parameters are influenced by contrast media and are influenced differently by different contrast media. Thus, theoretically, the high-osmotic contrast media should, through their disaggregation and rigidification of the red blood cells, decrease blood viscosity at low shear rates, and increase blood viscosity at high shear rates. These effects are, however, also counteracted by the decrease in hematocrit, which also reduces the effect of the contrast media and reduces the increase in viscosity. Thus, in vivo in whole-blood viscosity measurements, different contrast media affect whole-blood viscosity very little [14]. The viscosity is mostly influenced by the decrease in hematocrit and the changes between different contrast media are most likely to be of minor clinical importance. Of high clinical importance might, however, be the rigidification of the single red blood cells. This might be of great importance in any microcirculation where the red blood cells have to deform to get through the capillaries which have a smaller diameter than the red blood cells. The rigidified red blood cells might, for example, be one major explanation for the rise in pulmonary arterial pressure that has been shown to occur after the injection of high-osmotic contrast media, and this possible circulation-blocking mechanism of rigidified red blood cells might thus occur in every circulation where a contrast medium of high osmolality and high concentration is injected into the microcirculatory bed [1].

White Blood Cells

The interactions between white blood cells and contrast medium have not been shown to affect the blood circulation, but instead the function of the leukocytes [27]. High-osmolar contrast media also shrink the leukocytes and have been shown to induce a relase of histamine, serotonin, and kinin [19, 24, 29, 31]. Some of these effects may be responsible for the more general side effects experienced by patients after exposure to contrast media, such as "pseudoallergic symptoms" [13].

Studies have also shown that contrast media have a direct inhibitive effect on the chemotaxis of white blood cells [8]. This inhibitory effect that contrast media perform on the phagocytosis of leukocytes may have practical consequences. The reduction is mainly explained by the osmolality and that ionic high-osmotic contrast media reduce the phagocytosis more than nonionic contrast media and that NID induce the least inhibition in iodine-equivalent doses.

Platelets

Platelets are also influenced by contrast media, both in morphology and function [18, 33, 36]. Normally the platelets, like the red blood cells and the leukocytes are shrunk by high-osmotic contrast media and because of this a rapid decrease in platelet aggregation is observed by contrast media in humans. This inhibition in platelet aggregation is reversible within a few minutes to a few hours and is related to the dose; it is more marked for ionic contrast media. The eventual effect this has on the anticoagulant properties of contrast media will be dealt with in more detail in the chapter on contrast media and coagulation.

Contrast Media and In Vivo Coagulation

This subject is dealt with in more detail in Chap. IV "Clotting" and will only be briefly discussed here. As in vitro there is no proof that any contrast media in vivo have a procoagulant ability [20]. Also it is quite clear that the high-osmotic contrast media have a higher anticoagulant ability than the low-osmotic contrast media. The only importance and difference in contrast-media reactions that might exist are, of course, in interventional radiology, where blood is withdrawn into a syringe with contrast media and if an in vitro stimulation of thrombin in this syringe (reported in vitro) occurs [7]. The blood within this syringe does not coagulate because of the high concentration of contrast media, which means that the anticoagulant effect of fibrin is greater than the stimulating effect of thrombin. If, however, this contrast media/blood mixture is then injected into a closed volume of blood (distal to a stenosis etc.), theoretically the stimulated thrombin could induce increased coagulation. It has therefore been discussed whether the nonionic contrast media could be more dangerous than the ionic during, for example, percutaneous transluminal angioplasty (PTA). Clinically there are no clear reports supporting this theory and further studies are necessary.

Renal Toxicity

In recent years there have been an increasing number of reports on the renal toxicity of contrast media [30]. This has followed with the extensive use of interventional radiology. Thus, nowadays several procedures containing large doses of contrast media may follow within a couple of days.

The toxicity on the kidney from the injection of contrast media can be due to effects on the kidney circulation (hemodynamic disturbances and ischemia), intratubular obstruction, tubule cell damage, or immunologic mechanisms. Concerning overall renal toxicity, there has, however, been no certain proof that the new low-osmolar contrast media are superior to the high-osmolar ones [10, 11, 30].

Concerning renal hemodynamic disturbances and ischemia, a reduction in renal blood flow and increased blood viscosity have been reported and these are more pronounced with a high-osmolar contrast media [16]. When intratubular obstructions have been reported, however, the low-osmolar contrast media have not shown any advantage. On the contrary, the low-osmolar NID have been reported to increase tubular pressure and prolonged exposure of the contrast media to the tubular cells has also been reported [34]. Any drawbacks clinically of these effects have not been proven, however. Tubular cell damage, mostly enzymuria, has been reported and is more pronounced with a high-osmolar contrast medium. Very little is known of the immunologic mechanisms and no significant differences between different contrast media have been reported.

General Toxicity

The amounts of contrast media used in interventional radiology exceed those used in diagnostic procedures many times. In large arteriovenous malformations, contrast media dosages of 500–1000 ml containing 300 mg I/ml might occur. This has led to the agreement that in all procedures in which large amounts of contrast media are used, the least toxic contrast medium should be used. General toxicity is often expressed as LD_{50} and the LD_{50} of nonionic contrast media is much higher (less toxic) than that of ionic contrast media. LD_{50} differs between different species but the following figures could serve as bench marks:

- IM 6 mg I/ml per kilogram body weight
- ID 10 mg I/ml per kilogram body weight
- NIM 15 mg I/ml per kilogram body weight
- NID 20 mg I/ml per kilogram body weight

It is also important to know that the LD_{50} of contrast media is dependent upon the injection rate as well, thus the higher the injection rate, the lower the LD_{50}. The general effects of contrast media on the organs are less with low-osmolar contrast media and also the nonionic contrast media are more biocompatible with the body and body fluids than the ionic contrast media. In general, the nonionics are regarded as less toxic and better tolerated by the human body. The general intravascular effects of contrast media are associated with general peripheral arterial vasodilatation, transient tachycardia, and increased cardiac output. These effects are mostly related to the direct effect of the contrast media on the smooth vascular muscles and are mostly correlated to the osmolality of the contrast molecules. The vasodilatation and increased blood flow generally last 1–2 min and then return to normal. The subsequent hypoten-

Table 1. In vitro and in vivo effects of contrast media

	Ionic monomer	Ionic dimer	Nonionic monomer	Nonionic dimer
In vitro:				
Red blood cell	–	×	(×)	(×)
Coagulation	×	(×)	(×)	(×)
Viscosity	×	(×)	(×)	–
In vivo:				
Endothelium	–	(×)	×	×
Red blood cell	–	×	(×)	(×)
White blood cell	–	×	×	?
Platelets	–	×	×	?
BBB	–	–	×	×
Blood coagulation	×	(×)	(×)	?
Adverse reactions	–	(×)	×	×
General toxicity	–	(×)	×	×

×, preferable; (×), can be used; ?, not been tested; BBB, blood brain barrier

sion is generally counterbalanced by an increased blood volume. A feeling of warmth and sometimes pain is partly related to the degree of vasodilatation, but also a direct toxic effect on the endothelium may be the explanation. The pain can be reduced by the simultaneous injection of local anesthetics, suggesting that the pain is under neural control. In this regard, the low-osmolality contrast media are preferable to those with high osmolality.

Conclusion

The choice of a contrast medium in radiology and particularly in interventional procedures is dependent upon the type and number of procedures to be done, the total volume of contrast media that has to be used, and then all has to be correlated to the price of the contrast medium.

Generally there is, however, no doubt that the most biocompatible and for the body (the patient) least toxic products are the nonionic substances. The difference between different brands of nonionic contrast media is probably of little importance. There are, however, instances in which, for example, ID contrast media can be used. The use of ionic contrast media in interventional procedures is not usually recommended and the NID contrast media need further clinical evaluation before they can be generally recommended, especially with regard to their high price (Table 1).

References

1. Almén T, Aspelin P, Levin B (1975) Effect of ionic and non-ionic contrast medium on aortic and pulmonary arterial pressure. An angiographic study in rabbits. Invest Radiol 10:519–525
2. Aspelin P (1978) Effect of ionic and non-ionic contrast media on whole-blood viscosity, plasma viscosity, and hematocrit in vitro. Acta Radiol Diagn 19:977–989
3. Aspelin P (1988) Do nonionic contrast media increase red-cell aggregation and clot formation? Invest Radiol 23 [Suppl 2]:326
4. Aspelin P, Schmid-Schönbein H (1978) Effect of ionic and nonionic contrast media on red-cell aggregation in vitro. Acta Radiol Diagn 19:766–784
5. Corot C, Perrin JM, Belleville J, Amiel M, Eloy R (1989) Effect of iodinated contrast media on blood clotting. Invest Radiol 24:390
6. Dawson P, Hewitt P, Mackie IJ, Machin SJ, Amin S, Bradshaw A (1986) Contrast coagulation and fibrinolysis. Invest Radiol 21:248
7. Fareed J, Walenga JM, Saravia GE, Moncada RM (1990) Thrombogenetic potential of nonionic contrast media? Radiology 174:321–325
8. Georgsen J, Rassmussen F, Pedersen JO (1988) The effect of radiographic contrast media on the chemotaxis of granulocytes. Invest Radiol 23:621
9. Grabowski EF, Kaplan KL, Halpern EF (1991) Anticoagulant effects of nonionic versus ionic contrast media in angiography syringes. Invest Radiol 26:417–421
10. Harris KG, Smith TP, Cragg AH, Lemke JH (1991) Nephrotoxicity from contrast material in renal insufficiency: ionic versus nonionic agents. Radiology 179:849–852
11. Katzberg RW (1989) What do we really know about contrast medium-induced acute renal failure? Invest Radiol 24:219–220
12. Laerum F (1985) Injurious effects of contrast media on human vascular endothelium. Invest Radiol 20 [Suppl]:98
13. Lasser EC (1968) Basic mechanisms of contrast-media reactions. Theoretical and experimental considerations. Radiology 91:63
14. Lloyd DA, Stein J, Rowe MI (1991) The effects of a hyperosmolar intravenous contrast medium on blood viscosity. Invest Radiol 26:220–223
15. Michelet A (1987) Effects of intravascular contrast media on blood-brain barrier. Acta Radiol 28:329
16. Nygren A, Ulfendahl HR, Hansell P, Erikson U (1988) Effects of intravenous contrast media on cortical and medullary blood flow in the rat kidney. Invest Radiol 23:753
17. Nyman U, Almén T (1980) Effect of contrast media on aortic endothelium. Experiments in the rat with nonionic and ionic monomeric and monoacidic dimeric contrast media. Acta Radiol Diagn 362 [Suppl]:65
18. Parvez Z, Moncada R, Fareed J, Messmore HL (1984) Antiplatelet action of intravascular contrast media. Implications in diagnostic procedures. Invest Radiol 19:208
19. Parvez Z, Moncada R, Messmore HL, Fareed J (1982) Ionic and nonionic contrast media interactive with anticoagulant drugs. Acta Radiol Diagn 23:401
20. Parvez Z, Moncada R, Fareed J (1982) Contrast-media-induced serotonin release in human blood. Acta Radiol Diagn 23:561
21. Parvez Z, Moncada R (1986) Nonionic contrast medium: effects on blood coagulation and complement activation in vitro. Angiology 37:358
22. Parvez Z, Moncada R, Fareed J, Messmore HL (1983) Effects of nonionic contrast media (CM) on the components of coagulation and complement systems. Invest Radiol 18:279
23. Parvez Z, Kha T, Moncada R (1985) Ultrastructural changes in rat aortic endothelium during contrast media infusion. Invest Radiol 20:407
24. Pinet A, Corot C, Eloy R (1988) Evaluation of histamine release following intravenous injection of ionic and nonionic contrast media. Invest Radiol 23:174
25. Raininko R, Ylinen SL (1987) Effect of ionic and nonionic contrast media on aggregation of red blood cells in vitro. Acta Radiol 28:87

26. Raininko R, Ylinen SL (1990) Prevention and dispersion of contrast-media-induced red-cell aggregates. An in vitro study. Acta Radiol 31:309–314
27. Rasmussen F, Georgsen J, Grunnet N (1988) Influence of radiographic contrast media on phagocytosis. Acta Radiol 29:589
28. Robertson HJF (1987) Blood clot formation in angiographic syringes containing nonionic contrast media. Radiology 162:621–622
29. Rockhoff DS, Kuhn C, Chraplyvy M (1971) Contrast media as histamine liberators: IV. In vitro mast-cell histamine release by methylglucamine salts. Invest Radiol 6:186
30. Schwab SJ, Hlatky MA, Pieper KS (1989) Contrast nephrotoxicity: a randomized controlled trial of a nonionic and an ionic contrast agent. N Engl J Med 320:149–153
31. Siegle RL, Lieberman P (1984) Leukocyte histamine release related to ionic and nonionic contrast material and similar molecules. Invest Radiol 19 [Suppl 1]:105
32. Stormorken H, Skalpe IO, Testart MC (1986) Effects of various contrast media on coagulation, fibrinolysis and platelet function, an in vitro and in vivo study. Invest Radiol 21:348
33. Stormorken H, Testart MC, Braekke G, Sveen K, Jakobsen R, Grande T, Andrew E (1987) Effect of iopentol on coagulation and platelet function in vitro and in vivo. Acta Radiol 370 [Suppl]:93
34. Ueda J (1991) Effect of contrast media on single nephron functions. Medical thesis, University of Uppsala, Sweden
35. Wieslander JB, Stjernquist U (1987) The influence of nonionic contrast media on the endothelium of small arteries. Acta Radiol 370 [Suppl]:73
36. Zir LM, Carvalho AC, Harthorne JW, Colman RW, Less RS (1974) Effect of contrast agents on platelet aggregation and 14-C serotonin release. N Engl J Med 291:134

Improving Contrast Media Tolerance – Pharmacologic Options and Treatment of Allergic Reactions

K. Lackner and R. Fischbach

Introduction

Intravascular contrast materials (CM) used in radiologic procedures are relatively safe drugs. Parenteral administration of the contrast media is sometimes followed by harmless side effects. In a few cases, however, severe adverse reactions do occur. Many studies demonstrate the prevalence of adverse reactions to intravascular ionic radiopaque as well as to nonionic radiopaque CM [12, 16]; several reports are listed in Table 1. Different definitions of adverse reactions have led to varying results.

The overall frequency of acute adverse reactions to conventional ionic media is 12%–4% and 3%–1% for low-osmolality nonionic CM [3, 12, 22, 28, 31]. The availability of nonionic low-osmolality CM has reduced the prevalence of adverse reactions over the last years; Fig. 1 illustrates this development. In the series quoted from Ostheim-Dzerowycz 1991, there had been an increase in angiographic examinations, whereas the number of observed adverse reactions had decrased remarkably [21].

Most of the reactions including nausea, limited vomiting, limited urticaria, or pruritus do not require specific treatment. Moderate to severe adverse reactions are defined as reactions requiring some form of treatment [12]. Symptoms of moderate reactions include severe vomiting, profound urticaria, dyspnea, facial edema, laryngeal edema, and mild bronchospasm.

Life-threatening situations may arise from hypotensive shock, severe bronchospasm, pulmonary edema, convulsions, and respiratory or cardiac arrest. Severe reactions associated with ionic CM occur in 0.05%–0.3% (Table 1).

Table 1. Adverse reactions of intravascular contrast media

Reference	Severity	Ionic %	Nonionic %
Katayama et al. [12]	mild	12.66	3.13
	severe	0.26	0.04
Wolf et al. [31]	mild	4.4	0.59
	severe	0.32	0.01
Shehadi and Toniolo [29]	mild	4.73	–
	severe	0.05	–
Schrott et al. [26]	mild	–	2.1

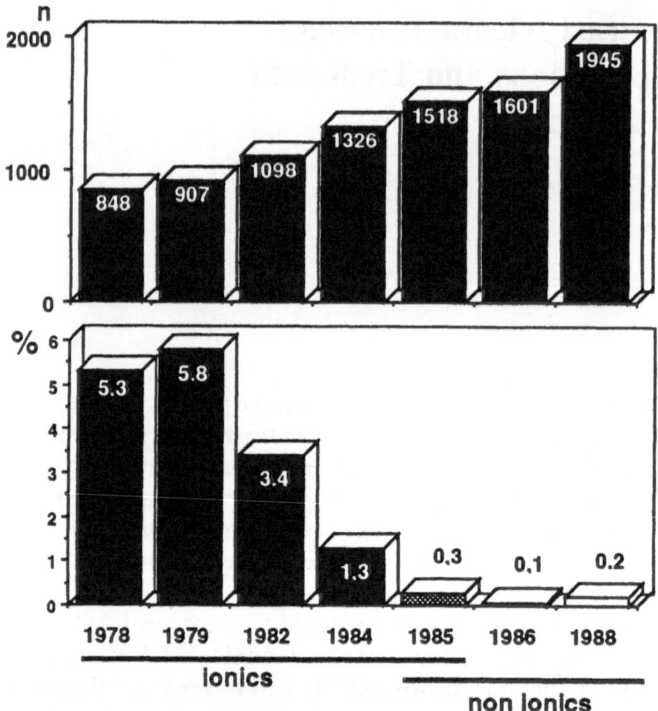

Fig. 1. Adverse reactions to intravascular contrast media in angiography of the extremities and number of examinations per year (From [21])

More than 100 randomized controlled trials comparing ionic and nonionic CM [16] and other major reports [3, 12, 22, 29, 31] showed that the use of nonionic CM reduced severe reactions by a factor of about five. Reported mortality rates for CM vary from 1 to 10000 to 1 in 169000 [12, 25, 28]. Nonionic CM seem to produce fewer fatal complications. A recent metaanalysis by Caro et al. 1991, however, did not yield a reduction in the risk of death with the use of nonionic contrast media compared to conventional substances [3]. Approximately ten fatal complications associated with the use of intravascular nonionic CM are registered in Germany each year [25].

Upper Volume Limits

In pediatric examinations nonionic CM should be used exclusively, since the frequency of adverse reactions is reduced and changes in serum osmolality and serum electrolytes can be minimized [13]. There are no studies clearly defining an upper limit in adults or children. Recommended upper volume limits for

CM application in the pediatric age group are based on clinical experience (Table 2).

In the adult patient, the administration of 300 ml CM generally seems safe according to vast clinical experience. Volumes exceeding 300 ml have been administered without considerable problems in many patients, but there are no controlled clinical studies providing sufficient data on adverse reactions to large volume contrast examinations.

The volume load due to high doses of contrast media is enhanced by the contrast media's osmotic effects [20]. In no-risk patients 25% change in the volume of circulating blood is tolerated without functional impairment [1]. In contrast-enhanced computed tomography (CT) examinations, we found a significant drop in hematocrit, indicating an increase in blood volume of about 1.5 l immediately after the injection of 300 ml nonionic CM (300 mg J/ml, injection time 5 min, [17]). Under normal conditions this effect normalized within 30 min (Fig. 2).

Table 2. Recommended upper volume limits for intravascular contrast media in children (300 mg J/ml)

Age	Upper volume limit
0–6 months	4.0 ml/kg body weight
6–12 months	3.5 ml/kg body weight
1–2 years	3.0 ml/kg body weight
3–7 years	2.5 ml/kg body weight
8–14 years	1.5 ml/kg body weight

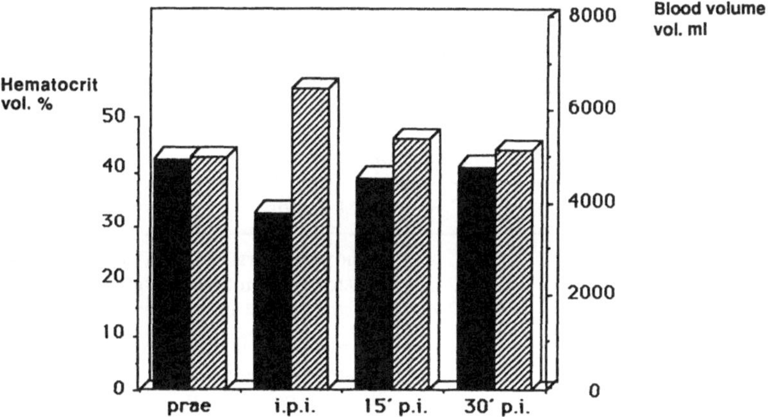

Fig. 2. Dynamics of hematocrit (■) and blood volume (▨) after administration of 300 ml nonionic contrast medium (300 mg J/ml, injection time 5–7 min). *prae*, preinjection; *i.p.i.*, immediately postinjection; *p.i.*, postinjection

High-Risk Patients

Several groups of patients (Table 3) are at high risk from adverse reactions [5, 30]. Generally, chemotoxic effects, which are directly dependent on dose and concentration, have to be differentiated from anaphylactoid (idiosyncratic) reactions, which in turn are unpredictable and independent of contrast dose above a certain threshold level [2, 30].

Patients with preexisting proteinuria, hypertension, diabetes, or dehydration do also have a higher risk of adverse reactions. The contrast agent's hyperosmolality, the potential for binding calcium ions, and the nature and concentration of the CM's cations are mainly responsible for chemotoxic adverse effects. We would like to emphasize that the underlying pathologic condition itself does not constitute a high risk, it is the administration of the CM.

Anaphylactoid reactions are governed by certain mediator substances. Contrast agents can cause the direct release of histamine from mast cells and basophils, and they can directly or indirectly activate the complement, coagulation, fibrinolytic, and kinin systems. At this point, it should be mentioned that patient anxiety is an important factor in allergy-like reactions. Lalli 1974 showed the importance of psychologic factors in contrast examinations [18]. Mainly young or inexperienced examiners tend to transfer their anxiety to the patient, thus increasing the risk of adverse reactions to the contrast media. Another factor increasing the patient's fear may result from today's demand to obtain the patient's informed consent before starting the contrast examination.

Kidney

The kidney must be recognized as a specific risk organ. Nephrotoxic effects are secondary to acute renal tubular necrosis and renal vascular damage. About 12% of hospital-acquired acute renal failures seem to be a result of contrast

Table 3. Increased risk of adverse reactions to contrast media

Reaction	Risk factor
Anaphylactoid	Known adverse reaction in previous examination History of multiple allergies History of asthma
Chemotoxic	Cardiovascular disease Renal dysfunction Renovascular disease Recent seizure Severe pulmonary disease Thyroid adenoma

nephrotoxicity [10]. A transient increase in creatinine, proteinuria, or hematuria was observed in one third of all patients after intravascular CM administration [4]. In almost all patients renal function is restored within 2–3 weeks. The comparison of the relative nephrotoxicity of ionic and nonionic CM in patients with abnormal renal function in a recent report revealed a lower rate of nephrotoxicity with nonionic CM [10]. A difference in clinically significant factors such as death or persistent renal dysfunction had not been observed. The combination of predisposing conditions like diabetes mellitus and renal insufficiency augments the relative risk of acute renal failure after CM administration [23].

There are several case reports on acute renal failure in patients with plasmacytoma. However, recent studies could not demonstrate a significant increase in renal failures in cases with proteinuria secondary to gammopathies [6]. Thus, plasmacytoma should not be regarded as an absolute contraindication of intravascular CM, but consensus with the nephrologists before, and close monitoring of the renal function parameters after the examination are mandatory.

In patients at risk from renal complications, the contrast dose should be kept minimal. The use of nonionic CM, sufficient hydration (1500 ml, 0.9% saline), and diuretics help reduce complications. Renal function impairment may produce severe problems in patients taking renally excreted drugs, e.g., oral antidiabetics and cardiac glycosides.

Thyroid Gland

Induction of hyperthyroidism is an important problem since about 5% of all patients from endemic goiter areas are affected [8]. Free inorganic iodine content in ionic CM ranges from 0.15 to 0.55 mg/100 ml CM and from 0.06 to 0.18 mg/100 ml CM in nonionic materials [7]. During the first week after the administration of conventional ionic contrast media, 6–100 mg free iodine accumulates. When using nonionic CM, free iodine accumulation is markedly reduced (3–6 mg), but it is still enough to induce hyperthyroidism or thyrotoxicosis in patients with a history of diffuse or localized adenoma, or latent immunogenic hyperthyroidism (M. Basedow).

To prevent iodine-induced hyperthyroidism, the administration of contrast media should be avoided in any patient with goiter whenever possible, until the thyroid risks have been excluded [11]. Prophylaxis in patients at risk when contrast examination is urgent includes the administration of perchlorate (1 g/day) and thyreostatics (carbimazole 20 mg/day) starting 2 days before the contrast media are given [27]. Perchlorate may be stopped 3 days and carbimazole 12 days after the CM administration. Thyroid-stimulating hormone (TSH), T_3, and T_4 levels are used to monitor thyroid function and turnover. Figure 3 shows a schematic diagram of the medication protocol. It has to be kept in mind that the effectiveness of prophylactic therapy has not been sufficiently documented in controlled trials [11].

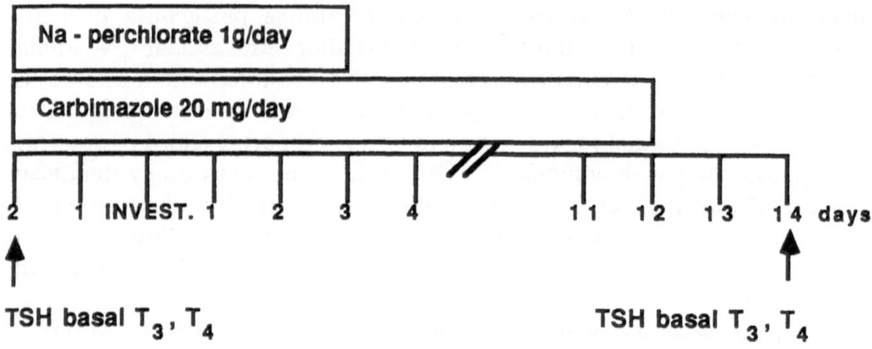

Fig. 3. Prophylaxis of iodine-induced hyperthyroidism in case of occult hyperthyroidism or adenoma. Medication and function parameters. *Invest*, investigation

Table 4. Pretreatment with H_1- and H_2 antagonists[a]

H_1	H_1	H_2	H_2
Clemastine (Tavegil) 2–6 mg	Diphenhydramine (Benadryl) 25–50 mg	Cimetidine (Tagamet) 200–400 mg	Ranitidine (Zantic) 50 mg

[a] Antagonists administered i.v., 20 min prior to CM administration

Premedication and Prevention

In patients at risk from severe anaphylactoid reactions, clinical experience, controlled studies, and pathophysiologic findings led to pretreatment protocols including steroids, H_1- and H_2-receptor antagonists, and sedation when alternative diagnostic procedures that do not require CM administration are not applicable (Table 4).

Lasser et al. 1987 demonstrated that premedication with a corticosteroid (32 mg methylprednisolone po, 12 h and 2 h before the examination) was able to reduce the prevalence of adverse reactions to ionic CM [19]. Notably, premedication with a single dose of a corticosteroid 2 h before CM administration did not yield a significant reduction in adverse reactions.

The value of systematic prophylaxis using H_1 and H_2 antagonists reported by several authors [9, 15, 24] has not been confirmed in large-scale controlled trials. Pathophysiologic and anesthesiologic data stress the efficacy of this concept. In the series by Reimann et al. 1986, adverse reactions to ionic CM were seen in 6% of high-risk patients after premedication, whereas 32% of high-risk patients developed symptoms without premedication. Greenberger and Patterson 1991 found adverse reactions in 0.5% of patients with a history of previous generalized adverse reaction after premedication with corticosteroids (50 mg prednisone, 13 h, 7 h, and 1 h before CM) and H_1 antagonist

(50 mg diphenhydramine, 1 h before CM) when using nonionic CM [9]. Pretreatment with diazepam (5–10 mg i.v.) is advised in patients with recent seizures [14], or in the very anxious patient.

Treatment of Acute Reactions

It is mandatory to have the necessary equipment and drugs immediately available. The patient's medical history including risk factors, current medication, and allergies should be known to the physician conducting the CM examination.

In case of an adverse reaction, contrast administration should be stopped immediately. Minor reactions usually are self limiting and not life threatening. It is important to provide psychologic support in reassuring the patient that a serious reaction is not occurring. Moderate to severe reactions require specific treatment. The radiologist must be familiar with the symptoms of the specific types of adverse reactions occurring so that the appropriate effective therapy can be started promptly. The administration of corticosteroids in acute adverse reactions does not seem indicated if the effects are mild; in severe reactions 250–1000 mg methylprednisolone i.v. can be given. Controlled clinical trials proving the effectiveness of this action are not available. Early specific treatment must be the aim of treating acute adverse reactions since lower doses of drugs are required in the early stages to reverse the reaction, thus minimiz-

Table 5. Treatment of acute reactions to contrast media

Reaction	Treatment
Nausea/vomiting	Supportive Dimenhydrinate, 65 mg i.v. (Vomex)
Urticaria	Supportive Clemastin, 4 mg i.v. (Tavegil and Ranitidine, 50 mg i.v. (Zantic)
Bronchospasm:	Oxygen
mild	Epinephrine, 0.1–0.2 mg SC (Suprarenin) 1:1000, or two inhalations orciprenaline (Alupent), or two inhalations terbutaline (Bricanyl)
Severe	Epinephrine, 0.1 mg i.v. (Suprarenin) 1:10000 or 0.5 mg orciprenalin i.v. (Alupent)
Hypotension:	
Tachycardia	Fluids, 1–3 l i.v. rapidly, e.g., hydroxyethyl starch 10% MW 200000 (HAES-steril) and Ringer's solution
Bradycardia	i.v. Fluids, 1–2 l i.v. rapidly and atropine 1 mg lv.
Seizures	Diazepam, 5–10 mg l.v. (Valium)
Severe reactions	Patient monitoring: Heart rate Blood pressure ECG monitor

ing potential drug-related side effects [2]. Symptoms and specific drugs are summarized in Table 5.

Conclusions

- Nonionic contrast media produce fewer chemotoxic effects and seem to have less potential to induce anaphylactoid reactions than conventional ionic high-osmolality CM.
- Severe adverse reactions are very rare, but even with nonionic CM fatal reactions do occur.
- The radiologist must be prepared for emergent treatment of acute reactions to stabilize the patient's condition until further measures can be undertaken.
- Alternative diagnostic procedures should be considered in high-risk patients. If CM administration is necessary, nonionic substances must be used. Depending on risk factors specific preventive treatments should be considered.
- The indication for the use of intravascular CM must be based on a benefit-risk analysis.

References

1. Albert SN (1963) Blood volume. Thomas, Springfield, pp 24–26
2. Bush WH, Swanson DP (1991) Acute reactions to intravascular contrast media: types, risk factors, recognition, and specific treatment. AJR 157:1153–1161
3. Caro JJ, Trindade E, McGregor M (1991) The risk of death and of severe nonfatal reactions with high- vs low-osmolality contrast media: a meta analysis. AJR 156:825–832
4. D'Elia JA, Gleason RE, Alday M, Malarick C, Godley K, Warram J, Kaldany A, Weinrauch LA (1982) Nephrotoxicity from angiographic contrast material. A prospective study. AJM 72:719–725
5. Fink U, Jung D, Fink KB (1991) Prämedikation bei Risikopatienten – Ergebnisse einer prospektiven Studie mit nichtionischen Kontrastmitteln. In: Peters PE, Zeitler E (eds) Röntgenkontrastmittel. Nebenwirkungen Prophylaxe Therapie. Springer, Berlin Heidelberg New York, pp 205–209
6. Gassmann W, Haferlach T, Schmitz N, Kayser W, Löffler H (1983) Zur Problematik der intravenösen Urographie bei Patienten mit Plasmocytom. Schweiz Med Wochenschr 113:301–304
7. Glöbel B, Glöbel H (1991) Die Schilddrüsenfunktion nach Applikation jodhaltiger Röntgenkontrastmittel. In: Peters PE, Zeitler E (eds) Röntgenkontrastmittel. Nebenwirkungen Prophylaxe Therapie. Springer, Berlin Heidelberg New York, pp 70–75
8. Grebe SF, Müller H (1984) Hyperthyreose-Risiko bei Kontrastmittelverabreichung. Digitale Radiographie. Schnetztor, Konstanz, pp 339–343
9. Greenberg PA, Patterson R (1991) The prevention of immediate generalized reactions to radiocontrast media in high-risk patients. J Allergy Clin Immunol 87:867–872
10. Harris KG, Smith TP, Craig AH, Lemke JH (1991) Nephrotoxicity from contrast material in renal insufficiency: ionic vs nonionic agents. Radiology 179:849–852

11. Herrmann J, Emrich D, Kemper F, Köbberling J, Pickardt RC (1984) Jodexzeß und seine Auswirkungen. Dtsch Med Wochenschr 109:1077–1080
12. Katayama H, Yamaguchi K, Kozuka T, Takashima T, Seez P, Matsuura K (1990) Adverse reactions to ionic and nonionic contrast media. A report from the Japanese committee on the safety of contrast media. Radiology 175:621–628
13. Kaufmann HJ (1985) Kontrastmittel in der Kinderradiologie. Workshop, 22–24 Aug 1985, Berlin. Schering, Berlin
14. Kelly JF, Patterson R, Lieberman P, Mathison DA, Svenson DD (1978) Radiographic contrast media studies in high-risk patients. J Allergy Clin Immunol 62:181–184
15. King J, Rothenberger K-H, Clauss W (1985) Prevention of anaphylactoid reactions after radiographic contrast media infusion by combined histamine H_1- and H_2-receptor antagonists: results in a prospective controlled trial. Int Arch Allergy Appl Immunol 78:9–14
16. Kinnison ML, Powe NR, Steinberg EP (1989) Results of randomized controlled trials of low- versus high-osmolality contrast media. Radiology 170:381–389
17. Lackner K, Köster O, v Uexküll V, Broich H (1984) Nebenwirkungen nach hochdosierter intravenöser Injektion nierengängiger Kontrastmittel. ROFO 141:447–452
18. Lalli AF (1974) Urographic contrast media reactions and anxiety. Radiology 112:267–271
19. Lasser EC, Berry CC, Talner LB, Santilini C, Lang EK (1987) Pretreatment with corticosteroids to alleviate reactions to intravenous contrast material. N Engl J Med 317:845–849
20. Mann S, Zeitler E (1975) Verhalten der Serumosmolarität bei hohen Kontrastmitteldosen im Rahmen der Angiographie. ROFO 122:135–137
21. Ostheim-Dzerowycz W (1991) Extremitätenangiographie. In: Peters PE, Zeitler E (eds) Röntgenkontrastmittel. Nebenwirkungen Prophylaxe Therapie. Springer, Berlin Heidelberg New York, pp 103–109
22. Palmer FJ (1988) The RACR survey of intravenous contrast media reactions final report. Australas Radiol 32:426–428
23. Parfrey PS, Griffiths SM, Barrett BJ, Paul MD, Genge M, Withers J, Farid N, McManamon PJ (1989) Contrast material-induced renal failure in patients with diabetes mellitus, renal insufficiency, or both. N Engl J Med 320:143–149
24. Reimann HJ, Tauber R, Kramann P, Gmeinwieser J, Schmidt U, Reiser M (1986) Prämedikation mit H_1- and H_2-Rezeptorantagonisten vor intravenöser Kontrastdarstellung der ableitenden Harnwege. ROFO 144:164–167
25. Schmiedel E (1989) Reduzieren nichtionische Kontrastmittel das Untersuchungsrisiko? Rontgenpraxis 42:335–337
26. Schrott KM, Behrends B, ClaußW, Kaufmann J, Lehnert J (1986) Iohexol in der Ausscheidungsurographie. Ergebnisse des Drugmonitoring. Fortschr Med 7:153–156
27. Schumm-Draeger P-M, Usadel KH, Senekowitsch FD, Maul HJC, Wenisch HJC, Böhm BO, Pickardt CR, Schöffling K (1987) Effekt einer thyreostatischen Therapie bei jodinduzierter Hyperthyreose – Untersuchungen an xenotransplantierten Geweben immunogener sowie nichtimmunogener Hyperthyreoseformen. In: Pickardt CR, Pfannenstiel P, Weinheimer B (eds) Schilddrüse 1987. Thieme, Stuttgart, pp 253–258
28. Shehadi WH (1975) Adverse reactions to intravascularly administered contrast media. AJR 124:145–152
29. Shehadi WH, Toniolo G (1980) Adverse reactions to contrast media. Radiology 137:299–302
30. Soyer P, Levesque M (1990) Prévention des accidents d'intolerance aux produits de contraste iodés. Presse Med 19:562–565
31. Wolf GL, Mishkin MM, Roux SG, Halpren EF, Gottlieb J, Zimmerman J, Gillen J, Thellman C (1991) Comparison of the rates of adverse drug reactions. Ionic contrast agents, ionic agents combined with steroids, and nonionic agents. Invest Radiol 26:404–410

19. [illegible]
20. [illegible]
21. [illegible] (1983) [illegible] Radiology [illegible]
24. [illegible]
25. [illegible] Radiology [illegible]
27. [illegible]

Discussion

on the papers by P. Aspelin and K. Lackner

In response to a question, Aspelin first went into the tolerance of larger doses of contrast medium. He pointed out that the dose tolerance is not only dependent on kidney function and state of hydration, but also on the time course of the contrast medium injection. With good kidney function and satisfactory hydration via infusion, large amounts of contrast medium, up to 600–1000 ml, can be tolerated. In the clinical context, the often inadequate information on kidney function and state of hydration is particularly critical. So in all patients over 60 years of age the creatinine level is required. Furthermore, radiologists are often not informed about previous contrast medium injections, for instance on the day before, which in the presence of risks can lead to kidney failure. According to Aspelin, a general tendency to administer larger amounts of contrast medium can be discerned, which might well be particularly due to the better tolerance of nonionic contrast media. This results in a danger of kidney failure, particularly in patients with risk factors, because there are no definite differences in nephrotoxicity between ionic high-osmolarity and ionic and nonionic low-osmolarity contrast media. In general, in Aspelin's view, it is mostly ignorance of the patient's condition and the risk factors that led to kidney failure after giving contrast medium.

A clear creatinine limit for patients with deficient kidney function regarding administration of contrast medium does not exist. Here, too, adequate hydration is necessary, and dialysis should be ordered if appropriate. Strict attention shall also be paid to the indications. Lackner then pointed out the effects of larger amounts of contrast medium on cardiac function. With fast injections in particular there is risk of cardiac volume overload, which can lead to left ventricular failure and subsequently to pulmonary edema.

During a discussion of experimentally observed endothelium-damaging effects of contrast media, the question of their reversibility was raised. Aspelin said that less serious effects can be reversed within a few hours. By contrast, repair processes after definitive endothelial damage last for days or weeks. The extent of endothelial damage due to the contrast medium depend strongly on the flow. In particular, the risk of endothelial damage increase greatly with standing columns of contrast medium. In vascular interventions, however, the endothelium-damaging effect of the contrast medium is much less important than the catheter-induced damage. It thus represents at most a relative risk. Existing contrast medium columns can sometimes be eliminated by washing out with saline.

Treatment of Emergencies During Radiologic Interventions

Type and Incidence of Serious Complications During and After Interventional Radiologic Procedures

E. ZEITLER

In the past few years interventional radiology has become a main part of radiology. More and more radiologists spend at least half their time in fluoroscopically controlled diagnostic and therapeutic interventions.

The results of the German Working Group of Interventional Radiology in the German Radiological Society (148 members), with the help of centralized documentation (answers from 35 departments), give basic information about complications arising during various interventional radiological procedures (Table 1).

In 1990, 6477 interventions were documented. Independent of the type of intervention, it is clear that in many diagnostic and therapeutic procedures the application of contrast medium is necessary to achieve better accuracy. Without question, it is necessary to apply contrast medium in all vascular interventions. Of all the interventions in the hands of radiologists in the 35 departments, 75% were of a vascular nature.

Briefly, I can demonstrate that out of 399 urogenital interventional radiological procedures, complications occurred in 6%. The treatment of varicoceles accounted for 46% of all interventions in the urogenital system, whereas stent application was performed in only 5%. Serious complications occurred in two patients with hypertension and in three patients with local thrombophlebitis out of these 399 patients.

Of the 457 embolizations most were necessary in the abdomen, 47% of them in the urogenital system. A typical complication was pain; serious complications encountered were in the embolization of a Gianturco coil in the lung, in balloon ruptures, and tissue necroses.

Table 1. Risks of general complications in interventional radiology

Type	Incidence (%)	Prevention
Severe heart insufficiency	0.5–2	I.v. access $H_1 + H_2$ premedication in patients at risk
Pulmonary embolization	0.1	AK at and after IR, leg compression "foot pumping"
Renal insufficiency	0.53	Creatine control, special premedication, special follow – up in patients

IR, interventional radiology; AK, anticoagulation

Angioplasty was the most commonly applied interventional procedure in the 35 departments in 1990. 63% of them were performed in femoropopliteal arteries, 30% in iliac, and 5% in renal arteries.

Table 2. Complications after interventional radiology (PTA) in 3791 patients in 1990

Complications	*n*	%
Bleeding/hematoma	56	1.48
Thrombus/occlusion	41	1.1
Embolism	29	0.8

Table 3. Typical complications of angioplasty and their incidence

Complications	Incidence
During PTA:	
Dissection	90/4*
Embolization	1–3
Arterial rupture	0.2
After PTA:	
Bleeding/hematoma	3–15
Thrombosis	4– 8

* 4 needed treatment.

Table 4. Complications after PTA during the period 1979–1990 (from [1])[a]

Complication	*n*
Peripheral embolism	28
Dissection	15
Perforation	10
Bleeding/hematoma	22
Aneurysm	9
Reocclusion	61
	145

[a] The total number of patients treated during this period was 7361, the incidence of complications therefore being 1.97%.

Table 5. Repeated leg surgery after PTA: complications during the period 1979–1990 (from [1])

Surgery	*n*	%
Vascular reconstructions:	113	1.56
Aortofemoral	10	
Axillofemoral	3	
Femoropopliteal	61	
Femorocrural	39	
Leg amputations (despite the above interventions)	6	0.08

Table 6. Prevention and treatment of PTA – complications

Complication	Prevention	Treatment
Dissection	DSA roadmapping	Stent application
Embolization	AK/precise technique	Aspiration Thrombolysis
Rupture	No overdilatation Small area ⟶ Large area ⟶ with blood pressure reduction	 Cuff compression Endoprotheses Surgery
Bleeding/hematoma	Good compression: "Sputnik" + bandage, patient control 4–24 h	95% conservative 5% surgery
Thrombus formation	Premedication with TFI + AK	Aspiration, thrombolysis, surgery

DSA, digital substraction angiography; AK, anticoagulation; TFI, thrombocyte function inhibitor.

In 5.8%, different types of complications were registered (Table 2), with several patients presenting more than one at a time. The most important ones were bleeding and hematoma, thrombotic occlusion, and clinically significant dissections. Five patients (0.14%) died within 2 weeks of the intervention, two of them following the combination of angioplasty with thrombolysis. Surgical correction within the first 2 weeks was needed in 0.4% of the complications.

According to the literature and our own experience (Table 3), the typical complications during percutaneous transluminal angioplasty (PTA) are dissection and embolization. Arterial rupture has a low incidence. After angioplasty, the most common and serious complications are bleeding, large hematomas, and thrombotic occlusions.

The prospective documentation within our department shows a rate of 1.2% for serious complications (without simple hematomas). In 0.8% surgical intervention was necessary.

Of the 171 patients undergoing angioplasty combined with local thrombolysis, complications occurred in 11.1%. Most of them were serious bleedings and large hematomas. In 3.5%, surgery was necessary to stop the bleeding or control the hematoma. One bleeding led to death within 10 days.

In the period from 1979 to 1990, computer statistics for the vascular surgeon at our clinic show a total of 145 complications after PTA (Table 4). During this period, 7361 patients were treated in our department. However, the patients recorded on the computer statistics of the vascular surgery department came from more than 15 clinics practicing angioplasty. In this group of patients, 113 needed vascular reconstructions and six out of them had to undergo amputation (Table 5).

Therefore, close cooperation between vascular surgeons and interventional radiologists is necessary, not only in the primary indication for interventional procedures (particularly for angioplasty) but also in the indication and control of complications and follow-up treatment. Today not all patients need surgery. The aspiration of embolisms and the local thrombolysis of thrombotic occlusions can take place, and special plastic occluders can be applied in patients with afterbleeding before it becomes necessary to submit the patient to surgical treatment.

Therefore, it is necessary to know how to prevent and treat complications which may occur in angioplasty as well as after all types of radiological intervention (Table 6).

We hope that with the centralized documentation, the German Radiological Society, together with its working group can help to provide clearer information about the low risk of interventional radiology. As semiactive treatment for many patients, it has a low-risk rate and is, at the same time, less expensive.

Reference

1. Raithel D (1991) Chirurgische Maßnahmen nach PTA, Indikationsstellung und Ergebnisse. Langenbecks Arch Chir: 529–533

Treatment of Cardiovascular Complications During Radiologic Interventions

M. Pfisterer

Introduction

Although the incidence of cardiovascular complications during radiologic interventions is low [2, 4, 5], they may occur and lead to life-threatening emergencies despite careful attention to detail and meticulous technique. This is particularly true if not only diagnostic, but also the newer therapeutic radiologic interventions are considered. This is nicely illustrated in a recent review of 2883 consecutive cardiac catheterization procedures performed during an 18-month-period [7], which showed that severe local vascular problems and neurologic events occurred at similar rates for diagnostic catheterization and percutaneous transluminal coronary angioplasty (PTCA), whereas severe cardiac complications such as cardiac arrest due to arrhythmias, myocardial infarction, the need for emergency coronary artery bypass graft surgery, or death occurred at least twice as frequently in conjunction with PTCA. In addition, investigator experience plays a major role in reducing severe complications as observed in the learning curves of such interventions, e.g., the recently published one of the Basel experience with PTCA [6].

Based on such analysis, patients at high risk for severe complications during cardiac catheterization have been identified [3]: infants below 1 year of age or patients older than 65 years, patients with unstable angina, those with left main coronary artery disease or severe left ventricular dysfunction (ejection fraction below 30%), as well as patients with combined valvular and coronary artery disease, or cardiac and severe noncardiac disease (renal insufficiency, insulin-dependent diabetes, advanced cerebral and/or peripheral vascular disease, or severe pulmonary insufficiency). For noncardiac radiologic interventions, the presence of significant heart disease per se is a relevant risk factor for cardiovascular complications.

In this overview of the treatment of cardiovascular complications during radiologic interventions, systemic hemodynamic and direct cardiac complications are discussed separately with regard to their principle causes, clinical presentation, and advised treatment. In addition, the principles of cardiopulmonary resuscitation and a list of emergency equipment and drugs are added in order to give the reader some practical guidelines for the treatment of such complications. It has to be stressed, however, that especially in conjunction with radiologic interventions, the main objective of each investigator has to be the *prevention* of cardiovascular complications.

Systemic Hemodynamic Complications (Table 1)

Vagovasal Reactions

This is the most frequent hemodynamic complication occurring in about 1% – 3% of patients. The major causes are local pain, mostly in association with a tense, anxious patient. Clinical manifestations are hypotension, bradycardia (rarely sinus arrest or high-degree AV block) resulting in nausea, dizziness, and sometimes loss of consciousness. This complication may be prevented by calm and assuring patient information before the procedure, thereby establishing a good patient–doctor contact, as well as by enough local anesthetics. Sometimes a mild sedative such as 5–10 mg diazepam perorally 1 h prior to the investigation may help to relax the patient. If a vagovasal reaction occurs, one should stop all catheter manipulations, tilt the patient by elevating the legs, and, if necessary, give 0.5–1.0 mg atropine intravenously. Very rarely it is necessary to use pressor substances. After 5–10 min, the procedure may usually be continued as planned.

Hypervolemia

Dye injection may lead to a marked increase in circulating volume which may be a problem in patients with congestive heart failure, cardiomyopathies, or significant stenotic valvular heart disease (mitral stenosis or aortic stenosis). Hypervolemia may be recognized if the patient becomes dyspneic, restless, and shows a high heart rate. Only in severe pulmonary edema, blood pressure may also fall. In this situation, nitroglycerine should be given immediately, 1–2 capsules sublingually (or as an intravenous infusion) to reduce the heart preload, followed by an intravenous injection of a diuretic drug (mostly furosemid 20–40 mg) to reduce the circulating volume. A sitting position and oxygen may help the patient subjectively and 5 mg morphine sulphate intravenously should be added in cases of pulmonary edema.

Table 1. Treatment of systemic hemodynamic complications

Complication	Treatment
Vagovasal reaction	Tilt, atropine
Hypervolemia	Nitroglycerin, diuretics
Hypovolemia	Volume infusion, tilt
Allergic reaction	Steroids, calcium, volume
Peripheral embolism	Heparin, PTA, surgery
Cerebral embolism	Dextran?, heparin
Local vascular	Compression, transfusion, surgery

Hypovolemia

Significant hypovolemia may be caused by unrecognized bleeding, be it in the groin, retroperitoneally, or gastrointestinally (stress ulcer!), or by dehydration due to limited fluid intake prior to the investigation or diuretics. Clinical symptoms are nausea/dizziness and cold sweating associated with hypotension and tachycardia. The treatment of this complication consists of tilting the patient to elevate his legs, replacing the lost volume by infusion, and stopping further bleeding after identification, and if possible, compression of the bleeding site. Sometimes, and only after the other measures have been taken, it may be necessary to apply pressure substances such as adrenaline or its analogues.

Hypotension

Hypotension may have different causes and has to be treated accordingly. Thus, it is important to make a quick differential diagnosis in such a patient to find out whether hypotension is due to myocardial ischemia, cardiac tamponade, severe heart failure, sustained ventricular tachycardia, bleeding, dehydration, or drug effects (note the vasodilatory effects of most contrast media!).

Hypertension

Like hypotension, hypertension has to be treated according to its cause. In an otherwise nonhypertensive patient, a high blood pressure is most often due to the stress of the investigation; hence, this stress should be prevented or relieved, and hypertension not treated with other antihypertensive drugs. In rare cases 10 mg nifedipine sublingually or a beta-blocking drug intravenously may have to be given to lower severe acute hypertension.

Other Noncardiac Emergencies

Other noncardiac emergencies during radiologic interventions are local vascular problems, peripheral or cerebral embolism, other neurologic events, as well as severe allergic and pyrogen reactions. All of them are directly due to the technique or the severity of the disease, may be expected, based on the patient's history and clinical examination, and may therefore be prevented in most instances. Local vascular problems such as bleeding, thrombosis, false aneurysm, or arteriovenous fistula formation may need compression, transfusion, and even vascular surgery, whereas neurologic events may lead to reversible or irreversible damage. They are therefore discussed in separate chapters. Allergic reactions have become much less important with newer contrast media; intravenous steroids, calcium, and volume infusions may be necessary to treat them. In cases of severe allergic reactions, no further dye should be injected.

Finally, contamination of catheters or fluids with sterile bacterial products or other foreign material may result in a pyrogen reaction characterized by rigors and temperature elevation. If this occurs, these catheters and fluids should be put aside for bacterial culture and the patient should receive 2–5 mg morphine sulfate intravenously. Again, prevention is better than treatment.

Direct Cardiac Complications (Table 2)

In most cases direct cardiac complications are related to cardiac catheterization or interventions, but they may also occur secondary to dye injection during noncardiac radiologic interventions. Tachy- and bradyarrhythmias, myocardial ischemia and infarction, as well as cardiac perforation and tamponade are discussed separately.

Tachyarrhythmias

Tachyarrhythmias occur quite frequently during cardiac catheterization due to catheter manipulations or dye injection in any of the heart chambers, especially if there is an elevated electric irritability of the heart such as in myocardial ischemia or after myocardial infarction. The patient may complain of palpitations or dizziness and in the case of a sustained tachycardia, hypotension may be present. In these cases the catheter has to be withdrawn immediately and further dye has to be injected slowly.

Supraventricular Tachyarrhythmias

Supraventricular tachyarrhythmias such as auricular flutter or fibrillation may be reverted to sinus rhythm by quinidine (500 mg sulphur quinidine perorally), digoxine (0.5 mg perorally initially, followed by additional doses if necessary), or direct current countershock. Since latent or manifest congestive heart fail-

Table 2. Treatment of cardiac complications

Cardiac complication	Treatment
Arrhythmias	
Tachy	Catheter ↗, antiarrhythmic drugs, countershock
Brady	Cough, atropine, pacemaker
Myocardial ischemia	Nitroglycerin, nifedipine
Myocardial infarction	nitroglycerin, aspirin, morphine
Cardiac tamponade	Pericardiocentesis (echo!)
Cardiac arrest	Cardiopulmonary resuscitation

ure is often the basis for new auricular fibrillation, a diuretic drug may facilitate conversion to sinus rhythm.

Ventricular Tachycardia

Ventricular tachycardia may be interrupted by a thump on the lower end of the sternum, by 50–100 mg lidocaine intravenously followed by pretylium or other antiarrhythmic drugs if lidocaine is ineffective, or by direct current countershock. In cases of ventricular tachycardia, serum concentrations of potassium and magnesium should be checked and these electrolytes replaced if levels are too low.

Bradyarrhythmias

Bradyarrhythmias may have the same causes and clinical presentation as tachyarrhythmias but their treatment is different. Therefore, electrocardiographic monitoring is essential in all rhythm disturbances. If extreme bradycardia is present, catheter and dye have to be removed immediately and the patient has to be encouraged to cough. Often this will be sufficient, especially if an obstruction of the sinus coronary artery during catheterization of the right coronary artery is the cause of this arrhythmia. Sometimes intravenous atropine, cardiac massage and intravenous adrenaline, or the placement of a temporary pacemaker may become necessary.

Myocardial Ischemia

Myocardial ischemia occurs during cardiac catheterization or coronary artery interventions due to coronary artery obstruction or spasm mainly in patients with unstable angina. They complain of typical chest pain associated with ST- and T-wave changes in the electrocardiogram. Withdrawal of the catheter from the coronary ostia is the first step to take. Nitroglycerin sublingually, intravenously, or directly into the coronary artery is the treatment of choice. A calcium channel-blocker such as nifedipine may be indicated to relieve coronary artery spasm whereas beta-blocking drugs are usually not given immediately in acute ischemia. If the coronary artery is totally occluded by a thrombus or due to a large dissection after PTCA, the patient will complain of severe chest pain and the electrocardiogram will show ST-segment elevation. These are typical signs of acute myocardial infarction. If this occurs during a noncardiac radiologic procedure, nitroglycerin is again the first drug followed by 250 mg aspirin intravenously or perorally. 5–10 mg morphine sulphate intravenously may be necessary to calm chest pain. In such a situation it has to be considered whether to install intravenous systemic thrombolysis (watch puncture-site bleeding!), or to perform acute coronary angiography in order to open the infarct-related artery by acute PTCA, or to send the patient for urgent coronary artery bypass graft surgery. In each case, a heparin infusion should be added. Of course, such a patient has to be monitored very closely.

Cardiac Perforation/Tamponade

During cardiac catheterization, especially of the right ventricle, the catheter may penetrate the ventricular wall into the pericardial space. This used to occur with relatively stiff pacemaker electrodes and may still occur today, in most cases without major sequelae. The patient may feel some pericardial pain and pericardial rub may be heard at auscultation. If cardiac perforation leads to drainage of blood into the pericardium, cardiac tamponade may be the consequence. This occurs more often in association with newer interventional therapies, such as valvuloplasty. In the presence of cardiac tamponade, the patient becomes hypotensive, has distended neck veins, a low pulse pressure, and the so-called pulsus paradoxus. It is important to recognize this unique situation, to verify it by immediate echocardiography, and to relieve it by pericardiocentesis. In most cases this can be done by direct transcutaneous puncture of the pericardium but sometimes a surgical approach is necessary. Heparin therapy should be stopped and lost blood volume replaced.

Cardiac Arrest and Cardiopulmonary Resuscitation

Cardiac arrest may either be due to ventricular fibrillation, asystole, or an electromechanical dissociation whereby ventricular fibrillation is by far the most common cause. The patient rapidly looses consciousness and starts to cramp, while no blood pressure can be measured. Immediate cardiopulmonary resuscitation is necessary. It is beyond the scope of this paper to describe all the steps necessary to perform effective resuscitation, although it is important that investigators doing radiologic interventions are familiar with external cardiac massage, artificial mouth-to-nose ventilation, the administration of epinephrine, and electrical defibrillation. Monitoring of the electrocardiogram to differentiate between ventricular fibrillation and asystole is essential, although, if no electrocardiogram is available it is more important to defibrillate without delay than to continue with massage and ventilation until the rhythm diagnosis is established. The electrocardiogram is, however, important for the diagnosis of electromechanical dissociation: in this situation there is a regular electrical activity but no mechanical pump function, be it due to global myocardial ischemia or cardiac tamponade (after myocardial rupture as in acute myocardial infarction). Here, only acute cardiac surgery may help in rare cases. Guidelines for cardiopulmonary resuscitation have been published in detail [1].

Emergency Equipment and Drugs

In view of the possibility of these life-threatening cardiovascular complications, certain minimal emergency equipment and some drugs should be available in a laboratory performing interventional radiologic procedures. These include:

1. Equipment
   - ECG/pressure monitor
   - Defibrillator
   - Temporary pacemaker
   - Suction apparatus
   - Oxygen supply
   - Ventilator bag
   - Laryngoscope/tubes
2. Drugs
   - Atropine
   - Epinephrine
   - Phenylephrine/isoprenaline
   - Nitroglycerin
   - Nifedipine
   - Morphine
   - Heparin
   - Sodium bicarbonate
   - Hydrocortisone
   - Aspirin
   - Calcium chloride
   - Guinidine sulfate
   - Digoxin

Most of them have been mentioned in the text or pertain to cardiopulmonary resuscitation. Since many of these drugs are used only infrequently it is important to check them at regular intervals. This is particularly true for the defibrillator which has to be tested every morning.

References

1. American Medical Association (1986) Standard guidelines for cardiopulmonary resuscitation (CPR) and emergency cardiac care (ECC). JAMA 255:2905
2. Folland ED, Oprian C, Giacomini J et al. (1989) Complications of cardiac catheterization and angiography in patients with valvular heart disease. Cathet Cardiovasc Diagn 17:15
3. Grossmann W, Baim DS (1991) Cardiac catheterization, angiography and intervention, 4th edn. Lea and Febiger, Philadelphia

4. Johnson LW, Lozner EC, Johnson S et al. (1989) Coronary angiography 1984–1987: a report of the Registry of the Society for Cardiac Angiography and Interventions. I.: Results and complications. Cathet Cardiovasc Diagn 17:5
5. Kennedy JW (1982) Complications associated with cardiac catheterization and angiography. Cathet Cardiovasc Diagn 8:5
6. Pfisterer M, Kiowski W, Schmitt HE, Burkart F (1991) Die perkutane transluminale Koronarangioplastie. Ther Umsch 48:567
7. Wyman RM, Safian RD, Portway V et al. (1988) Current complications of diagnostic and therapeutic cardiac catheterization. J Am Coll Cardiol 12:1400

Incidence and Treatment of Complications During Neuroradiologic Interventions

E. W. RADÜ, M. SCHUMACHER, and I. MADER

Interventional radiology is an area of neuroradiology which, owing to technological improvements and innovations, has greatly expanded the scope of its therapeutic application. It is now used in embolization of intra- and extracerebral aneurysms [61, 83], dural and intracerebral arteriovenous malformations [9, 50], tumour embolization [11, 31, 32, 76, 77, 79, 95, 97, 101, 114], fibrinolysis [13, 44, 105], vascular dilatation [7, 14, 17, 22, 30, 64, 87, 103] and intra-arterial chemotherapy.

For intra-arterial fibrinolysis and vascular dilatation no other treatment of comparable efficacy exists, and the indications for interventional procedures are quite clear [44, 103]. Embolization of tumours or arteriovenous malformations, on the other hand, is often regarded as a procedure preparatory to surgery and the decision to carry it out is made individually in each case.

Endovascular occlusion of aneurysms is only performed when the aneurysms are difficult to approach surgically or the patient's condition does not allow surgery. Neuroradiological treatment is almost always employed when the overall situation is difficult and alternative methods of treatment are burdened with high complication rates. Given this selection of cases which are complicated in the first place – often "problem cases" with a poor outlook – complications after neuroradiological treatment are to be expected. It is important to take particular notice of these complications when assessing the treatment; analysing them is the key to improvement.

The purpose of this paper is to survey the complications of neuroradiological treatment reported in the literature and formulate some recommendations for preventing them.

This goal may appear simple, but it is hard to achieve. In every area of application there are tools and materials specific to that area (balloon catheters, tissue adhesive, dilatation catheter), and corresponding specific complications (e.g. premature detachment of a balloon or the occurrence of emboli after dilatation) [67, 72].

In these technically demanding interventional procedures, the complication rate depends on both the materials used and the manual dexterity of the operator. Although publications often give detailed information about the materials and instruments used, they very rarely mention material defects and rarely make any statement about the experience of the operator or operators.

Almost all the serious complications are neurological deficits. Most publications are imprecise about the severity of signs and symptoms (usually merely dividing them up on a scale from "severe" to "slight") and about their duration – in various reports, "temporary deficit" can mean a deficit lasting anything between a few hours and several months.

Lastly, technical difficulties in manipulating the embolization materials are never mentioned unless neurological deficits result. Consequently, details are almost always lacking about embolization procedures that were aborted for medical or technical reasons.

Nevertheless, in this paper we will attempt to provide some overview of the published data on complications. First, the most commonly used catheters and embolization materials will be described; then the complications related to the various methods of embolization will be summarized according to pathology.

Catheters

Microcatheters (French 2–3) can be divided into two groups: those carried by the blood flow (flow-guided) and those that are pushed into place along a guidewire (flow-independent). Both are coaxially placed over a guiding catheter.

Among the *flow-guided* catheters, in addition to the very flexible, simple types with different tip designs [94], there is the calibrated leak microballoon catheter [67]. This catheter has a small, perforated balloon at its tip which, when inflated, is carried along by the blood flow, pulling the catheter behind it. Embolization material can be injected slowly through the catheter, not inflating the balloon, or injected faster, causing the balloon to swell and occlude the blood vessel, thus allowing the embolization material to leave the catheter into blood moving at a reduced flow. Because it is difficult to control balloon inflation, rupture of a vessel is always a risk, as is trapping the balloon in a small vessel and being unable to evacuate it.

Formerly, in order to shorten the route the catheter had to be manipulated along to the lesion, the internal carotid artery was punctured directly and the catheter introduced in the area of the throat [94]. The catheters themselves were pushed forward by a propulsion chamber, hydraulically, as it were, and a variety of different designs of catheter tip allowed them to reach the desired arteries. However, because of the amount of radiation during the manipulation and the uncomfortable patient position it requires, this route is seldom used now, the femoral access being preferred in almost all cases instead.

Microcatheters with guidewires vary in size, the stiffness of the guidewires, the flexibility of the distal part of the catheter, and their deformability [67, 72]. The difficulty in placing this kind of catheter is the high friction between catheter and guidewire, and the danger of perforating a vessel while pushing the guidewire forward.

Using either kind of catheter, fifth or sixth order arteries can be reached. Which catheter is chosen depends on the embolization material and the experience of the operator. For ectatic or tortuous vessels or where there is high blood flow, a flow-guided catheter will tend to be chosen; where blood flow is slower a manually guided one will more often be used.

Embolization Materials

Embolization materials available are: particles, fluids, coils and balloons.

Particles

Particles are either resorbable or non-resorbable. They are available in sizes from 50 μm to 2000 μm, so that the right size can be chosen for occlusion of capillaries or arterioles [29, 66, 91, 92, 96].

One well-known resorbable material is *Gelfoam,* which is used for preoperative embolization of pathological vessels or to temporarily occlude normal ones. Gelfoam particles can fragment and may then pass along collateral vessels between the external and the internal carotid artery. Of the non-resorbable materials, the best known are *Silastic balls.* These were first used by von Lussenhop in 1964 for devascularization of cerebral malformations [74].

More regular in form are *polyvinyl alcohol* (PVA) particles. Dissolved in fluid, these become very elastic and about 20% larger than when dry. They are manufactured with formalin and should be washed before use. Swollen in contrast medium, they form a suspension and are very easy to inject [72].

The manner of injection, the selectivity of catherization and the number of particles per millilitre determine the extent of the vascular occlusion. Although the particles are not resorbed, recanalization may be observed after some weeks, when endothelium wraps round the individual particles and makes room for renewed blood perfusion.

The best time for operation after particle embolization is after 3–6 days.

When carrying out particle embolization, the more vessels are occluded, the more one should bear in mind the possible formation of new collaterals, which can lead to unwanted occlusions in other vascular territories. Serial follow-ups are therefore essential, and should be carried out increasingly frequently as the embolization treatment proceeds.

Fluid Embolization Materials

Available fluid embolization materials are silicon, ethanol, *isobutylcyanoacrylate* (IBCA), *N*-butyl-cyanoacrylate (NBCA) and Ethibloc [2, 26, 78, 89, 106, 110]. Each of these substances has its own characteristic physical, chemical and biological properties.

The fluid most commonly used for intra- and extracerebral arteriovenous malformations is IBCA. This polymerizes on contact with ion-containing fluids (e.g. contrast medium, sodium chloride, blood or endothelium) within seconds. It is of low viscosity. The polymerization time can be varied by addition of Pantopaque: 0.2–0.5 ml Pantopaque per millilitre IBCA prolongs the polymerization time to 4–8 s. IBCA can be injected as a continuous column or by a "sandwich" technique with 5% glucose as transport medium [66].

When used in the territory of the external carotid artery, IBCA can occlude the blood vessels supplying the nerve sheets, causing cranial nerve deficits. For this reason, embolizations should be avoided in the area of the "dangerous vessels" [71].

Ethyl alcohol (ethanol) is a fluid with both occlusive and cytotoxic effects. It causes occlusion not directly but secondarily, by damaging the endothelium. It is used for obliteration of venous haemangiomas and for tumour embolization, and can also be administered percutaneously.

Ethibloc is a corn protein substrate containing 60% alcohol. It has a much higher viscosity than IBCA and a longer polymerization time, which can also be varied by using Pantopaque.

When fluid embolization materials are used, blood flow, embolization site and dilution must be precisely calculated. The occlusion site should be the capillary bed or the fistula of an arteriovenous malformation, to prevent the opening of new collaterals.

There is a danger that the embolizing substance may penetrate into the shaft of the vein, leading to thrombosis and possibly to a secondary haemorrhage.

Platinum Coils

In the last few years, *free microcoils* in various forms and sizes have come into use as embolization materials [84, 85, 93, 102]. In most cases these are made of platinum wire drawn into spirals of particular shapes and sizes. There are straight coils, bent coils and four-leaved-clover-shaped coils, obtainable in lengths of up to 40 mm. Their endovascular properties are largely unknown and consist chiefly in the induction of thrombosis. The thrombotic effect is due to the lattice work of the coil itself and can be increased by weaving threads into the coil. If the vascular lumen or aneurysm is not completely filled with coils, new aneurysms can be formed in the neck or the thrombus can undergo partial re-lysis.

A novelty still being tested is the Guglielmi detachable coil (GDC), in which the coil is connected to a guidewire by a special alloy [40, 42]. Once the coil has been correctly placed, it can be disconnected from the guidewire by an electric current. The current increases the thrombosis around the coil. This new form of coil has improved the safety of the procedure, since an incorrectly placed coil can be withdrawn again by the guidewire.

The main problem when using coils is to choose the optimal length and form of spiral. In addition, the size of the aneurysm and its neck must be very accurately measured.

Balloons

To occlude large-diameter arteries and eliminate aneurysms, *detachable and non-detachable balloons* are available. These are made of *latex or silicon. Latex balloons* come in many different shapes; their characteristic features are evenness of filling and great stretchability, meaning that they rarely tear. Their surface almost always reacts with the vascular or aneurysmal wall, resulting in increased thrombogenicity and the development of granulation tissue. They are light-sensitive and of limited durability. Latex balloons have to be fitted onto the catheter by the interventional neuroradiologist him- or herself, which requires a little practice. The structure of the latex can be altered by polymerizing materials (e.g. Hema A); this is not seen with Polymeran (Hema B).

Silicon balloons are less stretchable and have an internal closing mechanism which makes them easy to mount on a microcatheter [61]. Their surface reacts very little with the surrounding aneurysmal or vascular wall. The balloon is easy to mount and to detach [83, 86]. The latter property can be undesirable in high-flow fistulas, resulting in premature detachment.

To counter the risk of deflation of the balloon, it is filled with polymerizing material of the same osmolarity, Hema (2-hydroxyethylmethacrylate), a substance which at body temperature becomes markedly thickened within 15–20 min and then becomes unworkable. This substance initially has the viscosity of water. Small amounts of water-soluble contrast medium are added as a marker. This substance can be removed up to 15 min after administration if the balloon becomes displaced. With both latex and silicon balloons, only Hema B should be used as polymerization material [35, 60, 81].

One method of placing a balloon is to use a guide catheter, over which an outer catheter is used to detach the balloon when it has reached its definitive position. This requires a certain amount of pull, which can easily lead to dislocation of the balloon. Alternatively, a silicon balloon can be mounted on a catheter with a special tip. Assembly is easy, and so is detachment [86]. This balloon has an internal valve. To make detachment safer, various balloons are available with varying resistance at detachment, making it possible to prevent premature detachment in a high-flow fistula.

Since 1989 a catheter has been available for placing balloons which fulfills all the requirements of this difficult procedure [83]. It has high rotational stability in its proximal part for exact placement of the catheter, thermoplastic properties in its distal portion, to form the catheter tip, and allows simple detachment of the balloon. It has a double lumen with very little dead space, so that placement of polymerizing substances into the balloon lumen is easy.

During the placing of a balloon, difficulties can arise if the balloon slips into a small vessel and a kink occurs between the catheter and the balloon, making deflation impossible and provoking premature detachment. If a balloon inflates unevenly on being filled, it may rupture and the silver clips at the tip of some types of balloon may become dislocated.

Complications

This section will discuss complications arising in embolization and occlusion of aneurysms in the area of the extra- and intracranial cerebral circulation, carotid–cavernous sinus fistules, dural arteriovenous malformations, and intracerebral arteriovenous malformations.

Aneurysms of the Intracranial Cerebral Vessels

For elimination of aneurysms from the cerebral circulation, free and detachable platinum coils or balloons can be used, the latter primarily for vascular occlusion (occlusion of the carotid or vertebral artery) [25, 37, 59, 61, 63, 68, 82, 83, 99].

Coils

A summary of results of the use of *unfixed, free coils* for occlusion of aneurysms shows complete elimination of the aneurysm in 68% of patients and partial elimination in 28%. 3.2 percent suffered permanent and 14.7% temporary from or neurological deficits, and 6.5% died of complications [15, 35, 68, 84, 85, 90, 93] (Table 1).

The location of the aneurysm seems to be of no real significance in regard to the complications, since the catheter tip was optimally placed in the aneurysm in almost all cases (in only one patient this was reported to be impossible).

The most frequently reported complications were dislocations of the coil (16.2%), leading to neurological deficits, and perforation of the aneurysmal wall with subsequent haemorrhage (7%).

To avoid dislocation, imaging of the aneurysm by digital subtraction angiography in two planes is absolutely essential before detachment, and careful selection of the first and last coils is important [27]. The first should form a lattice preventing the following coils from dislocating, and the last should close off the aneurysm neck without touching the lumen of the artery. This last will

Table 1. Occlusion of intracranial aneurysms with coils

Ref.	No.	Occlusion			Complication			Technic
		total	partial	unclear	perm.	temp.	dead	
[85]	10	4	6			2		Disloc. 2
[84]	6	5			1		2	Disloc. 2
[25]	2		2				2	Disloc. 2
[93]	4	3	1			1		
[90]	16	11	4	1		3		Disloc. 3
[68]	7	7				2		Disloc. 1
[15]	16	12	4		1	1	0	
	61	42 (68%)	17 (28%)	1	2 (3.2%)	9 (14.7%)	4 (6.5%)	

always be an uncertain factor with unfixed coils, as the residual lumen cannot be estimated accurately even when imaged in several planes. In case of doubt it is better to leave a small remaining lumen and carry out follow-up angiography at intervals of a few months, with the option of adding more coils, than to run the risk of provoking a dislocation.

In large aneurysms, the main goal of preventing rupture by taking pressure off the aneurysm wall is achieved even by partial occlusion. However, if a residual lumen does have to be left, follow-up angiography is essential in order to pick up any renewed growth of the aneurysm.

Perforation of the aneurysm wall can be avoided by very careful manipulation of the coils. Magnetic resonance imaging before the embolization procedure can give clues to the presence of perforation risk sites and shows up existing thromboses in the aneurysm clearly.

The success rate for total occlusion of aneurysms using GD coils, including near-total (90–95%) occlusions, is a very promising 88% [10, 38–40]. Permanent neurological deficits caused by coil dislocation occur with a rate of 5%, temporary deficits with a rate of 6%. Mortality in publications to date is 5% (Table 2).

The placement of coils that are detached by electric current is safer than that of freely manipulable coils. They seem safer to use than any other kind, as if they are placed badly they can be withdrawn again. It is important not to twist the guidewire during placement, however, as kinking would prevent withdrawal of the coil.

Balloons

The elimination of aneurysms using detachable balloons has its own spectrum of complications. The main ones of these are rupture of the aneurysm with secondary haemorrhage, premature detachment and rupture of the balloon [12, 27, 57–59, 61, 62, 83, 99, 116] (Table 3).

Table 2. Occlusion of intracranial aneurysms with GDC coils

Ref.	Total Occl.			Complication			Technic
	No.	>95%	partial	perm.	temp.	dead	
[37]	58	53	5	4 (4)	5	1 [1]	Coil Mig. 3 Rupture 2 Thrombus Progress. 1
[40]	39	32	7	1 (1)	1	4 [3]	Thrombus Progress. 1 Rupture 1
[8]	4	4			–	–	
	101	89 (88%)	12 (12%)	5 (5) (5%)	6 (6%)	5 [4] (5%)	

( ) = mild neurological deficit; [ ] = Hunt Hess Grade V.

Table 3. Occlusion of aneurysms with detachable balloons

Ref.	No.	Occlusion		Complication			Technic
		total	partial	perm.	temp.	dead	
[82]	17	17		2		1	
[56]	25	17	9*	3	3	5 (R)	
[61]	25	25		3 (R)		1	
[55]	84	66	19	9		15 (10 R)	Disloc. 2
[62]	16	15	1	1	4	3	
[116]	1	1					
[83]	128	101	27 (1)	10		9 (5 R)	Impossibility to place balloon 36
[58]	88	77	11	9		16 (10 R)	Disloc. 2 Balloonrupture 1 Hema 1
	384	319 (83%)	67 (17.0%)	37 (9%)	7 (2%)	50 (13.0%)	

R = rupture of aneurysm; * = incomplete and occlusion of parent vessel.

Permanent neurological deficits are reported in 9% of patients, a figure markedly higher than when free or detachable coils are used. The reason for this is obvious, as an inadvertently detached or ruptured balloon can easily cause irreversible paresis. In addition, the polymerizing substances released when the balloon ruptures can disperse into branches of the middle or anterior cerebral artery.

The incidence of temporary neurological deficits when balloons are used is 2%, while the mortality is 12.1%, most deaths being due to rupture of the aneurysm or a balloon.

Only the polymerizing substances Polymeran or Hema B should be used with balloons, as these do not affect the tightness or surface qualities of either silicon or latex.

Although difficult to prove, a residual lumen at the aneurysm neck is important. Fox et al. [27, 28] found a 15% rate of aneurysm recurrence at the neck, while in a follow-up study of ten patients Higashida et al. [59] found one new aneurysm in this area and regarded this as an indication for placement of another balloon. In 11 cases of postembolization haemorrhage in their experience, this site was identified as the source of the bleeding. For this reason, regular follow-up angiography is advisable for all balloon-occluded aneurysms with a small residual lumen for about 3–5 years. If there is no change in appearance over this time, further follow-up does not appear necessary [27].

If a balloon becomes dislodged, a second, non-detachable balloon can be used to move it back into place. In the publications reviewed, only six cases of dislocation were reported as complications. However, Moret et al. [83] report 11 dislocations in their experience without classifying them as complications; ten were successfully brought back into place using a second balloon. Schumacher and Radü [98] describe a similar occurrence with a balloon at the basilar tip, the placement of which was corrected in the same way.

Overall, the success rate for balloon occlusion of aneurysms is 83% total occlusions and 17.4% partial occlusions, which is very high.

In most publications it is not apparent how many unsuccessful attempts were made to occlude the aneurysm. Only Moret et al. report a figure of 28% of aneurysms that could not be occluded by balloon. This is a notable proportion, indicating that difficulty in balloon placement is not rare [83].

The higher mortality (13.0%) associated with balloon occlusion compared to other methods is a sign of persisting technical difficulties which are obviously immanent to this system of occlusion.

At present, detachable coils seem to be the safest occlusion material, but the danger of a residual lumen is high. Follow-up angiography 3 months and 1 year after embolization is essential.

Giant aneurysms (>2.5 cm) of the internal carotid or vertebrobasilar artery, aneurysms without a neck or with a poorly formed neck, and fusiform aneurysms are suitable neither for balloon nor coil occlusion nor for surgery. The only possibility is occlusion of the feeding vessel [28, 56, 60, 62, 80, 88, 115]. For this, usually three balloons are released, one each immediately distal and proximal to the aneurysm, and a third proximally in the draining vessel. Placing the balloon distal to the aneurysm can be technically difficult and cause thromboembolism.

Taking together a total of 430 aneurysms, 422 (98%) were successfully eliminated by occlusion of the feeding vessel; an additional surgical procedure was necessary in the others.

Using this occlusion method, balloon rupture occurred in five patients (1.2%), permanent neurological deficits in 29 (7%), and temporary neurological deficits also in 41 (9.5%), 8 patients (1.9%) died. A reduction of balloon size occurred in 7 patients. The causes of the neurological deficits were balloon detachment and thromboembolism, although the patients were fully heparinized during the manoeuvre (Table 4).

Before the vascular occlusion, a test occlusion should always be carried out. In 40 patients this test occlusion showed the presence of a neurological deficit, so that an EC-IC bypass had to be instituted before embolization and occlusion of the artery.

The test occlusion should only be carried out when it has been definitely ascertained that the aneurysm cannot be approached surgically [28, 33]. In the clarification procedure, the entire circle of basilar vessels should be visualized with compression of the contralateral (nonaneurysm) side under close clinical observation and ^{133}xenon clearance of the brain. The angiogram shows, in the form of the subtlest indication of reduced perfusion on one side, a filling defect in the capillary phase.

The cerebral blood flow can show a reduction in perfusion of up to about 25% compared to the contralateral side without any clinical deficit appearing. Since there is a risk of neurological deficit from stress or a drop in blood pressure during surgery, a perfusion deficit of about 25% on one side should be taken as sufficient indication for an EC-IC bypass.

Table 4. Occlusion of aneurysms (Giant included) with occlusion of parent artery

Ref.	No.	Occlusion total	Complication			EC-IC-Bypass necessary	Technic
			perm.	temp.	dead		
[57]	68	68	3	7	1	2	Disloc. 2 Rupt. 1
[29]	58*	58 (11)	2	5		25	
[73]°	18	18	3	1	1	3	Deflat. 2
[60]	7	7	2			1	Deflat. 1
[58]	127	127	7	10	5	4	
[80]	6	6	1	3			Disloc. 2
[115]	21	21	2	1			
[19a]	8	8	2	2			Rupt. 4
[10]	15	14		3		3	
[60]	102⁺	95	7	9	1	2	
	430	422 (98%)	29 (7%)	41 (9.5%)	8 (1.9%)	40 (9.3%)	Rupt. 5 (1.2%) Deflat. 7 (1.7%)

* = only aneurysms of int. carotid artery; ( ) = ad. trapping; ° = only complications mentioned; ⁺ = 25 P balloon occlusion of aneurysms included.

The same procedure is followed for test occlusions of the vertebral artery [3, 62]. Here, however, the common carotid artery is compressed in order to test the patency of the posterior communication artery.

For the test occlusion the patient is fully heparinized. The test occlusion is carried out for 15–30 min using a detachable balloon. If occlusion for this period is tolerated without neurological deficit, the balloon is detached.

The usefulness of the investigation can be increased by arterial hypotension. EEG changes [72], which subtly indicate perfusion disturbances, evoked potentials [8] and cerebral blood flow [62] also help the examiner to recognize perfusion disturbances during the test occlusion.

After the definitive occlusion, the patient is kept under intense observation for 3 days, treated with aggregation inhibitors and low-dosed heparin, and blood pressure is kept slightly raised. If, despite these precautionary measures, ischaemia occurs, the systolic pressure should be raised at once and plasma volume expanders given [3, 53].

In none of the publications reviewed did permanent neurological damage arise from any test occlusion.

Carotid-Cavernous Sinus Fistulas

Traumatic and spontaneous fistulas from the internal carotid artery to the cavernous sinus can be well and safely treated through interventional neurological techniques [19, 34, 45, 47, 50, 55, 75, 108, 112, 118]. The treatment of choice is transarterial or transvenous placement of a balloon. Depending on the size of the fistula, more than one balloon may be necessary. The goal of treatment is to close the fistula without compressing the feeding vessel. Occasionally, however, an entirely satisfactory placement is not possible, and the internal carotid artery has to be occluded in the same session; its occlusion is also indicated if there is additional dissection.

A prerequisite of treatment is a full picture of the circulation of the brain by panangiography.

The success rate for complete elimination is very high, 94%. In 11 patients only partial occlusion was possible, and 8 (2%) were not treatable. Conservative treatment by compression of the fistula was also carried out, which in 8 patients (2% of the total number of patients) led to complete closure. No complications were seen after conservative treatment (Table 5).

Of the patients treated with occlusion, 3.8% developed permanent neurological deficits, 10.3% suffered temporary disturbances, and 4 patients (1%) died during treatment.

The complications were mostly due to difficulties in placing the balloon. Lylyk et al. [75] reported suboptimal placement of the balloon with secondary occlusion of the internal carotid artery as a technical difficulty in 27 out of 88 patients. Apart from poor placement, a problem in high-flow traumatic fistulas can be premature detachment or deflation of the balloon [45]. Rupture of the balloon or of the vessels themselves is a further complication and was seen in 5 patients.

In addition to arterial occlusion, one possibility is to close the fistula transvenously [23, 47, 50, 51]. To do this, the fistula itself and the cavernous sinus must be occluded, since occlusion of the fistula alone could lead to exophthalmos and proptosis. In the embolization procedure, the flow dynam-

Table 5. Occlusion of carotis-sinus cavernosus-fistula with balloons, coils or compression

Ref.	No.	Fist-Occlusion			Complication			Technic
		total	partial	un-changed	perm.	temp.	dead	
[107]	107	107			6	5	1	[27] Vessel
[34]	139	133			5	23	1	
		cons. 6						
[47]	14	12	1	1		1	1	
[112]	20	6	5	1	1	1		IBCA Retrograde → Thrombosis
[75]		cons. 2		6				
	88	traum. 67	1		1	6	1	[27]
		spont. 15	4		1	2		Deflat. Ball. 8
	368	348 (94%)	11 (3%)	8 (2%)	14 (3.8%)	38 (10.3%)	4 (1%)	

[ ] = patent artery occluded.

ics and neurological status should be watched for about 30 min after the balloon has been placed, before it is definitively detached.

The first choice treatment is transarterial placement of balloons or coils; the second choice is transvenous occlusion with the same [19, 45, 46, 48, 50, 52]. Unless the situation is urgent, conservative treatment with compression of the fistula is recommended, which after all has a 16% chance of success in direct fistulas and a 30% chance in indirect cavernous sinus fistulas [46].

Urgent treatment must be the option when bleeding occurs or there is progressive loss of vision, increasing proptosis or retro-orbital pain. The presence of a pseudoaneurysm with extension into the sinus, cortical venous drainage or obstruction of venous outflow should be regarded as increasing the risk of interventional procedures.

If the balloon detaches itself too early and migrates into the middle cerebral artery, the patient's blood pressure must be raised at once, plasma expander given and heparinization begun, to improve perfusion and gain time. One should then attempt to remove the balloon surgically [100].

Despite the possible complications, the interventional neurological procedure is the treatment of choice for cavernous sinus fistulas. Every surgical procedure has a lower success rate and a higher complication rate.

Dural Arteriovenous Malformations

Dural malformations probably arise as a result of a sinusal thrombosis. They consist of a network of branches of the cerebral arteries, predominantly from the territory of the external carotid artery, the ipsi- and contralateral cerebral arteries being not infrequently involved [4–6, 69, 108, 112]. The malformations drain into the sinus via multiple fistulas (rarely a single one); usually the transverse sinus, sinus rectus, and/or cavernous sinus are involved, more rarely the sagittal sinus. The extent and anatomy of the venous drainage determine what neurological deficits, if any, arise; these may occur in the form of epileptic attacks, increased intracranial pressure and intracerebral haemorrhage [6]. The therapeutic approach to these malformations may be from the arterial or the venous side. Particles, IBCA, Ethibloc or coils are used (Table 6).

The complicated structure of the malformations limits the possibilities of neuroradiological intervention; only half of the interventions undertaken led to complete occlusion. For this reason, additional surgery was required in 31% of cases. Combined surgery and embolization led to complete occlusion in 74% of cases and to marked reduction of blood flow in 24%.

Permanent neurological deficits occurred in 7 patients (4.9%). Causes were obstruction of venous outflow and one unintended embolization. Temporary deficits were seen in 13 patients (9.1%). Here, too, obstruction of venous outflow was the main cause of disturbance. Since the transverse sinus is often involved in venous thromboses, occipital and infratentorial infarcts or even cranial nerve palsies can result [70]. These last can occur during embolizations in the territory of the external carotid artery (ascending pharyngeal artery, posterior auricular artery).

Table 6. Occlusion of dural malformations

Ref.	No.	Therapy	Occlusion		Complication			Technic
			total	partial	perm.	temp.	dead	
[113]	14	Ch/+E	9	4 (1)$^{+}$				
[5]	7	Ch/+E	7					Sinus thromb. (1)
[6]	16	E/+Ch	14	2	1	2		Sinus thromb. (1)
[49]	11	E/+Ch venous	7	4		2		Sinus thromb. (1) Vestibular Deficit (1)
[46]	28	cons./E+Ch	16 [2/ 9]	11 (1)°	3			Sinus thromb. (1)
[50]	30	cons./E+Ch	26 [7/23]	4	1	3		Catheter glued (1)
[4]	6	E	4	2	1	2		Venous Infarctions
[73]*	30	E			1	4		Venous Infarctions
	142		83 (74%)	27 (24%)	7 (4.9%)	13 (9.1%)		[9/34]

[ ] = improvement after conservative therapy alone; Ch = surgery; E = embolisation; * = only complications mentioned; ( )$^{+}$ = refused therapy; ( )° = unchanged.

As the treatment is both surgically and neuroradiologically demanding, strict indications should be set for active treatment.

The most frequent main symptom of pulse-synchronized tinnitus is not, enough to justify active treatment unless it is very disturbing. The formation of cortical venous drainage is a significant risk factor for intracerebral haemorrhage and is therefore the main indication for treatment [45, 55]. Neurological deficits, particularly in the area of the cranial nerves, and intracerebral haemorrhage require endovascular treatment and, operation if embolization is unsuccessful.

Because of the high risk of recanalization, IBCA or Ethibloc are recommended embolization materials. To avoid complications, the arteries that could form collateral circulation (dangerous vessels) must be particularly watched:

1. Lingual and facial arteries — End branches to the face and orbit
2. Proximal maxillary artery — Anastomoses to ophthalmic and internal carotid arteries, end branches to skin
3. Distal maxillary artery — Anastomoses to ophthalmic and internal carotid arteries
4. Ascending pharyngeal artery — Anastomoses to vertebral and internal carotid arteries
5. Occipital artery — Anastomoses to vertebral artery

The embolization site should always be the nidus. If the occlusion is too far proximal, collateral circulation quickly develops; if the occlusion is too far distal, venous thrombosis occurs. In a malformation draining into the sagittal sinus, the distance from the tip of the catheter to the nidus may be consider-

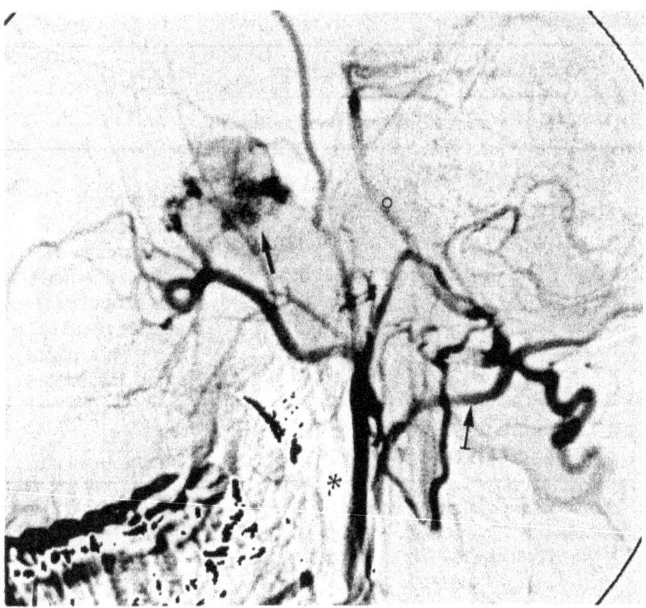

Fig. 1. Injection into the external carotid artery (*). Collateral circulation into the basilar artery (o) via the occipital artery (↦). Tumor blush of a juvenile angiofibroma (→).

able long, so that the latter cannot be reached in an optimal manner. Embolizations in the area of the vertebral artery are often difficult as well. If only partial embolization of a dural fistula is possible, elimination must be completed by surgery.

Malformations located temporal, infratentorial or in the anterior fossa lead to an increased incidence of haemorrhage and should therefore receive priority of treatment [72].

In cases of thrombosis in the area of the cavernous sinus, secondary thrombosis of the superior ophthalmic vein with secondary proptosis can result. This should be treated immediately with cortisone and heparin, which usually brings about a reduction of the symptoms within a few days. The presence of cortical venous drainage, however, constitutes a contraindication for heparin treatment.

For the management of dural arteriovenous malformations the following is recommended: in the absence of neurological deficits and any cortical venous drainage, conservative treatment should be pursued. If there is intracerebral haemorrhage and neurological deficit together with cortical venous drainage or obstructed outflow, active, aggressive treatment is indicated, first choice being an arterial approach using fluid embolization material (*cave* dangerous vessels), second choice a venous approach. If occlusion is incomplete, surgery to complete it is essential.

Intracerebral Arteriovenous Malformations

The goal of neuroradiological interventional therapy in intracerebral arteriovenous malformations is superselective catheterization of all feeding vessels and occlusion of the nidus while sparing all normal vessels [1, 9, 18, 20, 78, 89, 92, 96, 107, 109, 117, 119]. Although microcatheterization of all vessels is almost always possible, complete elimination of the malformation is attainable in only about 10% of cases. In addition, this appears only to hold when there are no more than three feeding vessels [107]. In cases where the malformation is large, partial embolization is regarded as a precondition or preparation for surgery or radiotherapy [49, 89, 92]. Rarely does embolization succeed in halting progressive neurological deficits.

Of the total of 516 intracerebral arteriovenous malformation in the publications surveyed, complete occlusion was achieved in only about 10% (several authors gave no details about the extent of occlusion). Complications were temporary neurological deficits in 10.6% and permanent deficits in 13.5%. Seventeen patients (3.2%) died of complications (Table 7). The most frequent causes were intracerebral haemorrhages resulting from unintended venous thromboses of catheter peforations. Vascular rupture was seen in 11 patients (2.2%), and fixation of the catheter with embolizing, adhesive fluid occurred in 7 patients.

Vascular rupture can be prevented only by extreme care and the use of fine catheters; the calibrated leak balloon – with one or two exceptions – is now

Table 7. Occlusion of intracerebral arteriovenous malformations

Ref.	No.	Material	% Occlusion				Complication			Hemorrhage	Technic
			100	<80	<50	n.c.	perm.	temp.	dead		
[88]	15	IBCA		8	6	1	3	2			2C fix.
[92]	51	PVA+Coils		nc			4	7	1	1	2C Perf.
[1]	12*	PVA	7^S		5^S		3			3	n.c.
[96]	35	PVA, Silk et. al.	3	12	20		3	5		4	3C Perf.
[78]	67	IBCA	6	21^R	33^J	7	7 (5)	12	4	5	2C Perf.
[18]	22	IBCA		nc			1		2	1	n.c.
[9]	202	IBCA		nc			35 (28)	25	9 [7]		5C fix.
[119]	11	PVA		1	7	3	1	4			2C Perf.-Particles Disloc. 10
[111]	101°	IBCA+Ch	31	50	14	3	13 (7)$^+$		1$^+$	4	2C Perf.
	516						70 (13.5%)	55 (10.6%)	17 (3.2%)	18 (3.2%)	

n.c. = no comment; ( ) = mild; [ ] = with little experience; fix. = glued; Perf. = Perforation of artery; $^+$ = any complication after embolisation; ° = 97 completely removed with surgery; S = inclusive neurosurgery; * = 12/28 had embolisations alone; R = after embolisation radiation therapy; J = after embolisation surgery; Catheter glued 7; Rupture 11.

obsolete [53]. In one institution, technical innovations in catheter materials and particles improved morbidity by about 50% and reduced mortality to zero [21].

The first step in embolizing an arteriovenous malformation is always to carry out superselective angiography [36]. Suitable catheters are the very flexible microcatheter (progressive suppleness pursil catheter), which is flow-guided, or a free catheter on a guidewire. Once cortical vessels have been reached, the catheter must be pushed forward only with the greatest of care. At this point, flow-guided catheters seem to move distally more quickly and easily.

If very large feeding vessels are present, proximal balloon embolization can be carried out preoperatively, particularly in order to prevent the serious complication of break-through haemorrhage [1, 49, 96]. Coils can also be used.

In case of doubt before a planned embolization, an Amytal (amobarbital) test is recommended (50 mg Amytal per injection). If normal vessels supplying the cortex are involved, administration of the barbiturate will lead to neurological deficits. Since collaterals can develop during embolization of a blood vessel, the Amytal test should be repeated, especially in case of doubt, after every embolization in the same vessel.

Available materials for partial embolization are Gelfoam, silk [54], PVA and microfibrillary collagen. Of these, Avitene seems to be the safest in use [20]. While silk threads do have a strong thrombotic and inflammatory effect, they are not radiopaque and may pass via fistulas into the lungs, causing pulmonary embolism.

A suitable fluid occlusion material is IBCA, which shows the lowest tendency to recanalization. A vessel that has been partly or almost entirely occluded using particles or an embolization fluid can for safety be finished off with a coil.

Difficulties are often encountered in the embolization of proximal aneurysms and distal arteriovenous malformations. If this combination is present, the recommended course is to first occlude the arteriovenous malformation and then await spontaneous thrombosis.

Since spasm can occur, especially during distal vascular embolization, treatment with calcium antagonists during the procedure seems indicated [16, 22]. EEG monitoring with superselective Amytal testing seems the best way to avoid neurological deficits and gross cerebral defects [113].

Summary

Despite the enormous technological progress in materials, occlusion of arteriovenous malformations by interventional radiology is regarded almost exclusively as an adjunct to or preparation for neurosurgery or radiotherapy. The great improvements in the quality and ease of handling of the embolization materials seem to be leading to a reduction in complications.

References

1. Andrews BT, Wilson CB (1987) Staged treatment of arteriovenous malformations of the brain. Neurosurgery 21:314–323
2. Apsimon HT, Khangure MS (1986) Improved technique of bucrylate embolisation in brain arteriovenous malformation. Acta Radiol 369:618–620
3. Aymard A, Gobin YP, Hodes JE, Bien S, Rüfenacht D, Reizine D, George B, Merland JJ (1991) Endovascular occlusion of vertebral arteries in the treatment of unclippable vertebrobasilar aneurysms. J Neurosurg 74:393–398
4. Barnwell SL, Halbach VV, Higashida RT, Hieshima GB, Wilson CB (1989) Complex dural arteriovenous fistulas. Results of combined endovascular and neurosurgical treatment in 16 patients. J Neurosurg 71:352–358
5. Barnwell SL, Halbach VV, Dowd CF, Higashida RT, Hieshima GB (1990) Dural arteriovenous fistulas involving the inferior petrosal sinus: angiographic findings in six patients. AJNR 11:511–516
6. Barnwell SL, Halbach VV, Dowd CF, Higashida RT, Hieshima GB, Wilson CB (1991) A variant of arteriovenous fistulas within the wall of dural sinuses. Results of combined surgical and endovascular therapy. J Neurosurg 74:199–204
7. Beck A, Ott D (1989) Percutaneous transluminal angioscopy of supraaortic branches and angioscopical control of PTA. In: Nadjmi M (ed) Imaging of brain metabolism, spine and cord. Springer, Berlin Heidelberg New York, pp 329–332
8. Berenstein A, Ransohoff J, Kupersmith M, Flamm E, Graeb D (1984) Transvascular treatment of giant aneursyms of the cavernous carotid and vertebral arteries. Functional investigation and embolization. Surg Neurol 21:3–12
9. Berenstein A, Choi IS, Kupersmith MJ, Benjamin V, Mardrid M (1989) Complications of endovascular embolization in 202 patients with cerebral AVMs. Presented at the American Society of Neuroradiology, Orlando, FL
10. Berenstein A, Choi IS, Jafar J, Kupersmith MJ (1991) Endovascular treatment of intracranial aneurysms with GDC electrocoil. Neuroradiology 33 (Suppl):145
11. Biondi A, Bien S, Cervigon E, Merland JJ (1989) Endovascular treatment of hemangioblastomas. In: Nadjmi M (ed) Imaging of brain metabolism, spine and cord. Springer, Berlin Heidelberg New York, p 318
12. Brassel F, Solymosi L, Lins E, Wappenschmidt J, Bekker W (1992) Embolization of large aneurysms with detachable balloons. In: Piscol K, Klinger M, Brock M (eds) Advances in neurosurgery. Springer, Berlin Heidelberg New York, p 58
13. Brückmann H, Ferbert A (1989) Putaminal haemorrhage after recanalization of an embolic MCA occlusion treated with tissue plasminogen activator. Neuroradiology 31:95–97
14. Brückmann H, Ringelstein EB, Zeumer H (1989) Long-term follow-up after percutaneous transluminal angioplasty (PTA) of the subclavian artery. In: Nadjmi M (ed) Imaging of brain metabolism, spine and cord. Springer, Berlin Heidelberg New York, pp 333–336
15. Casasco A, Rogopoulos A, Aymard A, Gobin YP, Hodes JE, Reizine D, George B, Merland JJ (1991) Endovascular treatment of surgical and nonsurgical intracerebral aneurysms with metallic coils. Neuroradiology 33 (Suppl):145
16. Castaings L, Moret J, Picard L, Per Z (1986) Sodium nitroprusside for the control of arterial spasm during embolization in the territory of the external carotid artery. J Neuroradiol 13:32–43
17. Courtheoux P, Theron J, Tournade A, Maiza D, Henriet JP, Braun JP (1987) Percutaneous endoluminal angioplasty of post endarterectomy carotid stenoses. Neuroradiology 29:186–189
18. Cromwell LD, Harris AB (1983) Treatment of cerebral arteriovenous malformations: combined neurosurgical and neuroradiologic approach. AJNR 4:366–368
19. Debrun GM, Viñuela F, Fox AJ, Davis KR, Ahn HS (1988) Indications for treatment and classification of 132 carotid-cavernous fistulas. Neurosurgery 22:285–289

19a. Debrun GM, Fox A, Drake C, Peerless S, Girvin J, Ferguson G (1981) Giant unclippable aneurysms: Treatment with detachable balloons. AJNR 2:167–173
20. Dion JE, Viñuela FV, Lylyk P, Lufkin P, Bentson J (1988) Ivalon-33% ethanol-avitene embolic mixture: clinical experience with neuroradiological endovascular therapy in 40 arteriovenous malformations. AJNR 9:1029
21. Dion JE, Viñuela FV, Duckwiler GR, Martin N, Jordan S, Bentson J (1989) Impact of recent technological advances on endovascular therapy of brain arteriovenous malformations and fistulas. AJNR 10:882
22. Dion JE, Duckwiler GR, Viñuela F, Martin N, Bentson J (1990) Pre-operative microangioplasty of refractory vasospasm secondary to subarachnoid hemorrhage. Neuroradiology 32:232–236
23. Dowd CF, Halbach VV, Barnwell SL, Higashida RT, Edwards MSB, Hieshima GB (1990) Transfemoral venous embolization of vein of Galen malformations. AJNR 11:643–648
24. Forsting M, Sartor K (1991) Hema and latex: a dangerous combination? Neuroradiology 33:338–340
25. Forsting M, Kummer R von, Alber FK, Sartor K (1991) Risiken der endovaskulären Aneurysmata-Behandlung mit Platinspiralen. Klin Neuroradiol 4:209–211
26. Fournier D, Terbrugge K, Rodesch G, Lasjaunias P (1990) Revascularization of brain arteriovenous malformations after embolization with brucrylate. Neuroradiology 32:497–501
27. Fox AJ, Drake CG (1990) Endovascular therapy of intracranial aneurysms. AJNR 11:641–642
28. Fox AJ, Viñuela F, Pelz DM, Peerless SJ, Ferguson GG, Drake CG, Debrun G (1987) Use of detachable balloons for proximal artery occlusion in the treatment of unclippable cerebral aneurysms. J Neurosurg 66:40–46
29. Fox AJ, Lee DH, Pelz DM, Brothers MF, Deveikis JP (1988) A thrombotic mixture as a "polymerizing" agent. AJNR 9:1029
30. Freitag G, Freitag J, Koch RD, Wagemann W (1986) Percutaneous angioplasty of carotid artery stenoses. Neuroradiology 28:126–127
31. Garcia-Cervigon E, Bien S, Rüfenacht D, Thurel C, Reizine D, Tran Ba Huy P, Merland JJ (1988) Pre-operative embolization of naso-pharyngeal angiofibromas. Report of 58 cases. Neuroradiology 30:556–560
32. Garcia-Cervigon E, Bien S, Tran Ba Huy B, Merland JJ (1989) Pre-operative embolization of naso-pharyngeal angiofibromas. Report of 58 Cases. In: Nadjmi M (ed) Imaging of brain metabolism, spine and cord. Springer, Berlin Heidelberg New York, p 319
33. Gonzalez CF, Moret J (1990) Balloon occlusion of the carotid artery prior to surgery for neck tumors. AJNR 11:649–652
34. Goto K, Hieshima GB, Higashida RT, Halbach VV, Bentson JR, Mehringer DM, Pribram HF (1986) Treatment of direct carotid cavernous sinus fistulae. Acta Radiol 369:576–579
35. Goto K, Katsuya G, Halbach VV, Hardin CW, Higashida RT, Hieshima GB (1988) Permanent inflation of detachable balloons with a low-viscosity, hydrophilic polymerizing system. Radiology 169:787–790
36. Grzyska U, Freitag J, Zeumer H (1990) Selective cerebral intraarterial DSA. Neuroradiology 32:296–299
37. Guglielmi G (1990) Balloon embolization of a basilar bifurcation aneurysm. AJNR 11:653–655
38. Guglielmi G (1992) Endovascular therapy of intracranial aneurysms with GDC coils. Meeting of the American Society of Neuroradiology, St Louis, 1992. Abstracts, pp 335–338
39. Guglielmi G (1992) Endovascular treatment of intracranial aneurysms. Interventional Radiol 2:269–278
40. Guglielmi G (1992) Embolization of intracranial aneurysms with detachable coils and electrothrombosis. In: Viñuela F (ed) Interventional neuroradiology. Raven, New York, pp 63–75

41. Guglielmi G, Viñuela F (1991) Endovascular electrothrombosis of intracranial aneurysms. Experimental research and initial clinical applications. Neuroradiology 33 (Suppl): 137
42. Guglielmi G, Viñuela F, Sepetka I, Macellari V (1991) Electrothrombosis of saccular aneurysms via endovascular approach. Part 1: Electrochemical basis, technique, and experimental results. J Neurosurg 75: 1-7
43. Guglielmi G, Viñuela F, Dion J, Duckwiler G (1991) Electrothrombosis of saccular aneurysms via endovascular approach. Part 2: Preliminary clinical experience. J Neurosurg 75: 8-14
44. Hacke W, Zeumer H, Ferbert A, Brückmann H, Zoppo GJ del (1988) Intra-arterial thrombolytic therapy improves outcome in patients with acute vertebrobasilar occlusive disease. Stroke 19: 1216-1222
45. Halbach VV, Higashida RT, Hieshima GB, Goto K, Norman D, Newton TH (1987) Dural fistulas involving the transverse and sigmoid sinuses: results of treatment in 28 patients. Radiology 163: 443-447
46. Halbach VV, Higashida RT, Hieshima GB, Reicher M, Norman D, Newton TH (1987) Dural fistulas involving the cavernous sinus: results of treatment in 30 patients. Radiology 163: 437-442
47. Halbach VV, Higashida RT, Hieshima GB, Hardin CW, Yang PJ (1988) Transvenous embolization of direct carotid cavernous fistulas. AJNR 9: 741-747
48. Halbach VV, Higashida RT, Hieshima GB, Rosenblum M, Cahan L (1988) Treatment of dural arteriovenous malformations involving the superior sagittal sinus. AJNR 9: 337-343
49. Halbach VV, Higashida RT, Yang P, Barnwell S, Wilson CB, Hieshima GB (1988) Preoperative balloon occlusion of arteriovenous malformations. Neurosurgery 22: 301-307
50. Halbach VV, Higashida RT, Hieshima GB, Hardin CW, Pribram H (1989) Transvenous embolization of dural fistulas involving the cavernous sinus. AJNR 10: 377-383
51. Halbach VV, Higashida RT, Hieshima GB, Mehringer CM, Hardin CW (1989) Transvenous embolization of dural fistulas involving the transverse and sigmoid sinuses. AJNR 10: 385-392
52. Halbach VV, Higashida RT, Hieshima GB, Wilson CB, Hardin CW, Kwan E (1989) Treatment of dural fistulas involving the deep cerebral venous system. AJNR 10: 393-399
53. Halbach VV, Higashida RT, Dowd CF, Barnwell SL, Hieshima GB (1991) Management of vascular perforations that occur during neurointerventional procedures. AJNR 12: 319-328
54. Hecht ST, Horton JA (1989) Silk suture embolization of high flow vascular malformations. In: Nadjmi M (ed) Imaging of brain metabolism, spine and cord. Springer, Berlin Heidelberg New York, p 303
55. Higashida RT, Hieshima GB, Halbach VV, Bentson JR, Goto K (1986) Closure of carotid cavernous sinus fistulae by external compression of the carotid artery and jugular vein. Acta Radiol 369: 580-583
56. Higashida RT, Hieshima GB, Halbach VV, Goto K (1986) Cervical carotid artery aneurysms and pseudoaneurysms. Acta Radiol 369: 591-593
57. Higashida RT, Hieshima GB, Halbach VV, Goto K, Dormandy B, Bell J, Cahan L, Bentson JR (1986) Intravascular detachable balloon embolization of intracranial aneurysms. Acta Radiol 369: 594-596
58. Higashida RT, Halbach VV, Cahan LD, Hieshima GB, Konishi Y (1989) Detachable balloon embolization therapy of posterior circulation intracranial aneurysms. J Neurosurg 71: 512-519
59. Higashida RT, Halbach VV, Barnwell SL, Dowd CF, Dormandy B, Bell J, Hieshima GV (1990) Treatment of intracranial aneurysms with preservation of the parent vessel: results of percutaneous balloon embolization in 84 patients. AJNR 11: 633-640
60. Higashida RT, Halbach VV, Dowd CF, Barnwell SL, Dormandy B, Bell J, Hieshima GB (1990) Endovascular detachable balloon embolization therapy of cavernous carotid artery aneurysms: results in 87 cases. J Neurosurg 72: 857-863

60a. Higashida RT, Halbach VV, Dowd CF, Barnwell SL, Dormandy B, Bell J, Hieshima GB (1991) Interventional neurovascular treatment of intracavernous aneurysms. Neuroradiology 33[Suppl]:136–138
61. Higashida RT, Halbach VV, Dowd CF, Barnwell SL, Hieshima GB (1991) Intracranial aneurysms: interventional neurovascular treatment with detachable balloons – results in 215 cases. Radiology 178:663–670
62. Hodes JE, Aymard A, Gobin AP, Rüfenacht D, Bien S, Reizine D, Gaston A, Merland JJ (1991) Endovascular occlusion of intracranial vessels for curative treatment of unclippable aneurysms: report of 16 cases. J Neurosurg 75:694–701
63. Hodes JE, Fox AJ, Pelz DM, Peerless SJ (1990) Rupture of aneurysms following balloon embolization. J Neurosurg 72:567–571
64. Kachel R, Basche S, Heerklotz I, Grossmann K, Endler S (1991) Percutaneous transluminal angioplasty (PTA) of supra-aortic arteries especially the internal carotid artery. Neuroradiology 33:191–194
65. Katada K, Sano H, Katoh Y, Kanno T, Jain VK, Mashita S, Takeuchi A, Koga S (1986) Ethyl 2-cyanoacrylate as an embolic agent for cranial arteriovenous malformations. Acta Radiol 369:623–626
66. Kendall B (1986) Embolisation techniques in neuroradiology. J Neurol 233:323–335
67. Kerber CW (1976) Balloon catheter with a calibrated leak. Radiology 120:574–577
68. Kühne D, Nahser HC (1991) Staged endovascular treatment of cerebral aneurysms with coils. Neuroradiology 33 (Suppl):145
69. Kutluk K, Schumacher M, Mironov A (1991) The role of sinus thrombosis in occipital dural arteriovenous malformations – development and spontaneous closure. Neurochirurgia 34:144–147
70. Landman JA, Braun IF (1985) Spontaneous closure of a dural arteriovenous fistula associated with acute hearing loss. AJNR 6:448–449
71. Lasjaunias P, Berenstein A (1987) Surgical neuroangiography, vol 1: Functional anatomy of craniofacial arteries. Springer, Berlin Heidelberg New York
72. Lasjaunias P, Berenstein A (1987) Surgical neuroangiography, vol 2: Endovascular treatment of craniofacial lesions. Springer, Berlin Heidelberg New York
73. Lownie SP (1992) Therapeutic management of complications in the angiography suite. Meeting of the American Society of Neurosurgeons, St Louis, 1992. Abstracts, pp 287–292
74. Luessenhop AJ, Rosa L (1984) Cerebral arteriovenous malformations. Indication for and results of surgery, and the role of intravascular techniques. J Neurosurg 60:14–22
75. Lylyk P, Viñuela F, Campos J, Fox AJ, Pelz DM, Debrun G, Drake CG (1986) Diagnosis and endovascular therapy of vascular lesions in the cavernous sinus. Acta Radiol 369:584–585
76. Macpherson P (1991) The value of pre-operative embolisation of meningioma estimated subjectively and objectively. Neuroradiology 33:334–337
77. Merland JJ, Reizine D, Guimaraens L, Rüfenacht D, Melki JP, Riche MC, George B (1985) L'angiographie diagnostique et thérapeutique dans le bilan et le traitement des tumeurs du glomus jugulaire. A propos de 32 cas. Neurochirurgie 31:358–366
78. Merland JJ, Rüfenacht D, Laurent A, Guimaraens L (1986) Endovascular treatment with isobutyl cyano acrylate in patients with arteriovenous malformation of the brain. Indications, results and complications. Acta Radiol Suppl (Stockh) 369:621–622
79. Mironov A (1990) Meningeomembolisationen mit flüssigen Embolisaten. Fortschr Röntgenstr 153:327–334
80. Molyneux AJ (1986) Giant carotid aneurysms. Treatment by detachable balloons. Acta Radiol 369:597–599
81. Monsein LH, Debrun GM, Chazaly JR (1990) Hydroxyethyl methylacrylate and latex balloons. AJNR 11:663–664
82. Moret J (1992) Endovascular therapy of SAH and intracranial aneurysms with balloons. Meeting of the American Society of Neuroradiologists, St Louis, 1992. Abstracts, pp 311–319
83. Moret J, Boulin A, Mawad M, Castaings L (1991) Endovascular treatment of berry aneurysms by endosaccular balloon occlusion. Neuroradiology 33 (Suppl):135–136

84. Nadjmi M (1991) Mikrospiralen in der interventionellen Neuroradiologie. Eine prospektive Studie. Klin Neuroradiol 4:192–202
85. Nahser HC, Kühne D (1991) Okklusion von Aneurysmata mit Platincoils. Klin Neuroradiol 4:203–208
86. Nelson M (1990) A versatile, steerable, flow-guided catheter for delivery of detachable balloons. AJNR 11:657–658
87. Newell DW, Eskridge JM, Mayberg MR, Grady MS, Winn HR (1989) Angioplasty for the treatment of symptomatic vasospasm following subarachnoid hemorrhage. J Neurosurg 71:654–660
88. Pelz DM, Viñuela F, Fox AJ, Drake CG (1984) Vertebrobasilar occlusion therapy of giant aneurysms. J Neurosurg 60:560–565
89. Pelz DM, Fox AJ, Viñuela F, Drake CC, Ferguson GG (1988) Preoperative embolization of brain AVMs isobutyl-2 cyanoacrylate. AJNR 9:757–764
90. Pruvo JP, Leclerc X, Soto Ares G, Deramond H, Clarisse J (1991) Endovascular treatment of 16 intracranial aneurysms with microcoils. Neuroradiology 33 (Suppl):147
91. Purdy PD, Samson D, Batjer JJ, Risser RC (1990) Preoperative embolization of cerebral arteriovenous malformations with polyvinyl alcohol particles: experience in 51 adults. AJNR 11:501–510
92. Purdy PD, Batjer HH, Samson D (1991) Management of hemorrhagic complications from preoperative embolization of arteriovenous malformations. J Neurosurg 74:205–211
93. Rogopoulos A, Casasco A, Gobin YP, Paquis P, Grellier P, Roche JL, Houdart E, Aboulker C (1991) Endovascular treatment of small intracranial aneurysms with microcoils. Neuroradiology 33 (Suppl):144
94. Rüfenacht D, Merland JJ (1986) Superselective catheterization using very flexible, formed catheters. Acta Radiol 369:600–602
95. Rüfenacht D, Radü EW, Huber P (1987) Der Beitrag der diagnostischen und der therapeutischen Angiographie in der Hals-Nasen-Ohren-Heilkunde. Ther Umschau 44:93–101
96. Schumacher M, Horton JA (1991) Treatment of cerebral arteriovenous malformations with PVA. Results and analysis of complications. Neuroradiology 33:101–105
97. Schumacher M, Radür EW (1991) Interventionelle Therapie von Prozessen der Temporalregion. In: Kohlmeyer K (ed) Conscientia diagnostica: Der Temporallappen. Schnetztor, Konstanz, p 175
98. Schumacher M, Radü EW (1992) Endovascular treatment of basilar bifurcation aneurysms. In: Piscol K, Klinger M, Brock M (eds) Advances in neurosurgery. Springer, Berlin Heidelberg New York, p 52
99. Strother CM, Lunde S, Graves V, Toutant S, Hieshima GB (1989) Late paraophthalmic aneurysm rupture following endovascular treatment. J Neurosurg 71:777–780
100. Swann KW, Heros RC, Debrun G, Nelson C (1986) Inadvertent middle cerebral artery embolism by a detachable balloon: management by embolectomy. Case report. J Neurosurg 64:309–312
101. Teasdale E, Patterson J, McLellan D, Macpherson P (1984) Subselective preoperative embolization for meningiomas. J Neurosurg 60:506–511
102. Teng MMH, Chang T, Huang CI, Pan DHC, Hu HH, Luk YO, Chen CC, Guo WY, Lee LS (1991) Percutaneous reposition of dislodged coils in the treatment of a vertebral arteriovenous fistula – with CT follow-up. Neuroradiology 33, 3:195–199
103. Théron J, Courtheoux P, Henriet JP, Pelouze G, Derlon JM, Maiza D (1984) Angioplasty of supra-aortic arteries. J Neuroradiol 11:187–200
104. Théron J, Cosgrove R, Melanson D, Etheir R (1986) Embolization with temporary balloon occlusion of the internal carotid or vertebral arteries. Neuroradiology 28:246–253
105. Théron J, Courtheoux P, Casasco A, Alachkark F (1989) Local intraarterial fibrinolysis in the carotid territory. Risk factors. In: Nadjimi M (ed) Imaging of brain metabolism, spine and cord. Berlin Heidelberg New York, p 303
106. Vinters HV, Galil KA, Lundie MJ, Kaufmann JCE (1985) The histotoxicity of cyanoacrylates. Neuroradiology 27:279–291

107. Viñuela F (1987) Endovascular therapy of brain arteriovenous malformations. Semin Intervent Radiol 4:269–278
108. Viñuela F (1992) Endovascular therapy of arteriovenous fistulae in the adult population. Meeting of the American Society of Neuroradiologists, St Louis, 1992. Abstracts, pp 341–343
109. Viñuela F, Debrun GM, Drake CG et al. (1983) Progressive thrombosis of brain arteriovenous malformations after embolization with isobutyl-2-cyanoacrylate. AJNR 4:1233–1238
110. Viñuela F, Debrun GM, Fox AJ (1984) The role of the preembolization superselective angiogram in the treatment of brain arteriovenous malformations with isobutyl-2-cyanoacrylate (IBC). AJNR 5:765–769
111. Viñuela F, Fox AJ, Debrun GM, Peerless SJ, Drake CG (1984) Spontaneous carotid-cavernous fistulas; clinical, radiological and therapeutic considerations. Experience with 20 cases. J Neurosurg 60:976–984
112. Viñuela F, Fox AJ, Pelz DM, Drake CG (1986) Unusual clinical manifestations of dural arteriovenous malformations. J Neurosurg 64:554–558
113. Viñuela F, Dion JE, Duckwiler G, Martin NA, Lylyk A, Fox A, Pelz D, Drake CG, Girvin JJ, Debrun G (1991) Combined endovascular embolization and surgery in the management of cerebral arteriovenous malformations: experience with 101 cases. J Neurosurg 75:856–864
114. Wakhloo AK, Schumacher M, Velthoven V van, Scheremet R, Schwechheimer K, Hennig J (1991) Extended microembolizaton of cranial meningiomas. Neuroradiology 33 (Suppl):148
115. Weil SM, van Loveren JR, Tomsick TA, Quallen BL, Tew JM Jr (1987) Management of inoperable cerebral aneurysms by the navigational balloon technique. Neurosurgery 21:296–302
116. Willinsky R, Lasjaunias P, Pruvost P, Boucherat M (1987) Petrous internal carotid aneurysm causing epistaxis: balloon embolization with preservation of the parent vessel. Neuroradiology 29:570–572
117. Willinsky RA, Lasjaunias P, Terbrugge K, Burrows P (1990) Multiple cerebral arteriovenous malformations (AVMs). Review of our experience from 203 patients with cerebral vascular lesions. Neuroradiology 32:207–210
118. Wilms G (1990) Unilateral double carotid cavernous fistula treated with detachable balloons. AJNR 11:517
119. Wolpert SM, Stein BM (1975) Catheter embolization of intracranial arteriovenous malformations as an aid to surgical excision. Neuroradiology 10:73–85
120. Yang PJ, Higashida RT, Halbach VV, Hieshima GB, Wilson CB (1989) Intravascular embolization of a cerebellar arteriovenous malformation for treatment of hemifacial spasm. AJNR 10:403–405

Discussion

on the papers by E. Zeitler and M. Pfisterer

Regarding the avoidance of local complications around the puncture, the question was raised of whether it is recommendable to determine the clotting time before removing the sheath. Schmitt regarded this as useful in all vascular interventions where larger sheaths were used or where there are risks of local complications (antegrade puncture in obese patients), because the response to the 5000 U heparin routinely administered was subject to substantial individual variations. The optimum time for removal of the sheath can be more precisely determined in this way. Cannula systems left in place must, however, always be fitted with pressure rinsing to prevent peripheral embolization.

The use of collagen clots for local hemostasis have not yet gained general acceptance. According to Zeitler, as yet, insufficient experience has been gained to demonstrate definitively the benefit of this measure.

The incidence of aneurysmata spuria and AV fistulas in the groin have, thought Zeitler, been increasing because of the increase in more complicated interventions using larger sheath systems. The possibilities for conservative therapy of these complications were discussed, Roeren mentioning his positive experience with targetted compression under duplex sonographic control. The optimum time for this was, he said, the acute phase between the third and fourth day, so the diagnosis also needs to be made early. The majority of aneurysms and AV fistulas could be cured in this way. With persistent aneurysms, Zeitler did not think that embolization is indicated and preferred surgical treatment, because aneurysms in the groin are generally easily accessible and safe to operate by ligature.

Further questions concerned the cardiac complications of angiography and vascular interventions. Arrhythmias are not rare in pulmonary angiographies. First, they can be triggered by catheter manipulations at the ventricular septum and can accordingly be eliminated by careful handling of the catheter or, if necessary, by removing it. Secondly, they can arise because of volume overload of the right ventricle when pulmonary arterial pressure is already raised. In Pfisterer's view, antiarrhythmic premedication is not necessary and also treatment shall only be given for persistent arrhythmias. Effective here is not only antiarrhythmic therapy but also reducing the pulmonary arterial pressure using, for instance, nifedipine.

The risk of cardiac complications with PTA is low, thought Pfisterer, as long as patients with risk factors have previously been selected. In particular, any history of previous heart infarct, disturbances of left ventricular function, and manifest angina pectoris shall be noted. The risk of suffering a myocardial infarction inter- or peri-interventionally is certainly increased by the stress of the intervention, especially as in advanced arterial occlusive disease it can be assumed that up to 90% of cases also have existing stenoses of the coronary arteries. However, routine monitoring of patients undergoing PTA without any specific history of heart disease does not seem to be necessary. Zeitler mentioned the general necessity for ECG monitoring in PTAs in the supra-aortic vessels, in the renal arteries, and in aorta dilatations, but not in pelvis-leg angioplasies. Pfisterer supported this view, especially for aorta dilatations, as the aortic occlusion results in pressure overload of the left ventricle. Zeitler was more precise regarding monitoring for supraaortic vascular dilatation, saying that he regards permanent intraarterial monitoring of blood pressure as necessary, with pulse or ECG registration running in parallel. The same is true for dilatation of renal arteries to avoid cerebral infarcts with preexisting carotid stenoses.

More thorough pretherapeutic cardiac examinations are not, in Pfisterer's opinion, necessary in asymptomatic patients. This is, however, regularly done in Basel in patients who were about to have aortic surgery, because in comparison with PTA the risk of intra- or peritherapeutic myocardial infarction is clearly higher. Here, pyramidol thallium scintigraphy is routinely carried out.

Severe cardiac complications are extremely rare during radiological procedures. However, said Schmitt, staff should have had suitable first aid training and cardiac defibrillation shall be available at short notice.

Postinterventional Drug Treatment

Pathophysiology of Restenosis After Percutaneous Transluminal (Coronary) Angioplasty

R. M. WALTER

Introduction

The purpose of this paper is to discuss the known bioeffects of percutaneous transluminal angioplasty (PTA) and percutaneous transluminal coronary angioplasty (PTCA) under the special aspect of restenosis. The development of PTA and PTCA techniques will be briefly presented. Known biologic effects of these procedures and their relevance to the pathophysiology of restenosis are discussed.

Evolution of Angioplasty

Since the first publication of a successful transluminal dilatation by C. T. Dotter and M. P. Judkins in 1964 [7], PTA has been the subject of an enormous research effort and major technical improvements.

PTA was first performed by advancing coaxial catheters with increasing diameters across a stenotic lesion. The disadvantages of this technique (large, 12 F arterial puncture, shear forces at the stenosis with the risk of peripheral embolization of plaque material) could not be overcome by the development of van Andel [17]. His catheters with varying diameters (8–12 F) at the tip allowed adaption of the dilating catheters to different vessel diameters, however, the major disadvantages of this system were the same as in Dotter's.

The next major step was the introduction of the balloon catheter into PTA. Grüntzig and coworkers in 1974 built and used a balloon catheter that retained its shape up to 6 bars and was available with 3–10 mm balloon diameter. The main advantage of balloon dilatation is that a small-profile catheter can be advanced into the stenotic segment without damaging other vessel segments and then, by inflating the balloon, a radial dilating force can be applied to the stenotic segment. Axial shear forces can thus be avoided and the risk of peripheral embolization be diminished. Grüntzig was also the first author who published percutaneous treatment of coronary artery stenosis [10].

The major technical difficulty was building cylindrical balloons that retain their shape even at pressures >6 bars. Balloons that suffice to dilate hard stenoses were first designed by Olbert and Hanecka [14]. A special reinforcement of the balloon wall allowed working pressures up to 12 bars for an 8-mm balloon with a bursting pressure of 15.5 bars. The second advantage of their system was a snug fit of the balloon on the shaft before and after dilatation; thus, complications at the puncture site could be diminished.

Today, PTA is used in almost all anatomic regions including the aorta and the peripheral arteries of the extremities, the mesenteric and renal arteries, the coronary and the carotid arteries. The development of high-pressure balloons with large diameters has led to the successful application of the "balloon dilatation technique" in other fields such as valvuloplasty and the treatment of strictures in the gut and biliary and genitourinary systems.

Mechanisms of PTA

The early concept of Dotter and Judkins for the mechanisms of angioplasty was that of compressing and remodeling the atherosclerotic lesion. Liquid elements of the atherosclerotic lesion were thought to be compressed out of the lesion with reshaping of the residual material and, thus, the lumen. The idea of reshaping is best described when compared to driving a nail into wood and then removing it, thus leaving a hole.

In 1980 Castaneda-Zuniga et al. introduced their concept of arterial wall disrupture and plaque splitting. It was documented that further inflation stretches the media and leads to a loss of elastic properties, thus causing permanent arterial enlargement [5]. Other studies [4, 9] demonstrate similar findings; excentric plaques split at the junction of the plaque and arterial wall, while concentric plaques split at the weakest point or line.

There is experimental and clinical evidence of plaque desquamation with the embolization of endothelial cells and superficial plaque elements after successful angioplasties. However, animal studies have only demonstrated little embolization, therefore it is likely that desquamation is only a minor contributor to an increased diameter post-PTA [4].

In summary, the combination of plaque splitting and stretching of the media seems to be the major mechanism of successful angioplasty.

Natural History of Plaque Growth and Thrombus Formation

For the purposes of further discussion, the natural history of plaques will be discussed in a very short fashion.

After formation of a plaque, it may remain morphologically unchanged and clinically silent, grow in a slow fashion secondary to macrophage activity with a further uptake of lipids and a slow increase in clinical symptoms, or rupture secondary to a variety of factors (including plaque composition and configuration, hemodynamic forces etc.). Plaque rupture or fissuring exposes collagen, lipids, and smooth muscle cells (SMC), thus activating platelets and the coagulation cascade.

A resulting stable thrombus may lead to a marked reduction in or obstruction of perfusion with clinical symptoms, or become incorporated into the diseased vessel, potentially causing growth of the plaque. A labile thrombus may induce transitory symptoms. Release of vasoactive substances may lead to arterial spasm [9].

Role of Spontaneous or Iatrogenic Plaque Rupture

However, the mechanisms responsible for successful PTA and PTCA may be similar or equal to those inducing restenosis. A paper by Nagatomo et al. [13] indicates that certain specific coronary morphology suggestive of ruptured atheromatous plaque (poorly defined or hazy borders, outpouchings, sharp leading or trailing edges) may be a predictor of accelerated plaque growth without intervention. Ischinger et al. [12] have shown that PTCA of a coronary artery with less than 60% diameter loss accelerates the time course of stenosis.

These findings support the role of plaque rupture (and/or vessel wall damage), may it be spontaneous or iatrogenic, for the progression of stenosis.

Biologic Effects After Angioplasty

All physiologic mechanisms of traumatic vessel damage repair seem to be involved in the processes after PTA and are therefore briefly presented.

The immediate mechanism leads to vasoconstriction on the basis of the active contraction of the vessel wall SMC and plug formation by platelet aggregation. This is followed by fibrin production of the coagulation system. Platelets form the plug and stimulate thrombin production. The mechanisms of plug formation include adhesion (von Willebrand factor), release reaction, aggregation, and fibrin/platelet fusion. The latter interlink by fibrinogen at IIb/IIIa receptors. Thromboxane A_2 enhances platelet aggregation and induces vasoconstriction, while prostacyclin acts as an antagonist both by inhibiting platelet aggregation and by vasodilatation.

After angioplasty, platelet accumulation occurs, with a maximum at 2 h post-PTA. The amount of platelet accumulation seems to be related to the amount of vessel-wall dissection present. Comparison of platelet accumulation in two experiments with (a) intimal denudation only versus (b) media fissuring results in a tenfold greater accumulation for the latter. Exposure of highly thrombogenic media collagen induces platelet aggregation [18].

Further tissue response is characterized by a proliferation of macrophages and spindle-shaped cells, which carry the immunohistochemical characteristics of SMC [16]. Platelets have been shown to release a potent SMC (and fibroblast) mitogen, platelet-derived growth factor (PDGF), which may be an important regulator of the neointimal regrowth after angioplasty, and thereby an important determinant of restenosis [15].

There is experimental and human in vivo evidence, that restenosis is largely secondary to smooth muscle cell proliferation (SMCP). The effects of progression of atherosclerotic disease seem to be of minor importance. Samples from both peripheral and coronary primary lesions, and restenoses retrieved by percutaneous transluminal atherectomies using the Simpson catheter have been cultivated and studied; SMC were the predominant cell type in all samples. After cultivation, the in vitro migratory velocity of SMC from initial lesions and restenoses were compared and found to be 2.4 times higher for cell lines from restenoses. The authors conclude that increased SMC migratory activity may represent a basic biologic mechanism involved in human accelerated arteriosclerosis and restenosis formation [1].

The role of lesion type was studied by Ueda et al. 1991 [16]. Seven hearts of patients who died within 20 days after PTCA were studied. A different histologic response pattern was found for lacerations of preexistent media as opposed to atheromas with thin fibrous caps. Spindle-cell proliferation was already present on day 6 post-PTCA in a heart with media laceration. In contrast, after plaque rupture with washout of debris, macrophages lined the crater, probably not identical to the preexistent lipid-laden foam cells. The authors conclude that the type of response (and the likelihood of restenosis) may be largely defined by plaque morphology, not only "by dictating the most likely type of laceration, but even more so by exposing 'trigger happy' cells move".

Therefore, it should be stressed here that balloon dilatations do not only alter the plaque, but also the adjacent vessel wall proximal and distal to a concentric or opposite or next to an excentric lesion. In the light of the results of Ueda et al. [16], this may be of the utmost importance for the understanding of restenosis. Another reason for discussing this fact is that balloon dilatation is used experimentally to produce lesions. Whether or not the findings of Ischinger et al. [12], who described that PTCA accelerates stenoses <60% in coronary arteries, further support the importance of media injury, can only be speculated. In less severe stenoses and excentric stenoses, overdilatation of the "normal segment" may be more likely, leading to a higher rate of media fractures and restenoses.

Side effects of angioplasty on normal vessel segments have been studied experimentally; they include loss of vasoconstrictor response [19] in another experiment by Zollikofer et al. [20], and depending on dilatation time (15–60 s) and the degree of overstretching (25% and 50%) focal/complete denudation of intimal cell lining, stretching/dehiscence of the internal elastic lamina, damage to SMC with intercellular edema, and separation of myocytes for 50% overstretching. Also, platelet aggregation and fibrin deposition were observed over denuded endothelium of normal vessels after dilatation.

While experimentally, dilated segments of animal vessels loose their ability to contract, vasospasm has been observed in humans. Provoked vasoconstriction probably reflects SMC presence in lesions and predicts the likelihood of restenosis in humans. Ergonovine-induced spasm occurring in the dilated segment before PTCA and at follow-up 6 months after PTCA was associated with a restenosis rate of 58%. Patients with spasm of the dilated segment only at restudy had a restenosis rate of 43%. In contrast, if spasm could not be provoked before and after PTCA, the restenosis rate was 20%. Similarly, patients who had spasm before, but not after PTCA, had a rate of 19%. The authors conclude that the association of findings may be based on the presence of excentric lesions with viable, nondiseased segments of media tissue which, after iatrogenic damage, may induce restenosis [3]. Whether or not the change in elastic properties secondary to overstretching induces media (SMC) proliferation as observed in venous parts of dialysis fistulas in order to withstand the tensile forces of pulsatile flow, can again only be speculated.

Assessment of Restenosis

For both peripheral and coronary follow-up studies, observer-dependent and technical problems limit the accuracy of restenosis assessment.

Visual estimation of stenosis severity is associated with high-intraobserver variability. For coronary angiograms, average standard deviations for the estimation of any segmented stenosis by a single reader was 18%, disagreement about the number of major vessels with a 70% stenosis occurred in 31% of readings carried out by single observers [6]. Also the progression of the (re)stenosing process in adjacent "reference" vessel segments makes percentage diameter stenosis calculations less accurate [2].

Table 1. Factors associated with restenosis after PTCA [8]

Morphologic factors
Total occlusions
Lesion severity
LAD lesions
Proximal lesions
Bifurcation lesions
Length > 10–15 mm
Calcified lesions
Excentric lesions
Diffusely diseased vessels
Saphenous vein grafts
Procedural factors
Severity of residual stenosis
Final gradient > 15–20 mmHg
Absence of localized intimal tear
Large dissection

The published incidence of restenosis after PTCA is approximately 30%. A number of studies for the prevention of restenosis have been published. However, the comparison of different studies is difficult, as different definitions of restenosis have been used. The National Heart, Lung, and Blood Institute (NHLBI) of NIH alone has proposed four different definitions (NHLBI I–IV); the selection of patients for follow up (F/U) angiograms and the time interval to PTCA have an impact on the detection rate of restenosis (see Table 1) [8].

After PTCA, up to 92% of occurring restenoses are detected within the first 6 months [11]. Therefore, F/U angiograms after PTCA at 3 months are widely recommended. After peripheral PTA, (Color-) Doppler studies and clinical F/U be sufficient to detect restenosis.

For peripheral F/U angiograms, the biplane technique is not routinely performed in most institutions. Therefore lesions which are situated strictly at the anterior or posterior vessel wall, without a narrowing of the vessel as seen in anteroposterior projection, may be missed.

Conclusion

Restenosis remains a significant problem in both peripheral and coronary angioplasty. Proliferation of SMC seems to be the main common denominator and occurs in the early postprocedural course between 6 days and 6 months. While pharmacologic interventions will be discussed in "Pharmacological Prevention of Restenosis Following Angioplasty," this volume, the possible implications of new knowledge on techniques may be summarized.

The role of new devices such as laser angioplasty, cutting atherectomy, and stents is still under investigation. Rotational atherectomy is thought to be capable of ablating atheromatous tissue without damaging normal vessel-wall media. Percutaneous transluminal ultrasound probes and flexible low-profile angioscopes will provide new knowledge on plaque morphology and will probably have an impact on methods and instrumentation of PTA for different types of lesions.

Specimens from atherectomies and studies with derived cell cultures will enhance our understanding of regulatory mechanisms and the pathophysiology of restenosis.

References

1. Bauriedel G, Windstetter U, Brandl R, Plas E, Kandolf R, Höfling B (1991) Erhöhte In-vitro-Motilität humaner Gefäßwandmyozyten aus Restenose-Läsionen peripherer und koronarer Gefäße. Z Kardiol 80:494–499

2. Beatt KJ, Juijten HE, de Feyter PJ (1988) Change in diameter of coronary artery segments adjacent to stenosis after PTCA: failure of percent diameter stenosis measurements to reflect morphologic changes induced by balloon dilatation. J Am Coll Cardiol 12:315–323
3. Bertrand ME, LaBlanche JM, Fourrier JL, Gommeaux A, Ruel M (1988) Relation to restenosis after percutaneous coronary angioplasty to vasomotion of the dilated coronary arterial segment. Am J Cardiol 63:277–281
4. Block PC, Elmer D, Fallon JT (1982) Release of atherosclerotic debris after transluminal angioplasty. Circulation 65:950–952
5. Castaneda-Zuniga WR, Formanek A, Tadavarthy M et al. (1980) The mechanism of balloon angioplasty. Radiology 135:565–571
6. DeRouen TA, Murray JA, Owen W (1976) Variability in the analysis of coronary arteriograms. Circulation 55(2):324–328
7. Dotter CT, Judkins MP (1964) Transluminal treatment of arteriosclerotic obstruction: description of a new technique and a preliminary report of its application. Circulation 30:654–670
8. Fanelli C, Aronoff R (1990) Restenosis following coronary angioplasty. Am Heart J 119:357–368
9. Fuster V, Stein B, Ambrose JA, Badimon L, Badimon JJ, Chesebro JH (1990) Atherosclerotic plaque rupture and thrombosis. Evolving concepts. Circulation 82 [Suppl II]:47–59
10. Grüntzig A (1978) Transluminal dilatation of coronary artery stenosis (letter). Lancet 1:263
11. Guiteras Val P, Bourassa MG, David PR et al. (1987) Restenosis after successful PTCA: the Montreal Heart Institute experience. Am J Cardiol 60:50B–55B
12. Ischinger T, Grüntzig AR, Hollman J et al. (1983) Should coronary arteries with less than 60% diameter stenosis be treated by angioplasty? Circulation 68:148–154
13. Nagatomo Y, Nakagawa S, Koiwaya Y, Tanaka K (1990) Coronary angiographic ruptured atheromatous plaque as a predictor of future progression of stenosis. Am Heart J 119(6):1244–1253
14. Olbert F, Hanecka I (1977) Transluminale Gefäßdilatation mit einem modifizierten Dilatationskatheter. Wien Klin WSchr 89:281–284
15. Ross R, Glomset JA, Kariya B, Harker LA (1974) A platelet-dependent factor that stimulates the proliferation of arterial smooth muscle cells in vitro. Proc Natl Acad Sci USA 71:1207
16. Ueda M, Becker AE, Fujimoto T, Tsukada T (1991) The early phenomena of restenosis following percutaneous transluminal coronary angioplasty. Eur Heart J 12:937–945
17. Van Andel G (1987) Review of the results of the Dotter procedure. In: Zeitler et al. (Eds) Percutaneous vascular recanalization. Springer, Berlin Heidelberg New York
18. Wilentz JR, Sanborn TA, Haudenschild CC, Valeri CR, Ryan TJ, Faxon DP (1987) Platelet accumulation in experimental angioplasty: time course and relation to vascular injury. Circulation 75(3):636–642
19. Wolf GL, Lentini EA, LeVeen RF (1984) Reduced vasoconstrictor response after angioplasty in normal rabbit aortas. AJR 141:1023–1025
20. Zollikofer CL, Chain J, Salomonowitz E, Runge W, Bruehlmann WF, Castaneda-Zuniga WR, Amplatz K (1984) Percutaneous transluminal angioplasty of the aorta. Light and electron microscopic observations in normal and atherosclerotic rabbits. Radiology 151:355–363

Pharmacologic Prevention of Restenosis Following Angioplasty

K. JÄGER, B. FRAUCHIGER, and R. EICHLISBERGER

Introduction

Percutaneous transluminal angioplasty (PTA) is a valuable and accepted treatment for patients with occlusive arterial disease [1, 3, 17, 19, 24, 32, 50, 51]. Advances in technology and increased experience have improved the primary success rate and resulted in a lower complication rate [3, 4]. The value of this therapeutic procedure, however, is curtailed by early restenosis or reocclusion. Although the rate of restenosis varies from report to report because of methodological differences, it is generally accepted to be about 30% of initially successful PTA [1, 10, 17, 32, 50].

The failure of conventional balloon PTA to provide a lasting result has led to the development of other methods of catheter-associated interventional therapy, such as atherectomy, stenting and laser angioplasty [3, 18, 46]. The advent of these techniques improved the primary success rate, but the long-term patency rate is still unsatisfactory [60]. Despite considerable basic and clinical efforts to address the problem of restenosis after PTA, no effective preventive therapies have yet been developed and pharmacological attempts to inhibit restenosis have generally been unsuccessful [20, 25]. The reason for the occurrence of a clinically significant restenosis in only a minority of the treated vessels remains unclear.

Recurrent disease after PTA is not specific to peripheral vascular disease, but can also be observed after coronary angioplasty (PTCA, [6, 9, 25, 35, 53]), endarterectomy, and vein grafts [11, 34, 41]. Early reocclusion (within a few days) is usually caused by acute thrombus formation at the site of treatment [15, 16]. Restenosis involves elastic recoil and intimal hyperplasia, which develop slowly over weeks, usually occurring within the first 3–6 months after the procedure. Symptoms that appear later than 6 months may be caused by progression of the pre-existing atherosclerotic plaque.

Response to Injury and Development of Restenosis

Vascular disruption, produced by the angioplasty balloon, denudes endothelial cells and exposes subendothelial structures to the blood stream, thereby inducing platelets to adhere to subendothelial collagen [15, 16]. Mitogen factors that induce the migration and proliferation of the smooth muscle cells in the intima are released. The "response to injury" hypothesis explains the beginning of intimal hyperplasia formation as a necessary wound-healing response. It is not yet clear why, in some patients, the reactions of the endothelial cell, smooth muscle cell, and the coagulation system are so strong, causing luminal narrowing and ultimate failure of the treatment [15, 16, 20]. Since pharmacological control and prevention of restenosis has been largely unsuccessful, it is very important to minimize injury to the vessel during the procedure; this is caused mainly by rapid inflation of an oversized balloon with high pressures [3, 10, 48]. In addition, the shear stress of axial movement should be prevented.

Intimal thickening is also influenced by hemodynamic factors. Increased blood pressure and decreased blood flow intensify the process of intimal thickening. Higher shear forces and the biological response to shear stress increase the risk of restenosis and occlusion in inadequately dilated vessels. Angiotensin-converting enzyme (ACE) inhibitors, calcium channel blockers, beta-adrenergic blockers, and prostanoids may offer some benefit by improving the hemodynamic conditions [9, 10, 45, 49, 52]. The typical restenotic lesion differs from the usual atherosclerotic plaque in architecture and lipid content. Both contain a complex mixture of smooth muscle cells, fibrous tissue, and cholesterol; restenotic lesions, however, are much more fibrous in nature, with few cholesterol pools.

Since the factors responsible for restenosis may be similar to those that cause atherosclerosis, the well-known risk factors should be under strict control. Diabetes, high cholesterol levels, and smoking are patient-related variables associated with restenosis [5, 22]. Pharmacological control, mainly during the early postoperative period, seems to be very important.

Not only the endothelial cells but also the thrombocytes form a very active and very varied biochemical system [20]. Platelet activation involves the stimulation of several membrane glycoproteins, the release of dense granules and alpha granules, and interaction with subendothelial collagen, plasma protein, fibrin, thrombin, etc. This illustrates why the inhibition of one pathway, for instance with acetylsalicylic acid (aspirin), may not be sufficient to prevent a recurrence of the disease or to inhibit atherosclerotic progression of disease.

Protective Effect of the Endothelial Cell

Intact endothelium prevents platelet aggregation (Fig. 1). Arachidonic acid from the endothelial cell is converted into cyclic endoperoxide and prostacyclin. The naturally occurring prostacyclin is a potent vasodilator and platelet inhibitor, but administration of prostacyclin or prostacyclin analogues produced only an insignificant reduction in the risk of restenosis after PTCA (27% vs 32% and 31% vs 53%, [51]).

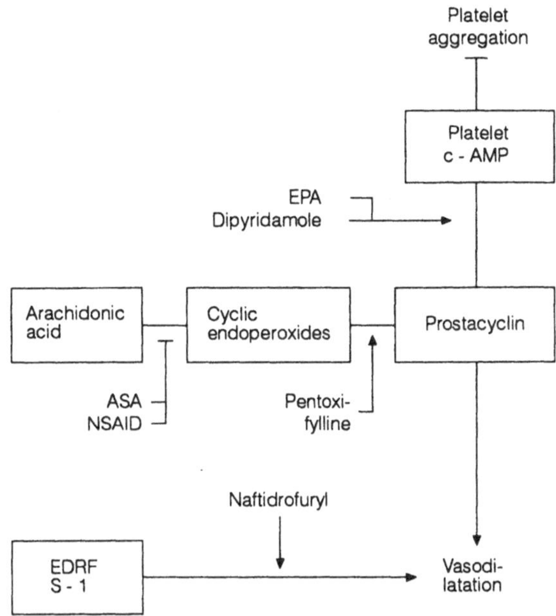

Fig. 1. Endothelial cells constitute a very active biochemical system. Substances, such as arachidonic acid, endothelial-derived relaxing factor (*EDRF*) and serotonin-1 (*S-1*) regulate vasodilatation and inhibit platelet aggregation. ⊣, inhibition; →; stimulation, activation; *ASA*, acetylsalicylic acid; *NSAID*, nonsteroidal anti-inflammatory drug; *EPA*, eicosapentanoic acid (fish oil); *c-AMP*, cyclic adenosine monophosphate

Endothelial-derived relaxing factor (EDRF) and serotonin-1 from the intact endothelial cell cause vasodilatation and inhibit platelet aggregation (Fig. 1). In contrast, serotonin-2 released during platelet degranulation at the time of vessel injury causes vasoconstriction (Fig. 2), and may directly stimulate proliferation of smooth muscle cell. S2 antagonists, such as naftidrofuryl, reduce vasoconstriction and inhibit smooth muscle cell proliferation. A study analyzing the effectiveness of naftidrofuryl after PTA is in progress and will be published in the very near future.

Dipyridamole is of limited benefit in the prevention of restenosis, although its addition may diminish the undesirable effect of high doses of aspirin, a reduction in the formation of prostaglandin. It has been shown that aspirin potentiates the effect of dipyridamole in a dose-dependent way, a higher dose giving better results [23, 24]. The effect, however, is not dramatic and not really reproducible from trial to trial.

Eicosapentanoic acid (EPA) is a naturally occurring fatty acid found in certain fish oils. We are not aware of any study done on peripheral arterial disease or after PTA, but several studies on its use after coronary angioplasty have been published [9, 36, 43, 44]. EPA seems to inhibit the formation of proaggregatory thromboxane A_2 (TXA_2) from arachidonic acid. In some studies its antimitogenic properties reduced the formation of intimal hyper-

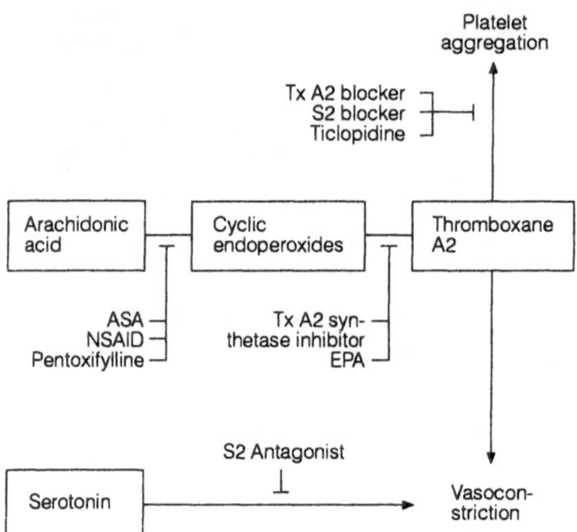

Fig. 2. Platelet-derived substances such as arachidonic acid and serotonin are responsible for platelet aggregation and vasoconstriction. ⊣, inhibition; →, stimulation, activation; *T A2*, thromboxane A_2; *S2*, serotonin-2

plasia. The results relating to a postulated favorable alteration in lipid profiles are not consistent and no consensus can yet be reached [36, 43, 44].

Inhibition of Platelet Activation

Platelet activity is stimulated by the conversion of platelet-borne arachidonic acid into cyclic endoperoxides and TXA_2 (Fig. 2). TXA_2 induces platelet aggregation and vasoconstriction [11]. Aspirin, the most often used acetylsalicylic acid, nonsteroidal anti-inflammatory drugs, and pentoxifylline irreversibly inhibit the enzyme cyclooxygenase, which is responsible in the platelet for the conversion of arachidonic acid to TXA_2 [37]. There is now good evidence that aspirin is an effective antithrombotic agent in patients with atherosclerotic disease, especially ischemic heart disease and cerebrovascular disease [2, 31]. A comprehensive meta-analysis, incorporating the trials of platelet-inhibiting drugs in almost 9000 patients with transient ischemic attacks (TIAs) or minor strokes, has established the efficacy of aspirin, with an estimated 22% reduction in the risk of vascular death [2]. The meta-analysis of nine placebo-controlled studies, including more than 16000 postmyocardial infarction patients, showed that aspirin significantly ($p<0.001$) reduces the risk of stroke, myocardial infarction, or vascular death by about 25% [2]. *The Second International Study of Infarct Survival* (ISIS-2), which included 17187 patients, showed that aspirin resulted in a risk reduction of 23% [31]. In patients with unstable angina, two studies showed that aspirin reduces the risk of cardiac death by 51% [2, 7, 57]. In peripheral arterial disease a delay in progression has not yet been documented but can be assumed [27, 59]. There are both theoretical and practical reasons for choosing the lowest effective dose of aspirin: the gastric side effects of aspirin appear to be dose dependent. Lower doses (100–325 mg/day) are as effective as higher doses (1000–1500 mg/day) in inhibiting cyclooxygenase-dependent platelet aggregation, while having a reduced influence on the synthesis of prostacyclin in vascular endothelial cells (Fig. 1). There is also good evidence that lower doses are effective in preventing stroke and myocardial infarction and it is reasonable to assume that they are of benefit in patients with peripheral arterial disease. Although effective, aspirin only partially inhibits platelet aggregation induced by adenosine diphosphate, collagen, or thrombin and, in addition, its influence on the more important adhesion of platelets is nil or only minimal. Consequently, platelet-derived growth factor (PDGF) and other mitogens may still affect the proliferation of smooth muscle cells.

Aspirin after PTCA has been tested in seven clinical trials. Control angiography was usually not evaluated quantitatively. When data from four clinical trials were studied in a meta-analysis, there was an insignificant (11%) reduction in the risk of restenosis with aspirin, compared with placebo [9]. Three trials compared high- and low-dose aspirin in the prevention of restenosis after angioplasty; two of these showed a trend towards a lower restenosis rate with low-dose aspirin [9].

After peripheral angioplasty most patients are treated with aspirin. The rationale for this regimen has been tested in only a few trials and is generally accepted by analogy with experience in coronary angioplasty and with studies analyzing the progression of atherosclerotic disease [23, 24, 42, 54]. It is clear from several studies that, although aspirin does not influence the incidence of intimal hyperplasia and restenosis, it definitely has a positive influence on acute complications during and after angioplasty, and at long-term follow-up, and for this reason long-term medication with aspirin can be recommended [26, 27, 29, 42].

Selective thromboxane synthetase inhibitors are under evaluation. In animal studies they were more effective than heparin or acetylsalicylic acid in inhibiting platelet deposition after balloon angioplasty. In a small post-PTCA study population, only 22% of the patients given TXA_2 synthetase inhibitor showed restenosis, compared with 53% in the placebo group. In addition to inhibiting the TXA_2 synthetase, it is also possible to block the TXA_2 receptor in the platelet [11].

Inhibition of Mitogenic and Chemotactic Substances

Several mitogens, including PDGF and fibrous growth factor (FGF) are released in response to balloon injury (Fig. 3). They activate the quiescent smooth muscle cells and induce intimal hyperplasia and restenosis through

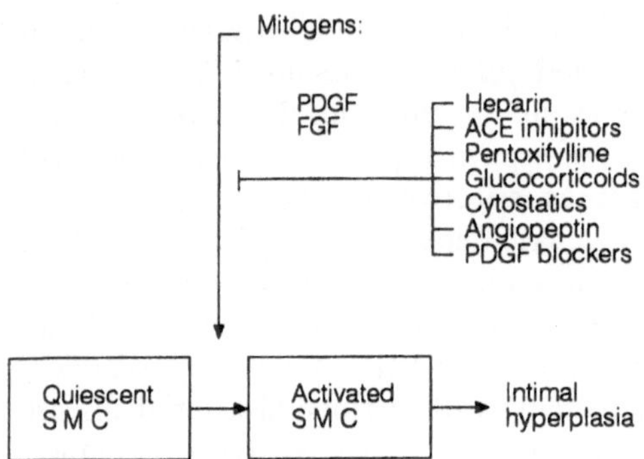

Fig. 3. Platelet aggregation mediates several chemotactic and mitogenic substances, such as platelet-derived growth factor (*PDGF*) or fibroblastic growth factor (*FGF*). Fibroblast and smooth muscle cell (*SMC*) migration and proliferation result in intimal hyperplasia. Drugs that modify platelet function may inhibit (⊣) intimal hyperplasia

proliferation and migration of smooth muscle cells. Interference with these growth factors may be most beneficial in inhibiting the recurrence of disease.

Angiotensin-converting enzyme (ACE) is a membrane-bound enzyme present in the walls of large arteries and veins. It has been shown that angiotensin II is a mitogen responsible for intimal hyperplasia after PTA. In rats, neo-intima formation was reduced by 80% when an ACE inhibitor was given. So far, captopril and cilazapril are the best-documented drugs. The effect seems to be dose dependent and synergistic with the effect of heparin. Heparin is a highly effective inhibitor of smooth muscle cell proliferation and migration. This effect is not dependent on the anticoagulant activity.

Damaged endothelial cells are capable of secreting chemotactic factors that increase the adhesion of monocytes, which give rise to macrophages. Activated macrophages in cultures secrete growth factors for fibroblasts, smooth muscle cells, and endothelium. It is recognized that not only platelets and endothelial and smooth muscle cells, but also monocytes/macrophages and neutrophils, are responsible for restenosis. The monocyte/macrophage-mediated events are sensitive to glucocorticoids, which influence the immunologically mediated inflammatory responses to injury. Hydrocortisone inhibits the growth of vascular smooth muscle cells in culture, but clinical studies have so far shown no significant improvement under glucocorticoid treatment [38]. It is possible that neutrophils activated after arterial wall injury play an important part in stimulating smooth muscle cell proliferation at the dilated site. Drugs that modulate neutrophil activation, such as pentoxifylline, may offer the possibility of a new therapeutic approach [37, 56].

Electron microscope findings showed that cytostatic agents prevented smooth muscle cell proliferation without damaging the normal smooth muscle cell. Because of the potential for serious side effects, however, no clinical data are available.

Angiopeptin, a new synthetic octapeptide, inhibits neo-intimal hyperplasia, as has been demonstrated in experimental vein grafts [8].

Trapidil is a PDGF antagonist which significantly inhibits intimal thickening in damaged carotid arteries of rabbits. Histological findings showed significantly less intimal hyperplasia.

Anticoagulation

Thrombin plays an essential role in the "reaction to injury" and in recurrent stenosis after PTA (Fig. 4). In addition to its function in the coagulation cascade, thrombin is an agonist for a number of cellular activators, such as those producing stimulation of endothelial and smooth muscle cells and proliferation of fibroblasts [12, 13, 55].

Hirudin, the anticoagulant agent from leeches, has been shown to be a very potent and specific thrombin antagonist, and to be more effective than heparin in preventing thrombosis [30, 40]. Hirudin binds strongly and specifically to thrombin. After complexing with hirudin, thrombin loses its effect on platelets, especially the thrombin-induced platelet aggregation. Hirudin is also able to inhibit the vasoconstrictor action of thrombin in de-endothelialized vessels. Recombinant hirudin and synthetic hirudin are currently under evaluation [30, 40, 47, 58].

When PTA was adopted as a therapeutic procedure for patients with peripheral vascular disease, anticoagulation with heparin and coumarin derivatives became an integral aspect [12, 14, 28, 34, 55]. Heparin binds reversibly with antithrombin, leading to increased antithrombin activity. The antithrombin – heparin complex then binds with factor Xa and factor II a, resulting in an anticoagulant effect. Low-molecular-weight (LMW) heparin has a more

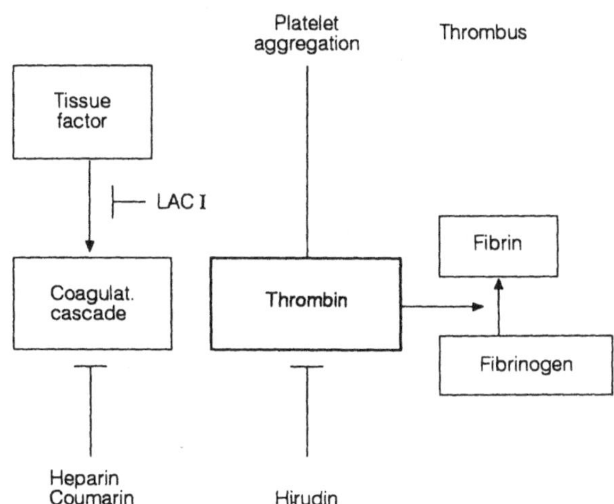

Fig. 4. Different processes involved in platelet aggregation and thrombus formation. *LACI*, lipoprotein-associated coagulation inhibitor

specific anti-Xa activity. In experimental studies it has been shown that LMW heparin inhibits both thrombosis after endothelial injury and proliferation of vascular smooth muscle cells [3, 15, 16]. In order to reduce the high thrombotic risk in the presence of residual mural thrombus, nonfractionated i.v. heparin is often used after PTA, especially after local lysis of fresh thrombi [4, 6, 33]. Bleeding complications are seen more often in patients treated with heparin (e.g., 8.2% vs 3.8%), but early thrombotic reocclusion can be prevented [25]. The optimum duration of heparin therapy is still unknown. On the basis of work done by Clowes, we concluded that 1 week is sufficient [15, 16]. In an early paper, published in 1973 by Zeitler and coworkers, heparin was used for 10 days and comparison groups of patients received heparin plus aspirin or aspirin alone [61]. Surprisingly, the reocclusion rate within 10 days was highest (21%) in the heparin group, followed by 7% in the aspirin plus heparin group, and 5% in the aspirin group.

Oral anticoagulation (AC) used to be the long-term treatment of choice after PTA [12]. The pioneers of PTA, Grüntzig and Zeitler, maintained their patients on AC for at least 1 year [19, 61]. The rate of stenosis in the group on AC was reported to be 21% by Grüntzig and 25% by Schmidtke und Zeitler [19, 50]. Both studies included a small group of patients receiving no specific treatment. These patients had restenosis rates of 45% and 48% respectively. Since it was an uncontrolled group representing a more or less negative selection with contraindications to AC, these patients do not constitute a true placebo group. We are aware of no prospective study conducted to compare oral anticoagulants with aspirin. Schneider compared AC and ticlopidine and Mahler compared AC and suloctidine, both thrombocyte-function inhibiting substances [39, 51]. In both studies the differences between the groups were insignificant.

Tissue-factor-induced coagulation, mediated by the extrinsic pathway, can be inhibited with lipoprotein-associated coagulation inhibitor (LACI). Activation of the extrinsic pathway plays a critical role in thrombotic reocclusion after vascular injury. It has been shown that the physiological inhibitor LACI prevents thrombotic arterial reocclusion after thrombolysis [21]. Endothelial tissue-factor activity may also be inhibited by pentoxifylline [56].

Summary and Conclusion

After angioplasty, "response to injury" leads to the development of intimal hyperplasia and thus to restenosis. At the present time, no reliable means of preventing this syndrome of accelerated arteriosclerosis is known. The problem continues to present a challenge to all angiologists, cardiologists, and radiologists involved in interventional therapy, as well as to vascular surgeons. This paper describes new approaches to pharmacological prevention of restenosis; some of these are very promising, but their efficacy remains to be proven in large-scale prospective studies. The treatment procedure employed by the authors and many other centers is summarized in Table 1.

Table 1. Pharmacological prevention of restenosis following angioplasty

Heparin

I: Beginning of procedure
S: Liquemin
D: 5000 U i.a. (add 2500 U. i.a. after 2 h)
I: – After local lysis
(until oral AC in therapeutic range)
– After stent implantation
S: Liquemin
D: Begin: 4 h after removal of catheter[a],
500 U/h i.v.
– After day 3[a],
1000 U/h i.v.: TT 2'/4–6[a]

LMW heparin

I: Bedridden (>3 d)
S: Sandoparin
D: 3000 U s.c./day

Oral anticoagulants

I: After local lysis
S: Marcoumar (Phenprocoumon)
D: Prothrombin time (Quick 20%–25%)
INR: 3.6–2.8

Platelet inhibitors

I: All patients (except AC)
S: Aspirin
D: 100 mg/day p.o., 6 months if aspirin contraindicated
S: Trental (Pentoxyphylline)
D: 400 mg p.o.; b.i.d.

Intimal hyperplasia

I: Restenosis (<6 months) hypertension
S: Inhibace (Cilacapril)
D: 1 mg → individual adjustment → 5 mg

I, indication; S, substance; D, dose

References

1. Adar R, Critchfield GC, Eddy DM (1989) A confidence profile analysis of the results of femoropopliteal percutaneous transluminal angioplasty in the treatment of lower-extremity ischemia. J Vasc Surg 10:57–67
2. Antiplatelet Trialists' Collaboration (1988) Secondary prevention of vascular disease by prolonged antiplatelet treatment. BMJ 296:320–331
3. Becker GJ, Katzen BT, Dake MD (1989) Noncoronary angioplasty. Radiology 170:921–940
4. Berridge DC, Gregson RHS, Makin GS, Hopkinson BR (1990) Tissue plasminogen activator in peripheral arterial thrombolysis. Br J Surg 77:179–182
5. Blankenhorn DH, Alaupovic P, Wickham E, Chin HP, Azen SP (1990) Prediction of angiographic change in native human coronary arteries and aortocoronary bypass grafts. Circulation 81:470–476
6. Bonnet JL, Bory M, Jau P, Joly P, D'Houdain F, Habib G (1990) Angioplastie coronaire précoce ou différée après thrombolyse intraveneuse pour infarctus du myocarde. Arch Mal Coeur 83:1375–1379
7. Cairns JA, Gent M, Singer J (1985) Aspirin, sulfinpyrazone, or both in unstable angina. N Engl J Med 313:1369–1375
8. Calcagno D, Conte JV, Howell MH, Foegh ML (1991) Peptide inhibition of neointimal hyperplasia in vein grafts. J Vasc Surg 13:475–479
9. Califf RM, Fortin DF, Frid DJ, Harlan WR, Ohman EM, Bengtson JR, Nelson CL, Tcheng JE, Mark DB, Stack RS (1991) Restenosis after coronary angioplasty: an overview. J Am Coll Cardiol 17:2B–13B
10. Capek P, McLean GK, Berkowitz HD (1991) Femoropopliteal angioplasty – factors influencing long-term success. Circulation 83 [Suppl I]:I70–I80
11. Castelli P, Basellini A, Agus GB, Ippolito E, Pogliani EM, Colombi M, Gianese F, Scatigna M (1986) Thrombosis prevention with ticlopidine after femoropopliteal thromboendarterectomy. Int Surg 71:252–255

12. Chesebro JH, Fuster V (1986) Antithrombotic therapy for acute myocardial infarction: mechanisms and prevention of deep venous, left ventricular, and coronary artery thromboembolism. Circulation 74 [Suppl III]: III1–III10
13. Chesebro JH, Zoldhelyi P, Badimon L, Fuster V (1991) Role of thrombin in arterial thrombosis: implications for therapy. Thromb Haemost 66:1–5
14. Clagett GP, Genton E, Salzman EW (1989) Antithrombotic therapy in peripheral vascular disease. Chest 95:128S–139S
15. Clowes AW, Reidy MA (1991) Prevention of stenosis after vascular reconstruction: pharmacologic control of intimal hyperplasia – a review. J Vasc Surg 13:885–891
16. Clowes AW (1991) Prevention and management of recurrent disease after arterial reconstruction: new prospects for pharmacological control. Thromb Haemost 66:62–66
17. Gallino A, Mahler F, Probst P, Nachbur B (1984) Percutaneous transluminal angioplasty of the arteries of the lower limbs: a 5-year follow-up. Circulation 70:619–623
18. Graor RA, Whitlow PL (1990) Transluminal atherectomy for occlusive peripheral vascular disease. J Am Coll Cardiol 15:1551–1558
19. Grüntzig A, Schneider HJ (1977) Die perkutane Dilatation chronischer Koronarstenosen – Experimente and Morphologie. Schweiz Med Wochenschr 107:1588
20. Harker LA (1987) Role of platelets and thrombosis in mechanisms of acute occlusion and restenosis after angioplasty. Am J Cardiol 60:20B–28B
21. Haskel EJ, Torr SR, Day KC, Palmier MO, Wun T-C, Sobel BE, Abendschein DR (1991) Prevention of arterial reocclusion after thrombolysis with recombinant lipoprotein-associated coagulation inhibitor. Circulation 84:821–827
22. Havel RJ (1990) Role of triglyceride-rich lipoproteins in progression of atherosclerosis. Circulation 81:694–696
23. Heiss HW, Mathias K, Beck AH, König K, Betzner M, Just H (1987) Rezidivprophylaxe mit Acetylsalicylsäure und Dipyridamol nach perkutaner transluminaler Angioplastie der Beinarterien bei obliterierender Arteriosklerose. Cor Vasa 1:25–34
24. Heiss HW, Just H, Middleton D, Deichsel G (1990) Reocclusion prophylaxis with dipyridamole combined with acetylsalicylic acid following PTA. Angiology 263–269
25. Hermans WRM, Rensing BJ, Strauss BH, Serruys PW (1991) Prevention of restenosis after percutaneous transluminal coronary angioplasty: the search for a "magic bullet". Am Heart J 122:171–187
26. Hess H, Müller-Fassbender H, Ingrisch H, Mietaschk A (1978) Verhütung von Wiederverschlüssen nach Rekanalisation obliterierter Arterien mit der Kathetermethode. Dtsch Med Wochenschr 103:1994–1997
27. Hess H, Mietaschk A, Deichsel G (1985) Drug-induced inhibition of platelet function delays progression of peripheral occlusive arterial disease. A prospective double-blind arteriographically controlled trial. Lancet 415–419
28. Hirsh J, Poller L, Deykin D, Levine M, Dalen JE (1989) Optimal therapeutic range for oral anticoagulants. Chest 95:5S–10S
29. Hirsh J, Salzman EW, Harker L, Fuster V, Dalen J, Cairns JA, Collins R (1989) Aspirin and other platelet-active drugs. Chest 95:12S–16S
30. Hubbard T, Olivier T, Bacher P, Walenga JM, Gala H, Fareed J, Pifarre R (1991) Use of recombinant hirudin to increase the patency rate of microanastomosis in a rabbit model. Blood Coagul Fibrinol 2:101–103
31. ISIS-2 (Second International Study of Infarct Survival) Collaborative Group (1988) Randomised trial of intravenous streptokinase, oral aspirin, both, or neither among 17187 cases of suspected acute myocardial infarction: ISIS-2. Lancet 349–360
32. Jäger K, Schlumpf M, Bollinger A (1987) 10 Jahre periphere transluminale Angioplastie (PTA): Schicksal der Patienten. Vasa [Suppl] 20:354
33. Jorgensen B, Bülow J, Jorgensen M, Tonnesen KH, Nielsen JD, Holstein P, Andersen E (1989) Femoral artery recanalisation with percutaneous angioplasty and segmentally enclosed plasminogen activator. Lancet 1106–1108
34. Kretschmer G, Wenzl E, Piza F, Polterauer P, Ehringer H, Minar E, Schemper M (1987) The influence of anticoagulant treatment on the probability of function in femoro-

popliteal vein bypass surgery: analysis of a clinical series (1970 to 1985) and interim evaluation of a controlled clinical trial. Surgery 102:453–459

35. Leisch F, Kerschner K, Harringer W, Schützenberger W (1990) Coronary angioplasty after intravenous streptokinase in acute myocardial infarction: influence of restenosis on clinical outcome and left ventricular function. Clin Cardiol 13:253–259
36. Levine PH, Fisher M, Schneider PB, Whitten RH, Weiner BH, Ockene IS, Johnson BF, Johnson MH, Doyle EM, Riendeau PA, Hoogasian JJ (1989) Dietary supplementation with Omega-3 fatty acids prolongs platelet survival in hyperlipidemic patients with atherosclerosis. Arch Intern Med 149:1113–1116
37. Lindgärde F, Jelnes R, Björkman H, Adielsson G, Kjellström T, Palmquist I, Stavenow L (1989) Conservative drug treatment in patients with moderately severe chronic occlusive peripheral arterial disease. Circulation 80:1549–1556
38. Mac Donald RG, Panush RS, Pepine CJ (1987) Rationale for use of glucocorticoids in modification of restenosis after percutaneous transluminal coronary angioplasty. Am J Cardiol 60:56B–60B
39. Mahler F, Schneider E, Gallino A, Bollinger A (1987) Combination of suloctidil and anticoagulation in the prevention of reocclusion after femoro-popliteal PTA. Vasa 16:381–385
40. Markwardt F (1991) Hirudin and derivatives as anticoagulant agents. Thromb Haemost 66:141–152
41. McCollum C, Alexander C, Kenchington G, Franks PJ, Greenhalgh R (1991) Antiplatelet drugs in femoropopliteal vein bypasses: A multicenter trial. J Vasc Surg 13:150–162
42. Minar E, Ehringer H, Ahmadi R, Dudczak R, Leitha T, Koppensteiner R, Jung M Stümpflen A (1989) Platelet deposition at angioplasty sites and its relation to restenosis in human iliac and femoropopliteal arteries. Radiology 170:767–772
43. Nye ER, Ablett MB, Robertson MC, Ilsley CD, Sutherland WHF (1990) Effect of eicosapentaenoic acid on restenosis rate, clinical course and blood lipids in patients after percutaneous transluminal coronary angioplasty. Aust NZ J Med 20:549–552
44. O-hara M, Esato K, Harada M, Kouchi Y, Akimoto F, Nakamura T, Wakamatsu T, Zempo N (1991) Eiocosapentanoic acid suppresses intimal hyperplasia after expanded polytetrafluoroethylene grafting in rabbits fed a high-cholesterol diet. J Vasc Surg 13:480–486
45. O'Keefe JH, Giorgi LV, Hartzler GO, Good TH, Ligon RW, Webb DL, McCallister BD (1991) Effects of diltiazem on complications and restenosis after coronary angioplasty. Am J Cardiol 67:373–376
46. Poredos P, Keber D, Videcnik V (1989) Late results of local thrombolytic treatment of peripheral arterial occlusions. Angiology 40:941–947
47. Sarembock IJ, Gertz DS, Gimple LW, Owen RM, Powers ER, Roberts WC (1991) Effectiveness of recombinant desulphatohirudin in reducing restenosis after balloon angioplasty of atherosclerotic femoral arteries in rabbits. Circulation 84:232–243
48. Sarembock IJ, LaVeau PJ, Sigal SL, Timms I, Sussman J, Haudenschild C, Ezekowitz MD (1989) Influence of inflation pressure and balloon size on the development of intimal hyperplasia after balloon angioplasty. Circulation 80:1029–1040
49. Schmidt E, Grützmacher P, Meyer T, Kaltenbach M, Schoeppe W, Bussmann W-D (1990) Einfluß von Verapamil auf die Restenosierungsrate nach transluminaler Angioplastie von Nierenarterienstenosen. Z Kardiol 79:441–445
50. Schmidtke I, Zeitler E, Schoop W (1978) Spätergebnisse (5–8 Jahre) der perkutanen Katheterbehandlung (Dotter-Technik) bei femoro-poplitealen Arterienverschlüssen im Stadium II. Vasa 7:4–15
51. Schneider E, Mahler F, Do D, Biland L (1987) Zur Rezidivprophylaxe nach perkutaner transluminaler Angioplastie (PTA): Antikoagulation versus Ticlopidin. VASA [Suppl] 20:355
52. See J, Shell W, Matthews O, Canizales C, Vargas M, Giddings J, Cerrone J (1987) Prostaglandin E_1 infusion after angioplasty in humans inhibits abrupt occlusion and

early restenosis. In: Samuelsson B, Paoletti R, Ramwell PW (eds) Advances in prostaglandin, thromboxane and leukotriene research. Raven, New York, pp 266–270
53. Simoons ML (1989) Reocclusion/restenosis after coronary artery bypass surgery, percutaneous transluminal coronary angioplasty and thrombolysis. Z Kardiol 78 [Suppl 3]: 35–41
54. Staiger J, Mathias K, Friederich M, Heiss HW, Konrad S, Spillner G (1980) Perkutane Katheterrekanalisation (Dotter-Technik) bei peripherer arterieller Verschlußkrankheit. Herz/Kreislauf 12: 383–386
55. Stead NW (1991) Therapeutic fibrinolysis. Circulation 84: 948–950
56. Steg PG, Paquier C, Huu TP, Chollet-Martin S, Juliard JM, Himbert D, Pocidalo MA, Gourgon R, Hakim J (1989) Does percutaneous transluminal coronary angioplasty activate neutrophils? Preliminary clinical result. In: Hakim J, Mandell GL, Novick WJ (eds) Pentoxifylline and analogues. Effects on leukocyte function. Karger, Basel
57. Théroux P, Quimet H, McCans J (1988) Aspirin, heparin, or both to treat acute unstable angina. N Engl J Med 319: 1105–1111
58. Walenga JM, Bakhos M, Messmore HL, Koza M, Wallock M, Orfei E, Fareed J, Pifarre R (1991) Comparison of recombinant hirudin and heparin as an anticoagulant in a cardiopulmonary bypass model. Blood Coagul Fibrinol 2: 105–111
59. Walsh DB, Gilbertson JJ, Zwolak RM, Besso S, Edelman GC, Schneider JR, Cronenwett JL (1991) The natural history of superficial femoral artery stenoses. J Vasc Surg 14: 299–304
60. Wholey MH (1990) Controversies in peripheral vascular intervention. Radiology 174: 929–931
61. Zeitler E, Reichold J, Schoop W, Loew D (1973) Einfluß von Acetylsalicylsäure auf das Frühergebnis nach perkutaner Rekanalisation arterieller Obliterationen nach Dotter. Dtsch Med Wochenschr 98: 1285–1288

Discussion

on the papers by R. M. Walter and K. Jäger

Zeitler emphasized specifically the point made in Walter's paper that angioplasty shall be limited to the stenoses and spare the normal sections of wall so as to avoid inducing intimal hyperplasia. In Roeren's view, this demand does not imply an overall superiority of techniques whose aim are to remove plaque material. At least, it has not yet been convincingly demonstrated that laser angioplasty, atherectomy, or rotation angioplasty are superior to the others.

Differential plaque evaluation by intravascular ultrasound or angioscopy can possibly improve our pathophysiological understanding regarding predispositions to developing residual stenoses, thought Jäger, but neither method have any great influence on immediate therapeutic decisions.

Regarding the formation of residual stenoses, according to Jäger it is still not clear why intimal hyperplasia arise in one third of the patients but not in the remainder. Although numerous individual factors were known, most study groups work with a more or less standardized procedure, and so there is few knowledge of how this pathomechanism might be avoided by modifying the procedure.

Regarding the avoidance of residual stenoses by medical therapy, Zeitler mentioned the controlled study, not yet complete, that was being carried out in several centers in Germany and Austria to compare aspirin, placebo, and anticoagulation. The use of heparin during the intervention is not generally disputed, even though there was only little clear evidence indicating a reduction in the risk of early occlusion or restenosis. The indication for post-treatment with heparin is in comparison less clear, even though it is not disputed that heparin has a proliferation suppressing action on smooth muscle cells. Here, the risk of restenosis in the immediate post-therapeutic period has to be balanced against the risk of bleeding. The discussion confirmed that in numerous centers heparinization is carried out post-therapeutically in complicated cases, such as dissections with slow flow. Recommended was 500 to 1000 U heparin per hour, intravenously. Roeren recommended continuing this therapy for at least 72 h, because after this period the intimal proliferative activity goes down considerably. Jäger then referred to animal studies that had shown the optimum duration of heparinization to be of the order of 6 days, but thought that in a clinical context heparinization for 3 days shall suffice.

Zeitler was of the opinion that heparinization is indicated after all aspiration therapies, thrombolysis, and stent applications.

In reply to a question about the dangers of vasospasm, Jäger responded that not only the risk of early reocclusion rises, but also that spasms increase the incidence of vascular hyperplasia and restenosis. Despite this, controlled studies have not yet shown that prostaglandins in the context of dilatations have any clear influence on the patency rate. This might, however, has been due in part to the prostaglandin therapy having been too short. The same is true of calcium antagonists, which also in theory help prevent intimal hyperplasia. A reduction in the occurrence of vasospasms and the antihypertensive actions was discussed as possible mechanisms of this effect.

Also mentioned was the risk of early occlusion due to excessive compression of the femoral artery in the groin after removal of the sheath. Zeitler commented that during the compression the simultaneous evaluation of the peripheral blood flow has to be part of patient evaluation. Decreasing the blood flow too strongly can thus be avoided. Basically, such compression should be specific and carefully dosed.

Subject Index